Evaluation and Assessment of Autism Spectrum Disorder

Evaluation and Assessment of Autism Spectrum Disorder

Editor: Collin Flowers

FOSTER ACADEMICS
www.fosteracademics.com

www.fosteracademics.com

FOSTER ACADEMICS

Cataloging-in-Publication Data

Evaluation and assessment of autism spectrum disorder / edited by Collin Flowers.
p. cm.
Includes bibliographical references and index.
ISBN 978-1-64646-623-8
1. Autism spectrum disorders. 2. Developmental disabilities. 3. Autism spectrum disorders--Diagnosis.
4. Autism spectrum disorders--Treatment. 5. Psychiatry. I. Flowers, Collin.
RC553.A88 E93 2023
616.858 82--dc23

Foster Academics,
118-35 Queens Blvd., Suite 400,
Forest Hills, NY 11375, USA

ISBN 978-1-64646-623-8 (Hardback)

Contents

Preface

It is often said that books are a boon to mankind. They document every progress and pass on the knowledge from one generation to the other. They play a crucial role in our lives. Thus I was both excited and nervous while editing this book. I was pleased by the thought of being able to make a mark but I was also nervous to do it right because the future of students depends upon it. Hence, I took a few months to research further into the discipline, revise my knowledge and also explore some more aspects. Post this process, I begun with the editing of this book.

Autism spectrum disorder (ASD) refers to a type of developmental disability caused by brain differences. ASD patients frequently struggle with social engagement and communication, as well as confined or repetitive activities or interests. Additionally, people with ASD have a distinct manner in which they learn, move or pay attention. Young adults and adolescents with ASD may struggle to develop and keep friendships, communicate with adults and peers, or comprehend the appropriate behaviors expected in the workplace or at school. There are several risk factors associated with ASD, including genetic, environmental and biological factors. There are no medical tests to diagnose ASD and the individual's development stage and behavior is assessed for diagnosis. ASD treatments aim to alleviate symptoms that affect quality of life and daily functioning. Treatment plans are typically collaborative and tailored according to the individual requirements. This book discusses the evaluation and assessment of autism spectrum disorder. A number of latest researches have been included herein to keep the readers up-to-date with the global concepts in this medical condition.

I thank my publisher with all my heart for considering me worthy of this unparalleled opportunity and for showing unwavering faith in my skills. I would also like to thank the editorial team who worked closely with me at every step and contributed immensely towards the successful completion of this book. Last but not the least, I wish to thank my friends and colleagues for their support.

Editor

1

Effortful Control and Prefrontal Cortex Functioning in Children with Autism Spectrum Disorder: An fNIRS Study

Karthikeyan Krishnamurthy [1], Michael K. Yeung [1], Agnes S. Chan [2] and Yvonne M. Y. Han [1,*]

[1] Department of Rehabilitation Sciences, The Hong Kong Polytechnic University, Hong Kong, China; karthikeyan.krishnamurthy@connect.polyu.hk (K.K.); kin-chung-michael.yeung@polyu.edu.hk (M.K.Y.)

[2] Department of Psychology, The Chinese University of Hong Kong, Hong Kong, China; aschan@psy.cuhk.edu.hk

* Correspondence: yvonne.han@polyu.edu.hk

Abstract: Effortful control (EC) is an important dimension of temperament, but is impaired in autism spectrum disorder (ASD). While EC is associated with the prefrontal cortex (PFC) functioning in typically developing (TD) children, it is unclear whether EC deficits are associated with PFC dysfunction in ASD. This study examines the relationship between EC and PFC activation and connectivity in children with high-functioning ASD. Thirty-nine right-handed children (ASD: $n = 20$; TD: $n = 19$) aged 8–12 years were recruited. The EC level was assessed with the Early Adolescent Temperament Questionnaire—Revised (EATQ-R), and PFC functioning, in terms of activation and connectivity during a frontal-sensitive (n-back) task, was assessed using functional near-infrared spectroscopy (fNIRS). Children with ASD showed a significant deficit in EC and its related constructs (i.e., executive, and socioemotional functions) compared to TD controls. They also showed significantly increased overall PFC activation and reduced right frontal connectivity during the n-back task. Among children with ASD, the EC level correlated significantly with neither PFC activation nor connectivity; it significantly correlated with social functioning only. This study demonstrated EC deficits and altered PFC functioning in children with ASD, but the exact neural basis of EC deficits remains to be determined.

Keywords: effortful control; executive function; autism spectrum disorder; connectivity; fNIRS

---

1. Introduction

Autism spectrum disorder (ASD) is a neurodevelopmental disorder characterized by socio-communicative dysfunction with the presence of repetitive or stereotypic behavioral patterns and interests [1]. These features are escalated in individuals with ASD, as a result of impaired temperamental effortful control (EC) [2–4]. EC is defined as "the efficiency of executive attention including the ability to inhibit a dominant response and/or to activate a subdominant response, to plan, and to detect errors" [5]. As human behavior comprises habitual or spontaneous actions, EC is mandatory to inhibit a dominant response and initiate a subdominant response [6]. Therefore, EC becomes a major component in controlling cognitive processes with their associated behavior [5], and serves as a defensive mechanism against compulsive thoughts, while regulating overarching emotions [7].

EC encompasses executive attention, flexibility, and inhibitory control components, which help activate, modulate, or withdraw tendencies pertinent to chosen behavior [5,8,9]. In contrast to EC, executive function (EF) consists of a set of higher-order cognitive processes, including updating (or working memory), inhibitory control, and set-shifting, which support goal-oriented actions [10]. Although EC and EF components conceptually overlap with each other in the self-regulation construct, EC differs from EF primarily in five key areas, including engagement in emotion-dependent contexts, working memory involvement, developmental patterns, adaptive function relationships, and underlying neural substrates [11].

The prefrontal cortex (PFC) has long been implicated in the top-down control of behavior [12]. In healthy children, tasks that engage the core EC components, such as flexibility and inhibitory control, typically activate parts of the PFC, anterior cingulate cortex, and parietal regions [12–14]. Additionally, the PFC synchronizes with neighboring regions, while regulating behavior associated with attention and inhibitory control in healthy individuals [15,16]. In the context of EC, one functional near-infrared spectroscopy (fNIRS) study found that parent-report temperamental EC was associated with better performance on a child version of the Stroop task, and with less activation in the dorsolateral PFC during task performance in healthy young children [14]. In another fNIRS study, Fekete and Beacher [17] found that a lower level of EC reported by parents was associated with a decrease in frontal network segregation during movie viewing. Altogether, the literature suggests a link between PFC functioning and EC in healthy children.

Extensive structural and functional imaging studies have implicated abnormalities in the brain, especially the PFC, in ASD [18–20]. Functional magnetic resonance imaging (fMRI) studies have found that, compared to typically developing (TD) individuals, individuals with ASD demonstrated altered activation in the PFC and other parietal regions during a variety of EF tasks [20,21]. These individuals also displayed altered connectivity within the frontal lobe and between the PFC and parietal regions. For example, some studies have found that individuals with ASD showed weaker functional synchronization between the cingulo-insular regions and the right lateral frontal and inferior parietal areas [22], between the frontal eye field and intraparietal sulcus [23], and between the right anterior PFC and left visual cortex [24] during inhibitory control and attention-orienting tasks. Notwithstanding the evidence that ASD can be conceived as a disorder of frontal lobe function or connection [18,25], the relationship between PFC functioning and EC in children with ASD is still not clear.

Convergent evidence from human lesion, fMRI, and fNIRS studies have shown that the *n*-back task, which requires participants to judge whether the stimulus they are currently seeing is identical to that presented *n* trials prior, relies critically on the PFC [26–28]. Although the *n*-back task is often considered a task for working memory, other cognitive processes, including executive attention and inhibitory control, are subsumed while responding to relevant stimuli and ignoring irrelevant stimuli, respectively [29,30]. The *n*-back task has been utilized to study a wide range of populations, including ASD [31]. Whereas the literature has reported inconsistent task performance results in individuals with ASD [32,33], almost all fMRI and fNIRS studies have found altered patterns of PFC activation and/or connectivity during the *n*-back task in adolescents and adults with ASD [34,35], suggesting that the *n*-back task is sensitive in revealing altered PFC functioning in ASD. Thus, we used the *n*-back task as a probe for PFC functioning in this study to clarify whether impaired EC is related to altered PFC functioning in children with ASD.

As an optical neuroimaging tool, fNIRS uses lights in the near-infrared spectrum (700–1000 nm) to measure changes in the concentration of oxygenated (HbO) and deoxygenated (HbR) hemoglobin that take place at the cortical surface [36,37]. This method has been validated against fMRI [38]. Over the past 10 years, this technique has been widely utilized in ASD research and has shown promise in understanding ASD [39]. As fNIRS is a relatively non-demanding neuroimaging modality for children, we used it to measure PFC activation and connectivity in this study. We hypothesized that, compared to TD children, children with ASD would demonstrate deficits in EC and its related functions (i.e., EF and socioemotional function). We predicted that these children would also exhibit altered PFC activation and connectivity during the *n*-back task (i.e., a frontal-sensitive task). Furthermore, we expected EC deficits to be associated with altered patterns of PFC activation and connectivity during the *n*-back task in children with ASD.

2. Materials and Methods

2.1. Participants

Participants were recruited from primary schools through an advertisement placed on campus, social media, and sent to schools by post. Consequently, 39 right-handed Chinese children, aged between 8 and 12 years, were recruited, with written informed consent obtained from children and their parents. Twenty children diagnosed with ASD by a psychiatrist and clinical psychologist using the Diagnostic and Statistical Manual of Mental Disorders—5th Edition (DSM-5; [1]) were included in the ASD group. Children with ASD receiving medications were excluded. In addition, 19 age-, handedness-, and IQ-matched children were recruited in the TD group. No children in the TD group had episodes of epilepsy, head trauma, developmental delay, or other neuropsychiatric disorders.

2.2. Procedure

The study was conducted in accordance with the ethical principles for medical research involving human subjects declared by Helsinki. The experimental protocol was approved by the Human Subjects Ethics Sub-Committee of the Hong Kong Polytechnic University (ethic approval code: HSEARS20170203004). All children were evaluated independently in two sessions (neuropsychological evaluation, and fNIRS data acquisition), which lasted about 2 h in total, including breaks. Simultaneously, the parents or caregivers of children were interviewed with standardized interviewing protocols, which included the short form of the Early Adolescent Temperament Questionnaire—Revised (EATQ-R), Social Responsiveness Scale—Second Edition (SRS-2), and Autism Diagnostic Interview—Revised (ADI-R). The assessments and interviews were conducted by a clinical psychologist, skilled research assistants, and graduate students.

2.3. Measures

2.3.1. Short Form of the Early Adolescent Temperament Questionnaire—Revised (EATQ-R)

The level of EC was measured using the short form of the EATQ-R, which is a standardized parent-rated instrument containing 16 items in three subscales (i.e., activation control, attention, and inhibitory control). The items are rated on a 5-point Likert scale, ranging from 1 (almost always untrue of you) to 5 (almost always true of you) for the direct items, and vice versa for the reversed items. A higher score in each domain indicates a greater ability in EC [40].

2.3.2. d2 Test of Attention

The d2 Test of Attention is a standardized paper-and-pencil test for attention, which involves cancelling out all target letters (i.e., the letter "d" with two dashes positioned above or below) interspersed with nontarget letters (i.e., the letter "d" without two dashes, and the letter "p" with any quantifiable dashes) [41]. The concentration performance index obtained by subtracting the sum of correct responses from the sum of commission errors was adopted as the primary measure [42]. The task takes 4.7 min to complete.

2.3.3. Cambridge Neuropsychological Test Automated Battery (CANTAB)

Three subtests from the Cambridge Neuropsychological Test Automated Battery (CANTAB) were administered via 10.5 inch Apple iPad. The reaction time (RTI) task assesses attention in terms of processing speed (motor and mental) and impulsivity. The task involves holding the response button at the bottom of the screen initially, and, as one of the five circles positioned at the top of the screen flashes yellow, participants are required to tap the highlighted circle (target button) as quickly as possible. The mean reaction times (i.e., mean duration of releasing the response button after stimulus presentation) of five-choice variants were calculated [43].

The multitasking test (MTT) measured selective attention (responds to task-relevant stimuli) and inhibition (ignores task-irrelevant stimuli). In each trial, a leftward- or rightward-facing arrow is either presented on the right or left side of the screen. Meanwhile, a cue is presented at the top of the screen, specifying the arrow's direction or location. Participants must press the right or left button at the bottom of the screen, in accordance with the arrow's location or direction, depending on the task cue. The switching block error, denoting the sum of incorrect responses during the block with intermixing task cues, i.e., mean duration of stimuli appearance to pressing button between congruent to incongruent stimuli and vice versa), was adopted as a prime measure in this study. The task included 40 practice and 120 test trials, lasting 8 min [44].

The emotion recognition task (ERT) evaluates the ability to distinguish basic facial expressions. The test requires participants to label photographs of male or female facial expressions presented for 200 ms each, using one of six labels (i.e., sadness, happiness, fear, anger, disgust, and surprise) shown on the screen. There is no time limit for responding. The total number of correct responses was adopted as the primary measure. This task included 5 practice and 90 test trials, lasting 9 min.

2.3.4. *n*-back Task

An *n*-back paradigm adopted from previous studies was employed as the activation task to probe PFC functioning [27,45]. It involved two loading conditions (low and high; 0- and 1-back). Trials were presented in 45 s blocks, interleaved with 30 s of rest, for a total duration of 330 s. Each condition was presented twice, and the two conditions were administered in alternating order (i.e., low–high–low–high; or high–low–high–low). The order was counterbalanced across participants to eliminate order effects. Each task block started with 5 s of a visual cue for a condition, followed by 20 (5 target and 15 nontarget) trials presented pseudorandomly. Each trial included a digit that appeared at the center of the screen for 500 ms, followed by an interstimulus interval of 1500 ms (Figure 1). The low-loading (0-back) condition required participants to left-click the mouse with their right index finger when the number "0" (target) was shown, but to right-click the mouse with their right middle finger when other numbers (nontargets) were shown. The high-loading (1-back) condition required participants to left-click the mouse when the number that appeared was the same as the number shown one trial before (i.e., target), but to right-click the mouse for other numbers (i.e., nontargets). E-prime 2.0 software (Psychology Software Tools, Pittsburgh, PA, USA) was utilized to present all stimuli. During task performance, the frontal brain activities were captured using an fNIRS machine.

2.4. *fNIRS Recording*

During the *n*-back task, fNIRS data acquisition was performed using the Hitachi ETG-4000 machine, which used two wavelengths (695 nm and 830 nm) and sampled data at a rate of 10 Hz. The machine included 33 optodes, including 17 sources and 16 detectors (52 channels), aligned in 3×11 montage with a 3 cm source-detector separation (Figure 2). During recording, participants sat on a chair 60 cm away from a 15′′ LCD monitor in a quiet dimly lit room. Participants' head dimensions (nasion-inion, left-right ear, and head circumference) were measured to facilitate offline spatial registration of NIRS channels [46], in which the channel positions were transformed into the Montreal Neurological Institute (MNI) space, and then projected onto the surface of a volume-rendered children brain template [47,48]. The probe placement regions (forehead) were disinfected with an alcohol pad for better signal quality. A custom-built headband mounted with probes was then placed on the participant's forehead (covering the PFC). As guided by the standardized reference point on the headband, the center of the bottom optode was anchored at Fpz according to the international 10–20 system. The spatial coordinates of 5 anatomical landmark points (nasion, inion, vertex, and left and right auricular points) and 33 optodes were digitized using a 3D digitizer. Based on the calibration procedure implemented in the acquisition software, good signal quality was ensured before the *n*-back task began.

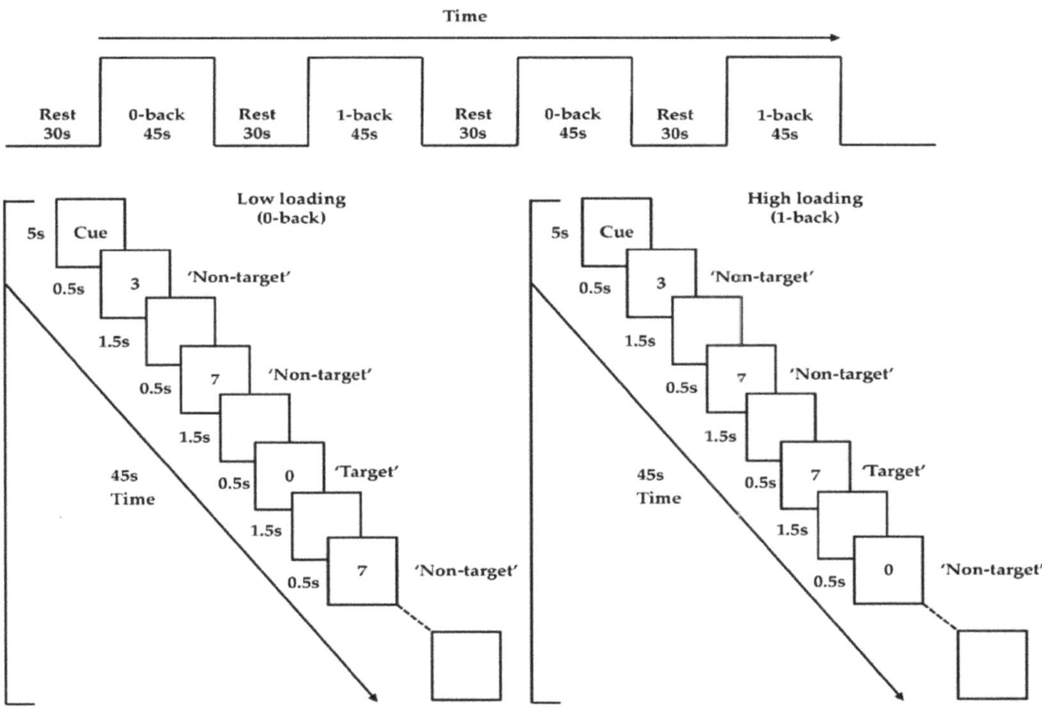

Figure 1. *n*-back task paradigm.

2.5. Data Analysis

Before analyzing the data, normality was checked through Shapiro–Wilk tests. Subsequently, any non-normal data were log-transformed for suitability for parametric testing. If the log-transformed variables still violated the normality assumption, then non-parametric tests were conducted. The data screening and analysis were performed using IBM SPSS Statistics 25 (IBM Corp., Armonk, NY, USA).

2.5.1. Questionnaires and Neuropsychological Measures

The SRS-2 total *T*-score, EATQ-R total score, and other behavioral measures fulfilled the normality assumption. Thus, independent-sample *t*-tests were used for group comparison. However, the behavioral measures of the *n*-back task did not meet the normality assumption even after log transformation. Hence, Mann–Whitney U tests were used to explore the group differences for these variables.

2.5.2. Preprocessing for fNIRS Data

Data preprocessing and analysis were performed using the AnalyzIR Toolbox [49] and Matlab 2019a (The Mathworks, Natick, MA, USA). First, the raw fNIRS data of the *n*-back task were derived in the integral mode after preprocessing with a 0.1 Hz low-pass and a 5 s moving average filter, using the inbuilt Hitachi machine software. The data were then input into the AnalyzIR Toolbox, in which the data were corrected for missing, flat, or saturated channel issues, using default functions. Next, the signals were resampled at 1 Hz, and a 0.1 partial pathlength factor was applied while converting optical density changes into HbO and HbR via the modified Beer–Lambert law [50]. Subsequently, first-level statistical analysis was conducted using the auto-regressive iterative reweighted least-squares (AR-IRLS) approach to estimate activation during task performance [51]. The robust auto-regressive whitened correlation method in the advanced general linear model was also used to estimate connectivity between possible channel pairs. The activation (beta value) and connectivity (*Z*-score) variables were then utilized for group analysis (second-level analysis). We focused on HbO, because, relative to HbR, it has been shown to have a higher signal-to-noise ratio and to correlate more strongly with the Blood Oxygenation Level Dependent (BOLD) signals measured by fMRI [38].

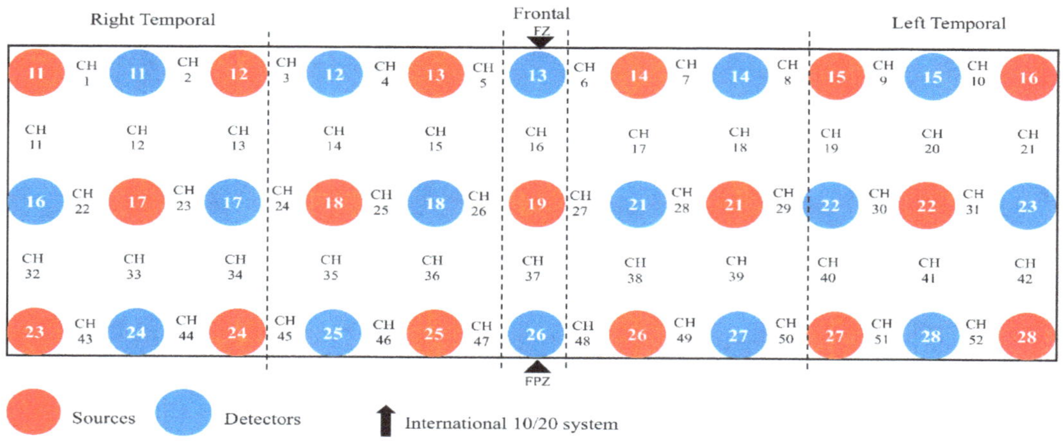

(a)

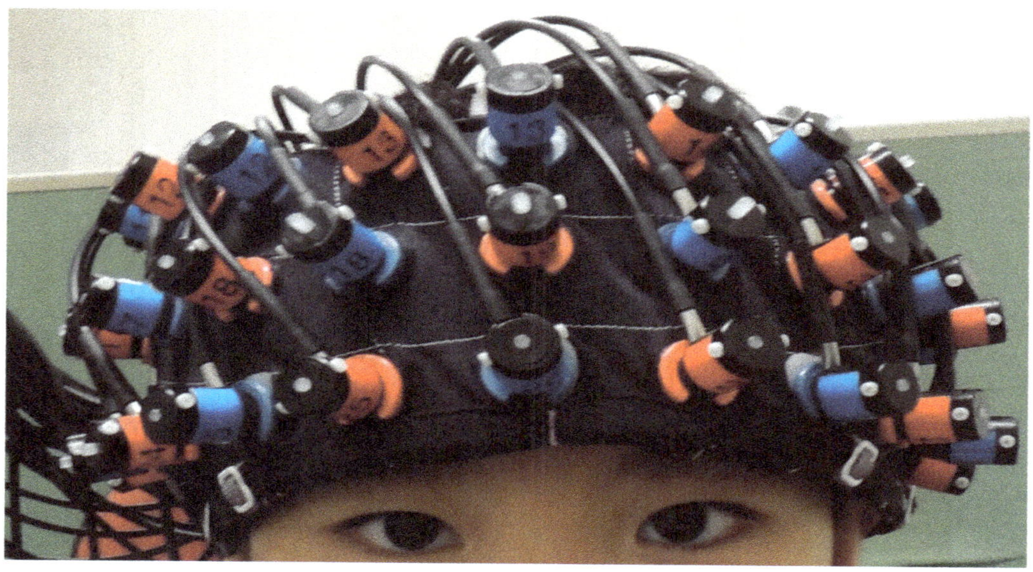

(b)

Figure 2. The 3 × 11 montage of the functional near-infrared spectroscopy (fNIRS) system: (**a**) 33 optodes and 52 channels (CH) arrangement; (**b**) placement on head.

Spatial registration of channels based on the digitized spatial coordinates (5 reference points and 33 optodes) was performed using Near Infra-red Spectroscopy-Statistical Parameter Mapping (NIRS-SPM; [52]). The output of individual MNI coordinates was further grouped together using BrainNet Viewer [53], and the mean composite estimation was obtained. Using an 80% registration probability, channels that fell in the inferior frontal gyrus (IFG), middle frontal gyrus (MFG), and superior frontal gyrus (SFG) on each side were determined, and the 6 anatomically defined PFC regions were defined as regions of interest (ROI; Figure 3; [54]). Note that some PFC channels were not classified into any ROI, because none of them fell into any ROI with an 80% registration probability, and that temporal lobe channels were not analyzed, because most of them yielded poor signal quality due to poor optode–scalp contact.

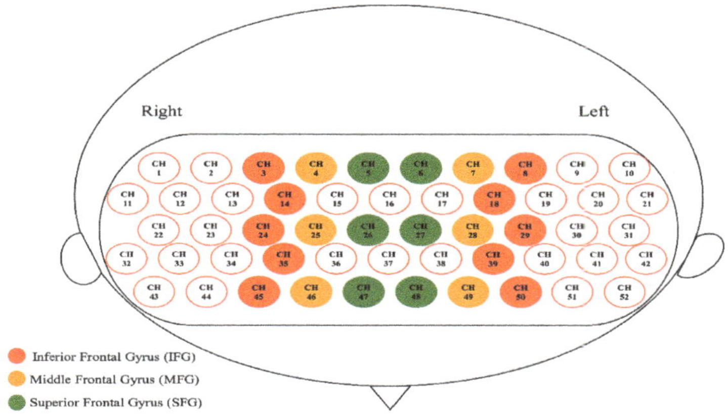

Figure 3. Six anatomically defined ROIs in the prefrontal cortex (PFC).

2.5.3. fNIRS Data Analysis

For activation, the beta values fulfilled the normality assumption. Hence, a $2 \times 2 \times 2$ mixed multifactorial analysis of variance (ANOVA) was utilized to analyze changes in HbO, in terms of beta values. The statistical model included two within-group factors, loading (low and high) and frontal side (left and right), and one between-group factor (TD and ASD).

For connectivity, 6 connectivity patterns were extracted based on the specified ROIs (Figure 4; [54]). Channel pairs were averaged for each connectivity pattern. All connectivity variables (i.e., mean Z-scores) fulfilled the normality assumption; hence, intrahemispheric connectivity was analyzed with a $2 \times 2 \times 2 \times 2$ mixed ANOVA, which included connectivity pattern (within and between ROI), loading (low and high), and frontal side (left and right) as within-subjects factors, and group (TD and ASD) as the between-subjects factor. Additionally, interhemispheric connectivity was analyzed with a $2 \times 2 \times 2$ mixed ANOVA, which included connectivity pattern (within and between ROI) and loading (low and high) as within-subjects factors, and group (TD and ASD) as the between-subjects factor.

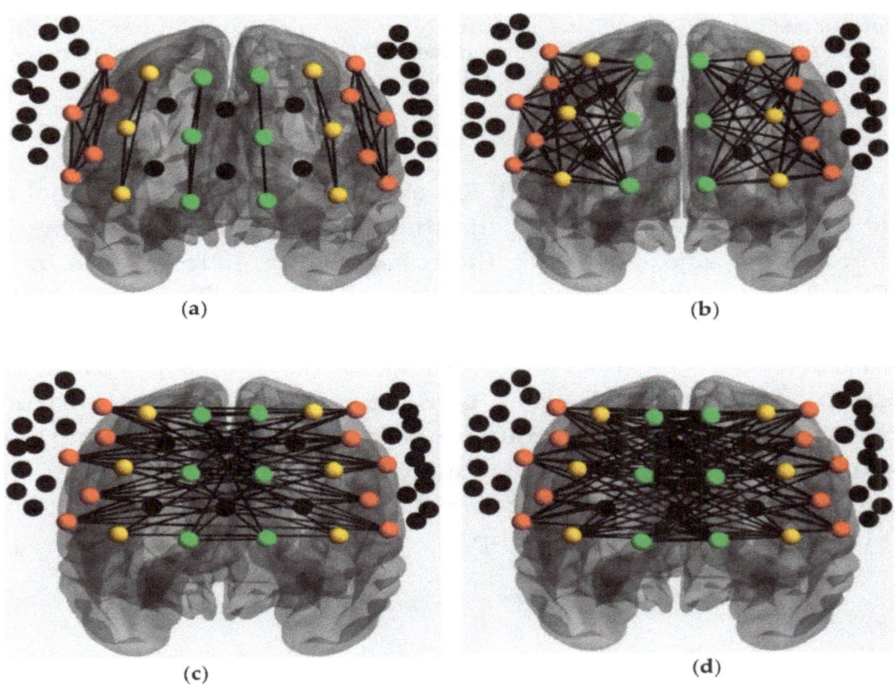

Figure 4. ROIs analysis for connectivity: (**a**) Intrahemispheric connectivity within ROI; (**b**) Intrahemispheric connectivity between ROIs; (**c**) Interhemispheric connectivity within ROIs; (**d**) Interhemispheric connectivity between ROIs.

2.5.4. Brain–Behavior Relationship

To explain individual differences in EC among children with ASD, we examined the relationship between measures of EC and measures of PFC functioning and EC-related constructs (i.e., EF and socioemotional measures) for the ASD group specifically. Variables that met and did not meet the normality assumption were analyzed using Pearson's correlations (r) and Spearman's correlation (r_S), respectively. To reduce the number of comparisons, only variables in which the two groups differed significantly were analyzed.

3. Results

3.1. Demographic, Intellectual, and Clinical Characteristics

Table 1 shows the demographic, intellectual, and clinical information of the TD and ASD groups. The two groups were matched in age, and IQ, $ts < 0.42$, $ps > 0.11$. Although gender was not matched between groups, $\chi^2(1) = 6.65$, $p = 0.01$, independent-sample t-tests revealed no significant differences between male and female TD children in any variable ($ps > 0.05$). As gender was not a confounding factor, it was not controlled for in any subsequent analyses.

Table 1. Demographic, intellectual, and clinical characteristics of the typically developing (TD) and autism spectrum disorder (ASD) groups.

	TD (n = 19)	ASD (n = 20)	$t/\chi^2/r$	p
	Mean (SD)	Mean (SD)		
Age (years)	10.28 (0.67)	10.16 (1.04)	0.42	0.68
IQ	108.79 (9.47)	101.65 (16.96)	1.63	0.11
Gender (Males:Females) #	12:07	20:00	6.65	0.010 **
ADI-R Social Interaction ##	-	14.20 (7.41)	0.052	0.83
ADI-R Communication ##	-	10.75 (5.70)	−0.32	0.18
ADI-R Restricted and Stereotyped Behavior ##	-	5.35 (2.70)	−0.30	0.21

Note: SD: Standard deviation; ADI-R: Autism Diagnostic Interview—Revised; # Groups were compared using the chi-squared test with Yates' correction of the Likelihood Ratio; ## Correlation with Early Adolescent Temperament Questionnaire—Revised (EATQ-R) (total score). ** $p < 0.01$.

3.2. EC, Executive, and Socioemotional Measures

The two groups differed significantly in all EC, executive, and socioemotional measures (Table 2), in which the ASD group showed more deficits than TD controls with a large effect size on the EATQ-R total score, t (36) = 2.83, p = 0.007, the concentration performance index on the d2 Test of Attention, t (37) = 2.69, p = 0.011, the mean score on the CANTAB reaction time, t (36) = 2.67, p = 0.011, the switch block error score on the CANTAB multitasking test, t (30.37) = 2.46, p = 0.019, the total score on the CANTAB emotion recognition task, t (35) = 3.48, p = 0.001, and the SRS-2 total T-score, t (35) = 6.22, $p < 0.001$. As the EATQ-R consisted of three discrete constructs, we performed independent-sample t-tests to compare the groups on each subscale after adjusting the p-value threshold to 0.017. Results showed that the ASD group had more deficits on the attention, t (36) = 2.79, p = 0.008, and inhibitory control subscales, t (36) = 3.05, p = 0.005, but not on the activation control subscale, t (36) = 1.39, p = 0.17, compared to the TD group.

Table 2. Effortful control, executive and socioemotional functions in the typically developing (TD) and autism spectrum disorder (ASD) groups.

Variables	TD (n = 19)	ASD (n = 20)	t	p	d
	Mean (SD)	Mean (SD)			
EATQ-R #					
Total	3.18 (0.50)	2.67 (0.61)	2.83	0.007 **	0.91
Attention	3.16 (0.68)	2.54 (0.67)	2.79	0.008 **	0.92
Inhibitory control	3.42 (0.48)	2.79 (0.76)	3.05	0.005 **	0.99
Activation control	2.97 (0.57)	2.68 (0.69)	1.39	0.17	0.46
D_2 Test of Attention					
Concentration performance index	141.2 (20.2)	121.5 (25.0)	2.69	0.011 *	0.86
CANTAB Reaction Time Task #					
Mean reaction time (ms)	421.8 (51.2)	468.0 (117.3)	2.67	0.011 *	0.51
CANTAB Multitasking Test #					
Switch block error	7.28 (4.39)	12.45 (7.86)	2.46	0.019 *	0.81
CANTAB Emotion Recognition Task #					
Total hit rate	23.72 (3.89)	19.00 (4.33)	3.48	0.001 **	1.15
SRS-2 #					
Total T-score	40.3 (17.4)	87.4 (26.8)	6.22	<0.001 ***	2.09

Note: SRS-2: Social Responsiveness Scale—Second Edition; * $p < 0.05$; ** $p < 0.01$; *** $p < 0.001$; # Missing data: The EATQ-R was uncompleted for 1 child with ASD; The Cambridge Neuropsychological Test Automated Battery (CANTAB) was not administered to 1 TD child; 1 ASD child did not complete the Emotion Recognition Task; The SRS-2 was uncompleted in 2 TD children.

Additionally, children with ASD were slower to respond than TD controls in the low loading condition of the n-back task ($U = 78.00$, $p = 0.001$; Table 3), despite comparable accuracy, $p = 0.79$. There was no significant difference in accuracy or mean reaction time between the two groups in the high loading condition, $ps > 0.074$. However, we noted a significant large correlation between accuracy and mean reaction time in the high loading condition among children with ASD ($r = -0.58$, $p < 0.01$), suggesting a speed–accuracy tradeoff. To control for this, the inverse efficiency score (IES) was calculated by dividing the mean reaction time by accuracy for each condition [55,56]. The IES score was also calculated for the low loading condition to facilitate comparison between conditions. The results indicated that the ASD group had significantly poorer performance, in terms of the IES, than the TD group in both loading conditions.

Table 3. n-back task performance in the typically developing (TD) and autism spectrum disorder (ASD) groups.

Variables	TD (n = 19)	ASD (n = 20)	Z	p	r
	Median (95% CI)	Median (95% CI)			
Mean reaction time (ms)					
Low load	445.1 (423.8–538.7)	502.1 (517.1–687.1)	3.15	0.001 **	0.50
High load	536.0 (505.0–644.4)	636.3 (603.9–811.6)	1.80	0.074	0.29
Accuracy					
Low load	0.97 (0.93–0.97)	0.95 (0.92–0.97)	0.27	0.79	0.043
High load	0.94 (0.87–0.95)	0.89 (0.83–0.93)	0.64	0.53	0.10
Inverse efficiency score					
Low load	496.1 (494.7–518.4)	633.8 (621.2–653.9)	5.36	<0.001 ***	0.86
High load	611.3 (608.8–664.8)	794.8 (761.2–875.0)	4.72	<0.001 ***	0.76

Note: ** $p < 0.01$; *** $p < 0.001$.

3.3. PFC Activation during the N-Back Task

The 2 × 2 × 2 (group × frontal side × condition) mixed ANOVA showed a significant main effect of group, $F(1,36) = 4.12$, $p = 0.050$, $\eta_p^2 = 0.10$, in which the ASD group exhibited more PFC activation ($M = 0.071$, $SE = 0.018$) than the TD group ($M = 0.019$, $SE = 0.018$). No other effects were significant ($ps > 0.05$).

3.4. PFC Connectivity during the n-Back Task

3.4.1. Intrahemispheric Connectivity

Results of the 2 × 2 × 2 × 2 (group × connectivity pattern × loading × frontal side) mixed ANOVA conducted for intrahemispheric connectivity (i.e., mean Z-scores) are presented in Table 4. The ANOVA demonstrated significant main effects of connectivity pattern, $p < 0.001$, loading, $p = 0.041$, and frontal side, $p = 0.037$. Whereas the main effect of group was not significant, $p = 0.26$, there was a significant interaction between frontal side and group, $p = 0.005$. Independent-sample t-tests showed a significant group difference in right intrahemispheric connectivity, $t(35) = 2.55$, $p = 0.015$, in which the TD group exhibited greater right frontal connectivity ($M = 0.22$, $SD = 0.083$) than the ASD group ($M = 0.15$, $SD = 0.088$). There was no significant group difference in left intrahemispheric connectivity, $p = 0.38$.

There was also a significant three-way interaction between connectivity pattern, loading, and group, $p = 0.024$. Follow-up independent-sample t-tests, exploring differences between the TD and ASD groups in within- and between-ROI connectivity in the two loading conditions, separately showed a significant difference between the two groups on between-ROI connectivity in the high-loading condition, $t(35) = 2.17$, $p = 0.037$, in which the TD group exhibited greater frontal connectivity ($M = 0.24$, $SD = 0.037$) than the ASD group ($M = 0.19$, $SD = 0.082$). The two groups did not differ significantly in between-ROI connectivity in the low-load condition, or in within-ROI connectivity in either load condition ($ps > 0.05$).

Table 4. Mixed ANOVA (group × loading × frontal side × connectivity pattern) results for intrahemispheric connectivity (i.e., mean Z-scores).

Main/Interaction Effects	Mean (*SE*)	*F*(1,35)	*p*	η_p^2
Connectivity pattern (within and between ROI)	Within: 0.18 (0.011) Between: 0.22 (0.012)	48.28	<0.001 ***	0.58
Loading (low and high)	Low: 0.21 (0.013) High: 0.19 (0.010)	4.50	0.041 *	0.11
Frontal side (left and right)	Right: 0.18 (0.014) Left: 0.22 (0.013)	4.68	0.037 *.	0.12
Group (TD and ASD)	TD: 0.21 (0.015) ASD: 0.19 (0.015)	1.29	0.26	0.036
Two-way interaction				
Connectivity pattern × loading		3.09	0.088	0.081
Connectivity pattern × frontal side		0.037	0.85	0.001
Loading × frontal side		2.42	0.13	0.065
Loading × group		0.61	0.44	0.017
Connectivity pattern × group		0.23	0.63	0.007
Frontal side × group		8.98	0.005 **	0.20
Three-way interaction				
Connectivity pattern × loading × frontal side		5.71	0.022 *	0.14
Connectivity pattern × loading × group		5.61	0.024 *	0.14
Connectivity pattern × frontal side × group		0.010	0.92	0.000
Loading × frontal side × group		2.99	0.092	0.079
Four-way interaction				
Connectivity pattern × frontal side × loading × group		0.006	0.94	0.000

Note: *SE: Standard error;* * $p < 0.05$; ** $p < 0.01$; *** $p < 0.001$.

3.4.2. Interhemispheric Connectivity

Results of the 2 × 2 × 2 (groups × connectivity pattern × loading) mixed ANOVA conducted for interhemispheric connectivity (i.e., mean Z-scores) are presented in Table 5. The ANOVA demonstrated a significant main effects of connectivity pattern, $p = 0.003$, and loading, $p = 0.026$. The main effect of group was not significant, $p = 0.15$, but there was a significant interaction effect between connectivity pattern and group, $p = 0.043$. Nevertheless, independent-sample *t*-tests revealed no significant difference in either within- or between-ROI connectivity between the two groups (*p*s > 0.05). This interaction effect was driven by the presence of higher between-ROI than within-ROI connectivity in the TD group, but not in the ASD group.

Table 5. Mixed ANOVA (group × loading × connectivity pattern) results for interhemispheric connectivity (i.e., mean Z-scores).

Main/Interaction Effects	Mean (*SE*)	$F(1,34)$	p	η_p^2
Connectivity pattern (within and between ROI)	Within ROI: 0.19 (0.014) Between ROI: 0.20 (0.013)	10.06	0.003 **	0.23
Loading (low and high)	Low: 0.21 (0.015) High: 0.18 (0.014)	5.43	0.026 *	0.14
Group (TD and ASD)	TD: 0.21 (0.019) ASD: 0.17 (0.018)	2.14	0.15	0.059
Two-way interaction				
Connectivity pattern × loading		0.75	0.39	0.021
Loading × group		1.44	0.24	0.041
Connectivity pattern × group		4.41	0.043 *	0.12
Three-way interaction				
Connectivity pattern × loading × group		0.14	0.71	0.004

Note: * $p < 0.05$; ** $p < 0.01$.

3.5. Individual Differences of EC in the ASD Group

We conducted correlation analyses to elucidate the basis of individual differences in EC among children with ASD. These children were found to have poorer performance in all EF and socioemotional measures, increased PFC activation across regions and conditions, and reduced right intrahemispheric connectivity across connection patterns and conditions, compared to TD children. Thus, we examined the correlation between the EATQ-R total score and each EF and socioemotional measure, overall PFC activation, and overall right intrahemispheric connectivity. The EATQ-R total score correlated significantly with the SRS-2 total *T*-score only, $r = -0.69$, $p = 0.001$. No other correlations were significant, *p*s > 0.05.

4. Discussion

The primary objective of this study was to elucidate the relationship between EC and PFC functioning in terms of activation and connectivity during a frontal-sensitive (*n*-back) task in children with ASD. We found that the ASD group demonstrated significantly lower levels of EC and its relevant EF and socioemotional measures, compared to TD controls. Children with ASD also exhibited altered PFC functioning, indicated by PFC hyperactivation and reduced right frontal connectivity across *n*-back conditions. We further showed that EC was associated with social skills but not with PFC processing or EF in the ASD group, suggesting that individual differences in EC among children with ASD may be explained by individual differences in social functioning only.

The current findings support our hypotheses. First, the children with ASD presented with more EC deficits than the TD group, such that the EATQ-R differentiated the two groups of children on the attentional and inhibitory control components. The result is consistent with previous findings, in which the parents of adolescents with ASD perceived lower attentional and inhibitory control abilities over a dominating response [3,57,58]. However, in contrast to Samyn and Roeyers's [57] report of an activation control deficit in ASD, the current finding showed a comparable effect of ASD on activation control, suggesting that the children from the TD and ASD groups had a similar ability to generate and persist with a novel action even when there is an urgency to terminate. The inconsistency may be due to age difference, as they [57] focused on adolescents with ASD, and activation control deficits may become more pronounced with age, due to underdevelopment in ASD.

Our fNIRS findings of reduced right PFC connectivity during the *n*-back task in the ASD group corroborate the "frontal disconnection syndrome" theory of autism, which postulates that frontal disconnection negatively influences the performance of higher-order cognitive tasks [59,60]. Our findings specifically support the underconnectivity theory of ASD, which bridges the neurophysiological basis of complex information processing impairment to its associated frontal lobe dysfunction in individuals with autism [61,62]. The *n*-back task used in our study required participants to monitor and hold onto a piece of information briefly, in accordance with specific loading conditions. It also required participants to respond to interchanging stimuli, involving activating, inhibiting, and switching elements, which necessitate a complex information processing system found to be defective in ASD [63]. As the right lateral frontal lobe has been shown to play an essential role in monitoring [64], hypoconnectivity in the right frontal lobe revealed that children with ASD had difficulty monitoring and processing complex information.

Our findings of a link between EC deficits and social impairment in ASD corroborate the hypothesized role of EC in social affect, empathy, and prosocial behavior, which together assist children in gaining adaptive function [4,65]. However, the present study did not yield significant relationships between EC and task measures of other related constructs (i.e., EF tests, ERT, and *n*-back behavioral measures) or between EC and PFC activation or connectivity. These findings suggest that EC may be a different construct from EF. In addition, questionnaires and behavioral measures may tap distinct response processes. That is, questionnaires include items on real-life behavior that requires individuals to respond using subjective perception or judgement in an open-ended environment and under noncompetitive circumstances, whereas the behavioral measures require individuals to respond on the basis of task performance in a structured setting and under competitive circumstances [66].

Notably, the absence of significant correlations between questionnaires and behavioral measures may be due to the methodological constraints of behavioral measures, which have poor reliability in general [67]. However, the test–retest reliability of the parent-report and behavioral measures used in the present study has been shown to be at least moderate-to-high and comparable with each other (e.g., CANTAB RTI five-choice reaction time in children: $r = 0.63$ [43]; d2 Concentration Performance in adolescents: $r = 0.74$ [68]; EATQ-R score in Chinese adolescents: *r*s from 0.62 to 0.72 [69]; SRS-2 total score in TD and ASD children/adolescents: *r*s from 0.72 to 0.95 [70]. Thus, poor reliability of behavioral measures is not a plausible explanation for the lack of correlations.

Although we found EC deficits and altered PFC functioning in the ASD group, there was a lack of a monolithic relationship between the two, suggesting that individual differences in EC deficits cannot be explained by the degree of overall PFC activation or right frontal underconnectivity among children with ASD. Temperamental EC refers to the ability to inhibit a dominant response to perform a subdominant response in emotionally salient settings [5]. In addition, emotion perception and behavior have been shown to heavily engage the amygdala and anterior cingulate cortex, as well as their interactions with the medial frontal cortex [71,72]. It has long been known that these regions exhibit structural and functional abnormalities in ASD [73]. Thus, it is possible that the EC deficits in ASD are better explained by disturbances in these brain regions and circuits, which remains to be determined.

This study is one of the first to explore EC and its relationship with brain theories and EF in children with ASD. The findings yield valuable evidence that EC deficits and altered PFC functioning are present in these children, but there is no evidence that individual differences in EC can be explained by the extent of altered PFC functioning among children with ASD. In addition, the current study demonstrates temperamental EC deficit and its strong link with social dysfunction in children with ASD, suggesting that EC intervention may be clinically useful to improve real-world social skills in these children. Furthermore, this study generates support for the application of fNIRS to understand ASD [39] and as a cost-effective and user-friendly tool to probe the functional coupling of cortical (but not subcortical) regions during cognitive tasks.

The study has several limitations. First, the small sample size and inclusion of only boys with high-functioning ASD, means that the findings may not be generalized to girls with ASD, low-functioning ASD, or other age groups. Nevertheless, we found that sex was not a confounding factor in any variables among TD children. Second, EC was measured using a parent-report questionnaire alone, and the possibility of parental bias that affects the estimation of the true EC status cannot be ruled out. Third, the *n*-back task had limited difficulty levels, in terms of working memory loading and interference [74], which is necessary to make it understandable to most, if not all, children. Thus, this task may lack optimal sensitivity to assess the level of PFC functioning to be correlated with the EC measure.

5. Conclusions

This study showed general deficits in EC and its related constructs (i.e., executive and socioemotional function), as well as altered PFC functioning in children with ASD. It also expands on the previous knowledge of PFC processing during working memory processing among these children and adds converging support for the model of frontal disconnection syndrome and information processing disorder as a neuropathological biomarker of ASD. The relationship between the EC deficit and social dysfunction observed in children with ASD implies that EC may be central to enhancing the social functioning of these children. The lack of a significant monolithic relationship between EC and PFC activation/connectivity among children with ASD warrants further research with the inclusion of a larger sample size and individuals with diverse autistic symptoms, examining the contribution of dysfunction in non-PFC (e.g., limbic) regions or circuits to EC deficits in ASD.

Author Contributions: Conceptualization, K.K., Y.M.Y.H., M.K.Y.; methodology, K.K., Y.M.Y.H.; software, K.K.; formal analysis, K.K.; data curation, K.K., Y.M.Y.H.; writing—original draft preparation, K.K.; writing—review and editing, M.K.Y.; visualization, K.K.; supervision, Y.M.Y.H., A.S.C.; project administration, Y.M.Y.H., A.S.C.; funding acquisition, Y.M.Y.H. All authors have read and agreed to the published version of the manuscript.

Acknowledgments: The authors would like to thank Sophia Sze, Ming Chung Chan, Winnie Cheung, and Issac Wong for their assistance in the recruitment of participants and the collection and management of data. Appreciation is extended to all the children and parents who participated in the research.

References

1. American Psychiatric Association. *The Diagnostic and Statistical Manual of Mental Disorders: DSM-5*; American Psychiatric Publishing: Washington, DC, USA, 2013.
2. Eisenberg, N.; Smith, L.C.; Sadovsky, A.; Spinarad, L.T. Effortful control: Relations with emotion regulation, adjustment, and socialization in childhood. In *Handbook of Self-Regulation: Research, Theory, and Applications*; Baumeister, R.F., Kathleen, D.V., Eds.; The Guilford Press: New York, NY, USA, 2004; pp. 259–282.
3. Konstantareas, M.M.; Stewart, K. Affect Regulation and Temperament in Children with Autism Spectrum Disorder. *J. Autism Dev. Disord.* **2006**, *36*, 143–154. [CrossRef]
4. Schwartz, C.B.; Henderson, H.A.; Inge, A.P.; Zahka, N.E.; Coman, D.C.; Kojkowski, N.M.; Hileman, C.M.; Mundy, P.C. Temperament as a Predictor of Symptomotology and Adaptive Functioning in Adolescents with High-Functioning Autism. *J. Autism Dev. Disord.* **2009**, *39*, 842–855. [CrossRef]
5. Rothbart, M.; Bates, J.E. Temperament. In *Handbook of Child Psychology: Social, Emotional, and Personality Development*, 6th ed.; Eisenberg, W.D., Lerner, R.M., Eds.; John Wiley & Sons, Inc: New York, NY, USA, 2006; Volume 3, pp. 99–166.
6. Goldstein, M.A.; Brendel, G.; Tuescher, O.; Pan, H.; Epstein, J.; Beutel, M.; Yang, Y.; Thomas, K.; Levy, K.; Silverman, M.E.; et al. Neural substrates of the interaction of emotional stimulus processing and motor inhibitory control: An emotional linguistic go/no-go fMRI study. *NeuroImage* **2007**, *36*, 1026–1040. [CrossRef]
7. Claes, L.; Vertommen, S.; Smits, D.; Bijttebier, P. Emotional reactivity and self-regulation in relation to personality disorders. *Pers. Individ. Differ.* **2009**, *47*, 948–953. [CrossRef]

8. Eisenberg, N.; Spinrad, T.L.; Eggum, N.D. Emotion-Related Self-Regulation and Its Relation to Children's Maladjustment. *Annu. Rev. Clin. Psychol.* **2010**, *6*, 495–525. [CrossRef]
9. Lengua, L.J.; Bush, N.R.; Long, A.C.; Kovacs, E.A.; Trancik, A.M. Effortful control as a moderator of the relation between contextual risk factors and growth in adjustment problems. *Dev. Psychopathol.* **2008**, *20*, 509–528. [CrossRef]
10. Miyake, A.; Friedman, N.P.; Emerson, M.J.; Witzki, A.H.; Howerter, A.; Wager, T.D. The Unity and Diversity of Executive Functions and Their Contributions to Complex "Frontal Lobe" Tasks: A Latent Variable Analysis. *Cogn. Psychol.* **2000**, *41*, 49–100. [CrossRef]
11. Zhou, Q.; Chen, S.H.; Main, A. Commonalities and Differences in the Research on Children's Effortful Control and Executive Function: A Call for an Integrated Model of Self-Regulation. *Child Dev. Perspect.* **2011**, *6*, 112–121. [CrossRef]
12. Miller, E.K.; Cohen, J.D. An Integrative Theory of Prefrontal Cortex Function. *Annu. Rev. Neurosci.* **2001**, *24*, 167–202. [CrossRef]
13. Kelley, W.M.; Wagner, D.D.; Heatherton, T.F. In Search of a Human Self-Regulation System. *Annu. Rev. Neurosci.* **2015**, *38*, 389–411. [CrossRef]
14. Quiñones-Camacho, L.E.; Fishburn, F.A.; Camacho, M.C.; Wakschlag, L.S.; Perlman, S.B. Cognitive flexibility-related prefrontal activation in preschoolers: A biological approach to temperamental effortful control. *Dev. Cogn. Neurosci.* **2019**, *38*, 100651. [CrossRef] [PubMed]
15. Seeley, W.W.; Menon, V.; Schatzberg, A.F.; Keller, J.; Glover, G.H.; Kenna, H.; Reiss, A.L.; Greicius, M.D. Dissociable Intrinsic Connectivity Networks for Salience Processing and Executive Control. *J. Neurosci.* **2007**, *27*, 2349–2356. [CrossRef] [PubMed]
16. Dosenbach, N.U.; Fair, D.A.; Miezin, F.M.; Cohen, A.L.; Wenger, K.K.; Dosenbach, R.A.T.; Fox, M.D.; Snyder, A.Z.; Vincent, J.L.; Raichle, M.E.; et al. Distinct brain networks for adaptive and stable task control in humans. *Proc. Natl. Acad. Sci. USA* **2007**, *104*, 11073–11078. [CrossRef] [PubMed]
17. Fekete, T.; Beacher, F.D.; Cha, J.; Rubin, D.; Mujica-Parodi, L.R. Small-world network properties in prefrontal cortex correlate with predictors of psychopathology risk in young children: A NIRS study. *NeuroImage* **2014**, *85*, 345–353. [CrossRef] [PubMed]
18. Courchesne, E.; Pierce, K. Why the frontal cortex in autism might be talking only to itself: Local over-connectivity but long-distance disconnection. *Curr. Opin. Neurobiol.* **2005**, *15*, 225–230. [CrossRef] [PubMed]
19. Ecker, C.; Bookheimer, S.Y.; Murphy, D.G.M. Neuroimaging in autism spectrum disorder: Brain structure and function across the lifespan. *Lancet Neurol.* **2015**, *14*, 1121–1134. [CrossRef]
20. Philip, R.C.; Dauvermann, M.R.; Whalley, H.C.; Baynham, K.; Lawrie, S.M.; Stanfield, A.C. A systematic review and meta-analysis of the fMRI investigation of autism spectrum disorders. *Neurosci. Biobehav. Rev.* **2012**, *36*, 901–942. [CrossRef]
21. Zhang, Z.; Peng, P.; Zhang, D. Executive Function in High-Functioning Autism Spectrum Disorder: A Meta-analysis of fMRI Studies. *J. Autism Dev. Disord.* **2020**, 1–17. [CrossRef]
22. Kana, R.K.; Keller, T.A.; Minshew, N.J.; Just, M.A. Inhibitory Control in High-Functioning Autism: Decreased Activation and Underconnectivity in Inhibition Networks. *Biol. Psychiatry* **2007**, *62*, 198–206. [CrossRef]
23. Fitzgerald, J.; Johnson, K.A.; Kehoe, E.; Bokde, A.L.; Garavan, H.; Gallagher, L.; McGrath, J. Disrupted Functional Connectivity in Dorsal and Ventral Attention Networks During Attention Orienting in Autism Spectrum Disorders. *Autism Res.* **2014**, *8*, 136–152. [CrossRef]
24. Solomon, M.; Ozonoff, S.J.; Ursu, S.; Ravizza, S.; Cummings, N.; Ly, S.; Carter, C.S. The neural substrates of cognitive control deficits in autism spectrum disorders. *Neuropsychologia* **2009**, *47*, 2515–2526. [CrossRef] [PubMed]
25. O'Reilly, C.; Lewis, J.D.; Elsabbagh, M. Is functional brain connectivity atypical in autism? A systematic review of EEG and MEG studies. *PLoS ONE* **2017**, *12*, e0175870. [CrossRef] [PubMed]
26. Owen, A.M.; McMillan, K.M.; Laird, A.R.; Bullmore, E. N-back working memory paradigm: A meta-analysis of normative functional neuroimaging studies. *Hum. Brain Mapp.* **2005**, *25*, 46–59. [CrossRef]
27. Yeung, M.K.; Sze, S.L.; Woo, J.; Kwok, T.C.Y.; Shum, D.H.K.; Yu, R.; Chan, A.S. Reduced Frontal Activations at High Working Memory Load in Mild Cognitive Impairment: Near-Infrared Spectroscopy. *Dement. Geriatr. Cogn. Disord.* **2016**, *42*, 278–296. [CrossRef]

28. Tsuchida, A.; Fellows, L.K. Lesion Evidence That Two Distinct Regions within Prefrontal Cortex are Critical for n-Back Performance in Humans. *J. Cogn. Neurosci.* **2009**, *21*, 2263–2275. [CrossRef]
29. Gajewski, P.D.; Hanisch, E.; Falkenstein, M.; Thönes, S.; Wascher, E. What Does the n-Back Task Measure as We Get Older? Relations between Working-Memory Measures and Other Cognitive Functions Across the Lifespan. *Front. Psychol.* **2018**, *9*, 2208. [CrossRef]
30. Di Martino, A.; Kelly, C.; Grzadzinski, R.; Zuo, X.-N.; Mennes, M.; Mairena, M.A.; Lord, C.; Castellanos, F.X.; Milham, M.P. Aberrant Striatal Functional Connectivity in Children with Autism. *Biol. Psychiatry* **2011**, *69*, 847–856. [CrossRef]
31. Barendse, E.M.; Schreuder, L.J.; Thoonen, G.; Hendriks, M.P.H.; Kessels, R.P.C.; Backes, W.H.; Aldenkamp, A.P.; Jansen, J.F. Working memory network alterations in high-functioning adolescents with an autism spectrum disorder. *Psychiatry Clin. Neurosci.* **2017**, *72*, 73–83. [CrossRef]
32. Lever, A.G.; Werkle-Bergner, M.; Brandmaier, A.M.; Ridderinkhof, K.R.; Geurts, H.M. Atypical working memory decline across the adult lifespan in autism spectrum disorder? *J. Abnorm. Psychol.* **2015**, *124*, 1014–1026. [CrossRef] [PubMed]
33. Williams, D.L.; Goldstein, G.; Carpenter, P.A.; Minshew, N.J. Verbal and Spatial Working Memory in Autism. *J. Autism Dev. Disord.* **2005**, *35*, 747–756. [CrossRef]
34. Koshino, H.; Carpenter, P.A.; Minshew, N.J.; Cherkassky, V.L.; Keller, T.A.; Just, M.A. Functional connectivity in an fMRI working memory task in high-functioning autism. *NeuroImage* **2005**, *24*, 810–821. [CrossRef] [PubMed]
35. Yeung, M.K.; Lee, T.L.; Chan, A.S. Right-lateralized frontal activation underlies successful updating of verbal working memory in adolescents with high-functioning autism spectrum disorder. *Biol. Psychol.* **2019**, *148*, 107743. [CrossRef] [PubMed]
36. Boas, D.A.; Elwell, C.E.; Ferrari, M.; Taga, G. Twenty years of functional near-infrared spectroscopy: Introduction for the special issue. *NeuroImage* **2014**, *85*, 1–5. [CrossRef] [PubMed]
37. Ferrari, M.; Quaresima, V. A brief review on the history of human functional near-infrared spectroscopy (fNIRS) development and fields of application. *NeuroImage* **2012**, *63*, 921–935. [CrossRef]
38. Cui, X.; Bray, S.; Bryant, D.M.; Glover, G.H.; Reiss, A.L. A quantitative comparison of NIRS and fMRI across multiple cognitive tasks. *NeuroImage* **2011**, *54*, 2808–2821. [CrossRef]
39. Zhang, F.; Roeyers, H. Exploring brain functions in autism spectrum disorder: A systematic review on functional near-infrared spectroscopy (fNIRS) studies. *Int. J. Psychophysiol.* **2019**, *137*, 41–53. [CrossRef]
40. Muris, P.; Meesters, C. Reactive and Regulative Temperament in Youths: Psychometric Evaluation of the Early Adolescent Temperament Questionnaire-Revised. *J. Psychopathol. Behav. Assess.* **2008**, *31*, 7–19. [CrossRef]
41. Bates, M.E.; Lemay, E.P. The d2 Test of Attention: Construct validity and extensions in scoring techniques. *J. Int. Neuropsychol. Soc.* **2004**, *10*, 392–400. [CrossRef]
42. José, H.L.; Elena, C.; María, P.F. Convergent validity of measures of attention and impulsivity from the trees simple visual discrimination test (divisa-uam). *An. Psicol. Ann. Psychol.* **2014**, *31*, 74–83.
43. Syväoja, H.J.; Tammelin, T.H.; Ahonen, T.; Räsänen, P.; Tolvanen, A.; Kankaanpää, A.; Kantomaa, M.T. Internal consistency and stability of the CANTAB neuropsychological test battery in children. *Psychol. Assess.* **2015**, *27*, 698–709. [CrossRef]
44. Wild, K.; Musser, E.D. The cambridge neuropsychological test automated battery in the assessment of executive functioning. In *Handbook of Executive Functioning*; Goldstein, S., Naglieri, J.A., Eds.; Springer: New York, NY, USA, 2014; pp. 171–190.
45. Ehlis, A.-C.; Bähne, C.G.; Jacob, C.; Herrmann, M.J.; Fallgatter, A.J. Reduced lateral prefrontal activation in adult patients with attention-deficit/hyperactivity disorder (ADHD) during a working memory task: A functional near-infrared spectroscopy (fNIRS) study. *J. Psychiatr. Res.* **2008**, *42*, 1060–1067. [CrossRef] [PubMed]
46. Singh, A.K.; Okamoto, M.; Dan, H.; Jurcak, V.; Dan, I. Spatial registration of multichannel multi-subject fNIRS data to MNI space without MRI. *NeuroImage* **2005**, *27*, 842–851. [CrossRef] [PubMed]
47. Sanchez, C.E.; Richards, J.E.; Almli, C.R. Age-specific MRI templates for pediatric neuroimaging. *Dev. Neuropsychol.* **2012**, *37*, 379–399. [CrossRef] [PubMed]
48. Xie, W.; Richards, J.E.; Lei, D.; Zhu, H.; Lee, K.; Gong, Q. The construction of MRI brain/head templates for Chinese children from 7 to 16 years of age. *Dev. Cogn. Neurosci.* **2015**, *15*, 94–105. [CrossRef]

49. Santosa, H.; Zhai, X.; Fishburn, F.; Huppert, T. The NIRS Brain AnalyzIR Toolbox. *Algorithms* **2018**, *11*, 73. [CrossRef]
50. Delpy, D.T.; Cope, M.; Van Der Zee, P.; Arridge, S.; Wray, S.; Wyatt, J. Estimation of optical pathlength through tissue from direct time of flight measurement. *Phys. Med. Biol.* **1988**, *33*, 1433–1442. [CrossRef]
51. Barker, J.W.; Aarabi, A.; Huppert, T.J. Autoregressive model based algorithm for correcting motion and serially correlated errors in fNIRS. *Biomed. Opt. Express* **2013**, *4*, 1366–1379. [CrossRef]
52. Ye, J.C.; Tak, S.; Jang, K.E.; Jung, J.; Jang, J. NIRS-SPM: Statistical parametric mapping for near-infrared spectroscopy. *NeuroImage* **2009**, *44*, 428–447. [CrossRef]
53. Xia, M.; Wang, J.; He, Y. BrainNet Viewer: A Network Visualization Tool for Human Brain Connectomics. *PLoS ONE* **2013**, *8*, e68910. [CrossRef]
54. Zhu, H.; Xu, J.; Li, J.; Peng, H.; Cai, T.; Li, X.; Wu, S.; Cao, W.; He, S. Decreased functional connectivity and disrupted neural network in the prefrontal cortex of affective disorders: A resting-state fNIRS study. *J. Affect. Disord.* **2017**, *221*, 132–144. [CrossRef]
55. Townsend, J.; Ashby, F. Methods of modeling capacity in simple processing systems. *Cog. Theory* **1978**, *3*, 199–239.
56. Townsend, J.; Ashby, F. *The Stochastic Modeling of Elementary Psychological Processes (Part 2)*, 1st ed.; Cambridge University Press: New York, NY, USA, 1983.
57. Samyn, V.; Eroeyers, H.; Bijttebier, P. Effortful control in typically developing boys and in boys with ADHD or autism spectrum disorder. *Res. Dev. Disabil.* **2011**, *32*, 483–490. [CrossRef] [PubMed]
58. Adamek, L.; Nichols, S.; Tetenbaum, S.P.; Bregman, J.; Ponzio, C.A.; Carr, E.G. Individual Temperament and Problem Behavior in Children with Autism Spectrum Disorders. *Focus Autism Other Dev. Disabil.* **2011**, *26*, 173–183. [CrossRef]
59. Geschwind, D.H.; Levitt, P. Autism spectrum disorders: Developmental disconnection syndromes. *Curr. Opin. Neurobiol.* **2007**, *17*, 103–111. [CrossRef] [PubMed]
60. Zeestraten, E.A.; Gudbrandsen, M.; Daly, E.; De Schotten, M.T.; Catani, M.; Acqua, F.D.; Lai, M.-C.; Ruigrok, A.N.V.; Lombardo, M.V.; Chakrabarti, B.; et al. Sex differences in frontal lobe connectivity in adults with autism spectrum conditions. *Transl. Psychiatry* **2017**, *7*, e1090. [CrossRef] [PubMed]
61. Just, M.A.; Keller, T.A.; Malave, V.L.; Kana, R.K.; Varma, S. Autism as a neural systems disorder: A theory of frontal-posterior underconnectivity. *Neurosci. Biobehav. Rev.* **2012**, *36*, 1292–1313. [CrossRef]
62. Frith, C. Is autism a disconnection disorder? *Lancet Neurol.* **2004**, *3*, 577. [CrossRef]
63. Minshew, N.J.; Goldstein, G.; Siegel, D.J. Neuropsychologic functioning in autism: Profile of a complex information processing disorder. *J. Int. Neuropsychol. Soc.* **1997**, *3*, 303–316. [CrossRef]
64. Stuss, D.T.; Alexander, M.P. Is there a dysexecutive syndrome? *Philos. Trans. R. Soc. B Biol. Sci.* **2007**, *362*, 901–915. [CrossRef]
65. Faja, S.; Dawson, G. Reduced delay of gratification and effortful control among young children with autism spectrum disorders. *Autism* **2013**, *19*, 91–101. [CrossRef] [PubMed]
66. Hedge, C.; Powell, G.; Sumner, P. The reliability paradox: Why robust cognitive tasks do not produce reliable individual differences. *Behav. Res. Methods* **2017**, *50*, 1166–1186. [CrossRef] [PubMed]
67. Dang, J.; King, K.M.; Inzlicht, M. Why Are Self-Report and Behavioral Measures Weakly Correlated? *Trends Cogn. Sci.* **2020**, *24*, 267–269. [CrossRef] [PubMed]
68. Brickenkamp, R.; Rump, G. Die Stabilität des Aufmerksamkeits-Belastungs—Tests (Test d2) über längere Zeitabschnitte. [Long-term, test-retest stability of the d2 Test of Attention.]. *Diagnostica* **1966**, *12*, 17–24.
69. Zhang, J.; Shen, L.; Gao, N.; Yan, C. The Revision and Application of the Revision of the Early Adolescent Temperament Questionnaire. *Chin. Ment. Heal. J.* **2008**, *22*, 439–443.
70. Bölte, S.; Poustka, F.; Constantino, J.N. Assessing autistic traits: Cross-cultural validation of the social responsiveness scale (SRS). *Autism Res.* **2008**, *1*, 354–363. [CrossRef]
71. Etkin, A.; Egner, T.; Kalisch, R. Emotional processing in anterior cingulate and medial prefrontal cortex. *Trends Cogn. Sci.* **2011**, *15*, 85–93. [CrossRef]
72. Phelps, E.A.; LeDoux, J.E. Contributions of the Amygdala to Emotion Processing: From Animal Models to Human Behavior. *Neuron* **2005**, *48*, 175–187. [CrossRef]
73. Baron-Cohen, S.; Ring, H.; Bullmore, E.; Wheelwright, S.; Ashwin, C.; Williams, S. The amygdala theory of autism. *Neurosci. Biobehav. Rev.* **2000**, *24*, 355–364. [CrossRef]

2

Natural Antioxidants: A Novel Therapeutic Approach to Autism Spectrum Disorders?

Luca Pangrazzi *, Luigi Balasco and Yuri Bozzi *

Center for Mind/Brain Sciences (CIMeC), Neurodevelopmental Disorders Research Group, University of Trento, 38068 Rovereto, Italy; luigi.balasco@unitn.it

* Correspondence: luca.pangrazzi-1@unitn.it (L.P.); yuri.bozzi@unitn.it (Y.B.)

Abstract: Autism spectrum disorders (ASD) are a group of neurodevelopmental syndromes with both genetic and environmental origins. Several recent studies have shown that inflammation and oxidative stress may play a key role in supporting the pathogenesis and the severity of ASD. Thus, the administration of anti-inflammatory and antioxidant molecules may represent a promising strategy to counteract pathological behaviors in ASD patients. In the current review, results from recent literature showing how natural antioxidants may be beneficial in the context of ASD will be discussed. Interestingly, many antioxidant molecules available in nature show anti-inflammatory activity. Thus, after introducing ASD and the role of the vitamin E/vitamin C/glutathione network in scavenging intracellular reactive oxygen species (ROS) and the impairments observed with ASD, we discuss the concept of functional food and nutraceutical compounds. Furthermore, the effects of well-known nutraceutical compounds on ASD individuals and animal models of ASD are summarized. Finally, the importance of nutraceutical compounds as support therapy useful in reducing the symptoms in autistic people is discussed.

Keywords: autism; inflammation; oxidative stress

1. Introduction

Autism spectrum disorders (ASD) represent a heterogeneous group of neurodevelopmental syndromes clinically characterized by deficits in social interaction/communication and repetitive/stereotyped behaviors, accompanied by a different degree of sensory deficits and other comorbidities [1]. The pathogenesis of ASD is complex and not fully disclosed. Research has identified both genetic and environmental factors, especially those involving fetal and early life development, in describing this complex condition.

Although studies performed in twins with ASD have revealed a high degree of heritability (38–54%), several meta-analyses studies have also shown that genetic-independent causes of ASD do exist [2]. In the last two decades, a consistent number of genetic modifications has been reported to increase the risk for developing ASD or autistic symptoms. Approximately 10% of ASD cases are of genetic etiology (Fragile X syndrome [3], tuberous sclerosis [4], Cowden syndrome [5], and Angelman syndrome [6]); of those, single genetic mutations account for only 1–2% of cases [7], with the majority of cases remaining idiopathic. Recent advances in genetics and genomics have allowed for the identification of an increasingly high number of ASD-associated gene variants, including chromosomal deletions or duplications (copy number variations, CNVs), de novo and familial mutations, and epigenetic in candidate as well as novel genes [8–10]. Many of these mutations and CNVs have been the subject of investigation in mouse models and some of them revealed to be promising for ASD research. Several genetic mutations in ASD have been associated with genes coding for proteins involved in synaptic functions, such as SH3 and multiple ankyrin repeat domains 3 (SHANK), contactin-associated protein-like (CNTNAP), neuroligin (NLGN), and neurexin

(NRXN). Some examples of CNVs associated with ASD include chromosomal loci 15q11-q13, 16p11.2, and the ubiquitin protein ligase E3A (UBE3A) genes. Moreover, a subset of single gene mutations associated with ASD are also responsible for other neurodevelopmental disorders, including fragile X mental retardation syndrome 1 (FMR1) in fragile X syndrome, tuberous sclerosis 1(TSC1) in tuberous sclerosis, and methyl-CpG binding protein 2 (MECP2) in Rett syndrome [11]. There is a strong evidence indicating that highly convergent cellular mechanisms underlie the genetic and functional complexity of autism spectrum disorders. Indeed, most of ASD-associated genes code for proteins involved in synaptic signaling, transcriptional/post-transcriptional mechanisms and cell adhesion, and function of excitatory and inhibitory neurons. These mechanisms crucially operate during nervous system development, controlling the birth, differentiation, and migration of neuronal subtypes, along with the formation and maintenance of their connections [8,9]. Several studies have identified mutations and chromosomal aberrations in genes that are involved in brain development from intrauterine life through childhood. As frequent mutations in genes involved in the cytoarchitectural organization and neuronal connectivity have been found, ASD has been proposed to be a synaptopathy [12]. However, several lines of evidence suggest a role of inflammation in the underlying mechanism of ASD, despite some concern about whether it causes ASD onset or regulates ASD pathogenesis and symptomatology.

Immunity takes a key role in neural development of both central and peripheral nervous system, regulating several aspects such as neuronal proliferation, synapse formation, and plasticity, together with the removal of apoptotic neurons; in addition, immune dysfunction has also been shown to contribute to large number of neurological conditions [13–15]. Several studies over the last decades have highlighted altered immune responses in individuals with ASD [16,17]. People with ASD have increased levels of pro-inflammatory markers while having decreased levels of anti-inflammatory markers [18]. Moreover, we recently discussed how oxidative stress may support brain inflammation and ASD-like behaviors [19]. In particular, the levels of reactive oxygen species (ROS) scavenging enzymes, such as superoxide dismutases (SODs), catalase, glutathione peroxidase (GPx), and antioxidant molecule glutathione (GSH) are lower in individuals with ASD, in comparison with healthy controls. Moreover, several studies reported how neuroinflammatory conditions may be present in ASD patients, which are commonly linked and supported by high levels of ROS. Furthermore, post-mortem brain samples from ASD individuals revealed increased levels of pro-inflammatory markers [20] and increased microglia activation [21,22]. Given the current pieces of evidence, solutions that target oxidative stress and inflammation could represent a valid strategy to tackle ASD.

In this review, we summarize the recent literature about impairments in the vitamin-based antioxidant network in the context of ASD. In addition, we describe how natural antioxidants present in plants and food may help in counteracting ASD-like behaviors.

2. Evidence of Inflammatory State in Animal Models of ASD

Experimental animal models represent a fundamental element for the understanding of the etiology and pathogenesis of any disease and human condition, including ASD. Animal models can be considered as reliable if (a) they show the same diagnostic markers of a human condition, demonstrating resemblance to the human situation (face validity); (b) they show similarity with the causes of the disease (construct validity); and (c) they show expected responses to treatments that are effective in the human disease (predictive validity). This can be achieved in a relatively simple way whenever there are distinct markers for a disease. For example, in animal models of hemophilia, one has to show similar coagulation defects. However, it is more difficult to prove that an experimental animal is the suitable model for ASD. Indeed, according to the Diagnostic and Statistical Manual of Mental Disorders 5 (DSM-V), diagnosis of ASD is solely based on behavioral changes, and the behavior of a mouse is not the same as the behavior of a child or adult [1]. Despite this obstacle, a variety of neurobehavioral tests have been used to demonstrate a behavioral pattern that mimics the core behavior of ASD in animal models. Among typical behaviors assessed in mice and rats, directly related to the core symptoms of autism, are deficits in social interaction (i.e., three-chamber social approach paradigm), deficits in communication (i.e., analysis of ultrasonic vocalizations), increased repetitive/stereotyped motor behaviors (i.e., self-grooming or marble burying), and persistence on sameness and restricted interests (i.e., perseveration in the T maze or water maze) [23,24]. Moreover, rodents can also be tested for a number of other behaviors aiming at testing sensory deficits, which are reported to be present in a large subset of ASD subjects [25]. Despite the evident heterogeneity of the clinical manifestation in ASD, animal research allows consistent investigations of different aspects of the condition, from circuitry to cellular and molecular processes affected in autism.

ASD models can be grouped in three large categories: (i) induced by genetic perturbations, mimicking the genetic alterations found in humans with ASD; (ii) environmentally induced, by exposure of the pregnant animals to certain chemicals or infectious/inflammatory agents; and (iii) inbred strains, analogous to idiopathic cases of autism in which no genetic mutations have been identified. According to the Simons Foundation Autism Research Initiative (SFARI) gene database (http://gene.sfari.org/, as of November, 2020), there are up to now 284 genetic, 45 pharmacologically-induced, and 8 inbred mouse models of ASD.

The progress made in identifying genetic modification associated with ASD [8–10] has resulted in the generation of a multitude of mouse models by knock-out and knock-in mutations in ASD candidate genes. Thanks to these, it was possible to infer the effect of single mutations, allowing researchers to advance in the understanding of the biological bases underpinning this complex syndrome. Given the heterogeneity of genetic mutations (which can take place in different positions along the DNA, thus in different genes) and the resulting increasing number of genetic mouse models that have been generated, different animal models reproduce various aspects of ASD symptomatology, with the best animal model keeping together all three types of validity criteria.

Despite the advancement in genetic screenings of ASD populations, for the majority of cases the exact etiology of ASD remains unknown. Novel technologies and large population-based studies have provided new insight into the risk architecture of ASD and the possible role of environmental factors in its etiology. If earlier studies on twins suggested heritability as high as 80–90% for ASD with little contribution from the environment [26], according to recent evidence, up to 40–50% of variance in ASD liability is determined by environmental factors [27,28]. Among the most documented environmental risk factors are maternal infection [29] and prenatal exposure to the anticonvulsant drug valproic acid (VPA) [30]. To this first category belong mouse models of maternal respiratory infection with influenza virus and maternal immune activation (MIA) with either polyinosine/cytosine (poly(I:C), a synthetic, double-stranded RNA that evokes an antiviral-like immune reaction), or lipopolysaccharide (LPS, which evokes an antibacterial-like immune reaction) [31]. Poly (I:C) MIA offspring exhibit behaviors similar to the core symptoms of autism—deficits in social interaction and communication (USVs) and increased repetitive/stereotyped motor behaviors [32]. Whereas maternal LPS administration yields offspring with some of the same features, and a few of the abnormal behaviors can be reversed by antipsychotic drug treatment [33]. To the second category belongs instead the mouse model of prenatal exposure to VPA. A single injection of VPA in pregnant mice results in behavioral abnormalities relevant to the core symptoms of autism in the offspring [34,35].

In addition to the genetically modified and environmentally induced models of ASD, several inbred mouse strains also incorporate face validity as ASD models since they display robust and well-replicated social deficits and repetitive behaviors. Between the most popular inbred strains are A/J, BALB/cByJ (BALB), BTBR T+Itpr3tf/J (BTBR), C58/J (C58), and 129S1/SvImJ mice, which exhibit lack of sociability, as compared to inbred mouse strains with high sociability, such as C57BL/6J (B6) and FVB/NJ mice. Of these, BTBR has been the most extensively characterized and well replicated for ASD-related behaviors [36,37]. However, one might wonder how adequate the above models are. Indeed, in these models, only certain aspects of ASD are reproduced and we know, at the same time, that autism is a multifactorial condition. In animal models, we can observe manifestations associated with "human" autistic disorders, but it is difficult to identify whether these manifestations are the reasons for these disorders and their consequences, whether they are different consequences of identical reasons, or whether these manifestations are interconnected by some other relations. Despite this, we and many other researchers believe that the heterogeneity of face validity in mouse models of ASD could be converted from a problem into an advantage as long as investigators exploit these differences to advance our understanding of autism.

Nonetheless, certain aspects of ASD symptomatology such as inflammation and oxidative stress seem to be shared by many ASD mouse models [19]. Although the link between immune system alteration and ASD has long been postulated [38], only in the last decades has the research looked more closely at the potential contribution of the immune system to ASD. Studies performed in ASD patients indicated that immune system dysfunction is often supported by a strong inflammatory state [39,40]. Moreover, signs of microglia activation as well as increased inflammatory cytokines and chemokines (i.e., interferon (IFN)γ, interleukin (IL)-1β, IL-6, tumor necrosis factor (TNF), and chemokine C-C motif ligand (CCL)-2) have been found in the brains and cerebrospinal fluid of ASD subjects [20,41]. Immunological studies on mouse models of ASD have classically focused on MIA and VPA mouse models. Maternal immune activation (MIA) mouse offspring have been reported with altered immune functions showing systemic deficits in $CD4^+$ $TCR\beta^+$ $Foxp3^+$ $CD25^+$ T regulatory cells and increased IL-6 and IL-17 cytokine production by $CD4^+$ T cells [42]. Moreover, central neuro-inflammation and altered inflammatory responses, together with synaptic alterations, have been shown in VPA rodent models [43,44]. However, inflammatory alterations have also been found in genetic and inbred mouse models of ASD [19,45,46], suggesting that increased production of pro-inflammatory molecules in ASD may represent a strong contributor to the pathogenesis and the severity of these disorders. In the following chapters, we focus on natural antioxidants and their anti-inflammatory activity as potential target to treat ASD symptomatology.

3. Vitamin E/Vitamin C/Glutathione Antioxidant Network Controls Oxidative Stress

Vitamin E is present in lipid-rich plant products and vegetable oils, such as wheat germ, rice bran, coconut, soybean, and olives. Eight different isoforms have been identified: α-, β-, γ-, δ- tocopherols and α-, β-, γ-, δ-tocotrienols. Vitamin E is incorporated into cellular membranes, in which it effectively inhibits the peroxidation of lipids, as both tocopherols and tocotrienols scavenge highly reactive peroxyl radicals. Vitamin E does not work in isolation from other antioxidants, but it is part of an interlinking set of redox antioxidant cycles known as the "antioxidant network" [47]. When all vitamin E isoforms react against free radicals, they are converted into their oxidized tocopheroxyl/tocotrienoxyl forms. In order to be active again, vitamin E is converted from its free radical form into its reduced native state after the interaction between water- and lipid-soluble substances, using both enzymatic and non-enzymatic mechanisms.

Reduced vitamin C (dehidroascorbate, DHA) can directly regenerate vitamin E after being converted into ascorbate, its oxidized form. Thiol antioxidants such as glutathione can convert ascorbate into DHA, which is then available for regenerating again vitamin E. Thus, vitamin C is particularly effective at reducing oxidative damage when it is used in conjunction with vitamin E [48,49]. When vitamin E, vitamin C, and glutathione systems act synergistically, low steady-state concentrations of vitamin E radicals and ascorbate are present in the cells, and the loss or consumption of vitamins is prevented. Vitamin C is a potent antioxidant that can neutralize and remove oxidants, such as highly reactive molecules generated in metabolic processes in the brain but also in other organs [49]. Vitamin C plays a vital role in tissue growth, synthesis of vasoactive agents, immune regulation, and many other metabolic functions [50,51]. Decreased vitamin C levels are known to support the pathophysiology of various diseases, such as cancer, endocrinopathies, and neurological disorders [52]. The biological significance of vitamin C in the brain is related to the development of neurons, their functional maturation, and antioxidant responses. When a vitamin C deficiency is present, neurons show decreased growth and activity, as well as increased susceptibility to oxidative damage [53].

Another important molecule within the antioxidant network, necessary for the reconversion of ascorbate into DHA, is glutathione. Glutathione is a tripeptide (cysteine, glycine, and glutamic acid) present in high levels in most cells, which exists in two forms, reduced (GSH) and oxidized (GSSG). The ratio of GSH to GSSG determines the cell redox status of a cell. Resting healthy cells show a GSH/GSSG ratio > 100, while the ratio drops to 1 to 10 when cells are exposed to oxidant stress. De novo glutathione synthesis is mainly controlled by the cellular levels of the aminoacid cysteine, the availability of which is the rate-limiting step. For this reason, administration of antioxidant N-acetyl L-cysteine (NAC), a precursor of cysteine, is known to boost the synthesis of intracellular glutathione [54,55]. Thus, the integration of several antioxidants within the antioxidant network is fundamental for counteracting the onset of oxidative stress within the body, a condition known to support the pathogenesis of diseases.

4. Vitamin E/Vitamin C/Glutathione Network is Impaired with ASD

Studies have shown that all players involved in the vitamin E/vitamin C/glutathione network are impaired with ASD. Alterations in the expression of major antioxidant enzymes of ROS scavenging system are present in both ASD mouse models and autistic patients, in the brain but also in the peripheral blood [19,56–61]. This indicates that levels of oxidative stress may be elevated with ASD.

It has been described that concentration of vitamin E in the blood was reduced and was associated with ASD-like behaviors in autistic people [57,62]. Future studies must assess whether vitamin E supplementation may attenuate ASD-like symptoms. Vitamin C deficiency has additionally been observed with ASD. Differently from lipid-soluble vitamin E, vitamin C is not stored in any reservoir within the body. As it is not endogenously produced, it is rapidly lost within the urine if not supplemented from the diet. Thus, plasma concentration of vitamin C is related to its dietary intake and it has a half-life of 12–24 h [63]. The consumption of very low amounts of food rich in vitamin C may lead to scurvy, a rare disease that is mainly present in people with unusual eating habits, suffering of alcoholism, or with mental disorders. Recently, increased prevalence of scurvy has been observed in children with ASD [64]. This situation may be caused by vitamin C malabsorption and/or low vegetable and fruit intake. In addition, low vitamin C levels have been observed in the blood of children with ASD, in comparison with healthy controls [65,66]. Another aspect which can typically be observed in ASD children is a decreased level of glutathione, particularly in its reduced form [56,67–69]. In parallel, the levels of oxidized glutathione are higher than in normally developing children. As reduced glutathione is needed to regenerate DHA from ascorbate (Figure 1), lower levels of vitamin C in its reduced form can be expected with ASD. Consequently, increased amounts of vitamin E in its oxidized tocopheroxyl/tocotrienoxyl form may be present in the presence of ASD.

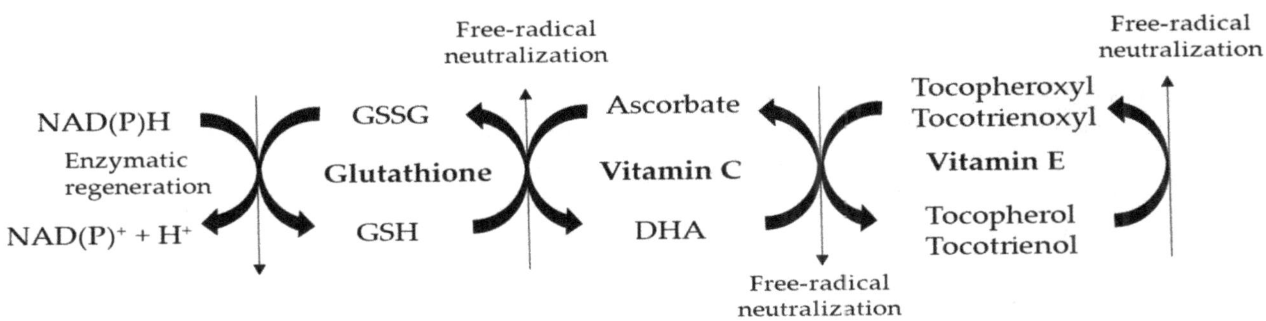

Figure 1. Schematic representation of vitamin E/vitamin C/glutathione antioxidant network involved in free-radical neutralization. GSSG: glutathione disulphide (oxidized glutathione); GSH: reduced glutathione; DHA: dehidroascorbate (reduced vitamin C).

Clinical trials have been planned in order to counteract this situation, with the aim of restoring vitamin E/vitamin C/glutathione antioxidant network in ASD individuals [70]. In a double-blind, placebo-controlled study, the safety and efficacy of glutathione alone or glutathione, vitamin C, and NAC treatment was evaluated in children with autism [70]. A placebo or one of the two treatments was administered to the participants for 8 weeks. The authors observed an improvement in both developmental skills and behavior with both glutathione or the combined therapy glutathione, vitamin C, and NAC therapy as compared to placebo therapy. A positive correlation between changes in behavior and GSH/GSSG ratio was additionally observed [70]. Thus, evidence exists that ASD-like symptoms may be improved by targeting the vitamin E/vitamin C/glutathione network. Whether nutritional interventions aiming at increasing the levels of vitamin E and vitamin C, both present within foods, may help in restoring an optimal functionality of the antioxidant network have not investigated yet but it can be expected. Thus, a careful evaluation of nutritional status should be performed in autistic patients before planning more elaborate testing. Indeed, as ASD are a very heterogeneous group of diseases, differences in the nutritional status of autistic people may be present. This may be very helpful to plan nutritional interventions to counteract ASD-like symptoms.

5. Functional Food and Nutraceutical Compounds

The first and fundamental role of food is to provide nutrients (i.e., carbohydrates, proteins, fats, vitamins, and minerals) to the body, which are necessary for growth, maintenance, and wellness. In addition, non-nutrients such as fibers, probiotics, antioxidants, and bioactive molecules are included in the food. Although they are not directly required to support the basic functions of organisms, their presence is beneficial to promote health and wellness. When a kind of food can provide health benefits in addition to its nutritional value, it is defined as functional food. Generally, a typical hallmark of these aliments is the presence of antioxidant molecules such as carotenoids, flavonoids, and phenols. Typical examples of functional foods are many kinds of fruits, vegetables, nuts, seeds, whole grains, legumes, and seafood. When functional compounds are isolated from the food matrix, they are called nutraceuticals. This term was coined by De Felice in 1989, combining the words "nutrition" and "pharmaceutics", to indicate "food or parts of food that provide medical or health benefits, including the prevention and treatment of diseases" [71]. In this way, when interesting molecules are identified within functional foods, they can potentially be enriched and sold as nutraceuticals on the market. Despite this, it is important to consider that bioactive compounds may be less effective when isolated from functional foods, and, in some cases, toxic effects may appear. Nevertheless, these molecules may be helpful in counteracting pathological conditions and supporting body health. Recently, many studies have started exploring the role of nutraceuticals in the context of chronic disorders such as cancer, diabetes, atherosclerosis, cardiovascular diseases, and neurological disorders, and interesting results have been achieved [72–76]. In addition, evidence exists that nutraceutical compounds may also play a beneficial role in individuals with ASD. In these studies, the antioxidant potential of nutraceutical compounds played a major role in improving the disease situation. Thus, functional food may represent a powerful tool for counteracting a broad spectrum of diseases thanks to the combination of several nutraceuticals, most of which are antioxidant compounds. As previously discussed, nutritional interventions may be important to counteract ASD-like symptoms in individuals with ASD. We next summarize recent studies describing how not only the antioxidant activity of vitamins (nutrients), but also how the antioxidant potential of functional foods/nutraceuticals (non-nutrients) may help in counteracting autistic-like behaviors.

6. Nutraceutical Compounds and ASD

6.1. Carotenoids

Carotenoids are a class of fat-soluble, red, orange, and yellow natural pigments synthesized by plants, bacteria, and fungi. These molecules present in and give the characteristic color to carrots, tomatoes, and pumpkins. Importantly, many carotenoids show antioxidant and anti-inflammatory properties [77]. Several studies showed that people consuming more carotenoids in their diets had reduced risk of chronic diseases, such as cardiovascular diseases, photosensitivity diseases, cataracts, and age-related macular degeneration [78]. In addition, carotenoids were shown to improve cognitive performance in middle-aged people, suggesting that these compounds can be helpful in supporting brain health [79]. The importance of carotenoids in the context of ASD has been described by the work of Krajcovicova-Kudlackova and colleagues, which reported that blood levels of lycopene, a type of carotenoid, were reduced in autistic patients [62].

Among all the carotenoids, astaxanthin, a carotenoid belonging to the family of terpenes, has shown promising effects in the context of neurodegenerative disorders. Like many carotenoids, astaxanthin is a lipid-soluble pigment with a red-orange color, and a strong capability of reducing reactive oxidizing molecules. Interestingly, astaxanthin has been shown to display the strongest antioxidant potential among all the carotenoids [80,81]. This compound is naturally produced by microalgae *Haematococcus pluvialis* and the yeast fungus *Xanthophyllomyces dendrorhous*. In particular, when the algae are stressed by increased salinity, lack of nutrients, or excessive sunshine, they create astaxanthin. Animals who feed on the algae, such as red trout, salmon, flamingos, and crustaceans (i.e., shrimps, crabs, and lobsters), subsequently acquire the red-orange astaxanthin pigmentation. Thus, a nutrition based on algae and red-colored seafood leads to a consistent astaxanthin intake. Several studies performed in the context of cardiovascular diseases, metabolic syndromes, and cancer have described that astaxanthin shows a strong anti-inflammatory potential [82]. More recently, it was documented that this molecule may additionally show a neuroprotective potential, particularly in the elderly and in the presence of neurodegeneration, as it displays a therapeutic role in preserving cognitive function [83]. In addition, astaxanthin may attenuate microglial activation and the release of pro-inflammatory cytokines. Furthermore, this molecule is known to protect neuronal integrity [84–86]. In a prenatal valproic acid (VPA)-induced mouse model of ASD, astaxanthin was shown to improve behavioral disorders and oxidative stress in the treated animals [87]. Thus, if these results are to be confirmed in humans, the consumption of astaxanthin-rich food may be proposed to autistic patients in order to attenuate ASD-like symptoms.

6.2. *Polyphenols*

In addition to carotenoids, polyphenols have been shown to play a beneficial role in ASD. Phenols are a class of nutraceutical compounds representing the most abundant group of secondary metabolites produced by plants. These molecules are spread throughout many foods, such as vegetables, fruits, and seeds. As they contain one or more hydroxyl groups attached to a benzene ring, they have the capability of donating electrons to oxidized molecules. For this reason, phenols are considered strong antioxidant molecules. Phenolic compounds are a very heterogeneous group, and they show different chemical properties. Several polyphenols have been shown to modulate sirtuin 1 signaling pathway and regulate key cell processes, such as cell cycle, DNA repair, protein aggregation, inflammation, and mitochondrial function [88]. In addition, this class of molecules can also interfere with other key cell signaling pathways (such as those controlled by activator protein 1 (AP-1), nuclear factor kappa-light-chain-enhancer of activated B cells (NF-kB), and signal transducer and activator of transcription 1 (STAT1), ultimately leading to protection against oxidative stress, inflammation, and cell proliferation [89,90]. Among the polyphenol class are flavonoids, which include quercetin and luteolin, both showing antioxidant and anti-inflammatory properties [91,92].

Recent studies have shown that dietary polyphenols can be promising molecules to alleviate ASD symptoms. Several studies reported that some polyphenols, including resveratrol, regulate mitochondrial activity and prevent mitochondrial dysfunction, typically present in individuals with ASD [93]. Furthermore, resveratrol was efficient in preventing the downregulation of cytochrome c oxidase and in suppressing the production of ROS within mitochondria in azide-stimulated primary hippocampal astrocytes [94]. It is important to consider that polyphenols may have low bioavailability within the brain, as not all of these compounds can cross the blood–brain barrier. Despite this, they are present at high concentrations in the intestinal lumen [95,96], and therefore they may modulate the microbiota, which is of great importance for ASD typically characterized by impairments in the microbiota–gut–brain axis [97]. To date, very few studies have investigated the potential benefits of dietary polyphenols in ASD patients.

Taliou and co-workers performed a pilot study including 50 children diagnosed with ASD [98]. An oral formulation including a combination of flavonoids (quercetin, luteolin, and quercetin glycoside rutin) was administered daily for 26 weeks. The results showed that ASD children receiving the polyphenols showed a significant improvement in communication and concentration, with reduced abnormal behaviors. More recently, it was shown that children treated with the same polyphenolic formulation improved autistic-like behaviors and, in parallel, the serum levels of pro-inflammatory cytokines IL-6 and TNF were significantly reduced when compared to the beginning of the study [99]. Thus, the administration of polyphenols may lead to decreased neuroinflammation, promoting an improvement in ASD-related symptoms in the children as a result. In addition, a single case report described that a 10-year-old ASD child who received microgranules including palmitoylethanolamide and luteolin twice a day for one year showed an improvement in ASD-like behaviors [100]. Similar effects were observed in VPA-induced autistic mice after the administration of the same formulation [100]. Taken together, evidence exists that polyphenols may represent a class of natural molecules important for counteracting ASD symptoms.

6.3. Omega-3

Omega-3, known also as n-3 or short-chain fatty acids, are a class of polyunsaturated fatty acids (PUFAs) extensively distributed in nature, very important constituent of lipid metabolism. Three main types of omega-3 fatty acids are fundamental for human physiology: α-linolenic acid (ALA), present in plant oils, and eicosapentaenoic acid (EPA) and docosahexaenoic acid (DHA), both commonly found in marine oils. The main sources of plant oils containing ALA are represented by seeds, walnut, and clary sage seed oil, while animal omega−3 fatty acids EPA and DHA are mostly included in fish, fish oils, and chicken eggs. As mammals are unable to synthesize ALA omega-3, this compound must be introduced through the diet. In addition, ALA is required for the synthesis of EPA and DHA, and thus deficits in the intake of ALA lead to an overall omega-3 reduction within the body. In contrast to long-chain, n-6 polyunsaturated fatty acids (n-6 PUFAs), which support inflammatory processes, omega-3 are anti-inflammatory molecules and thus they are fundamental for keeping inflammation under control [101].

Impaired fatty acid metabolism is known to affect normal brain function. Indeed, omega-3 play an important role in the structure of the neuronal cell membranes, as well as in the development of myelin sheath [102]. In particular, DHA constitutes 90% of the whole amount of omega-3 in the human brain and 10–20% of total lipids [103]. A link between abnormal fatty acid metabolism and the pathophysiology of ASD has been reported [69,104]. Increased DHA intake reduces the risk of bipolar disorder, schizophrenia, and depression, while low levels of this molecule are a potential risk factor for mental illness [105]. In keeping with these findings, children with ASD showed lower DHA and EPA levels and lower total omega-3 serum levels compared to healthy, age-matched children [106]. This condition may be caused by defects in enzymes involved in the DHA and EPA production from ALA, impairment in cell membrane incorporation, or dysfunction in mitochondrial PUFA oxidation [102,107]. More recently, a model linking ASD phenotype and DHA deficiency has been proposed [108]. The gut–brain axis was recently suggested as an alternative pathway for the omega-3 action against ASD. Indeed, n-3 fatty acid deficiency during perinatal period is known to alter intestinal microbial balance in offspring, leading to a reduction in bacterial density and a reduced proportion of Firmicutes to Bacteroidetes [109,110]. Omega-3 supplementation could increase the Lactobacillus and Bifidobacterium species in the gut and decrease the levels of potential pathobionts belonging to the Enterobacteriaceae family [109]. In addition, microbial overgrowth impaired the uptake and metabolism of PUFAs and other molecules. Taken together, omega-3 administration may improve ASD-like behaviors in autistic people, most-likely by reducing neuroinflammatory conditions within the brain and supporting the optimal functionality of gut–brain axis.

6.4. Plants as Sources of Nutraceutical Compounds to Treat ASD

Several compounds present in plants have been described to reduce brain inflammation and oxidative stress, and therefore these molecules may be very beneficial to treat ASD-like disorders [111]. Green tea (*Camellia sinensis*) extracts are an important source of polyphenols, such as flavonoids such as myricetin and quercetin [112]. When green tea extracts were daily administered to the VPA-treated mice from postnatal day 14 to day 40, the researchers documented an improvement of ASD-like behaviors [113]. The extracts were shown to reduce the expression of pro-inflammatory molecules TNF and C-reactive protein (CRP), and thus displayed evident anti-inflammatory properties [114]. One important ASD-related feature is the loss of Purkinje cell integrity within the cerebellum [115]. Importantly, treatment with 300 mg/kg green tea extracts lead to the regeneration of Purkinje cell layer in mice, suggesting that molecules present in the extract may potentially help in treating ASD [113].

The plants *Piper longum* and *Piper nigrum* (black pepper) are sources of another nutraceutical compound, piperine, a well-known anxiolytic, neuroprotective, antioxidant molecule [116,117]. In addition, piperine is used to treat seizures disorders and enhances memory and cognition [118]. In the VPA mice treated with 20 mg/kg piperine, antioxidant markers and behavioral abnormalities could be rescued in comparison to untreated mice [119]. Clinical trials have been started to assess whether piperine may additionally be beneficial for ASD children [118]. Another plant with well-known neuroprotective effects against neuropsychiatric disorders is turmeric (*Curcuma longa*), whose properties can be mainly attributed to curcumin. This molecule can target several signaling pathways, and thus the most important effects of curcumin include the increase of intracellular glutathione levels, and reduction of mitochondrial dysfunction, inflammation, oxidative stress, and protein aggregation [120]. In a VPA-induced rat model, a single curcumin supplement increased the expression of antioxidant enzymes [121]. Furthermore, rats that received curcumin showed reduced levels of pro-inflammatory cytokines IL-6 and IFNγ. In another study performed in old rats, increased synaptic plasticity after regular curcumin intake has been observed [122]. Future clinical studies must investigate the effects of curcumin on individuals with ASD. The standardized extract of *Ginkgo biloba* leaves, known as EGb 761 (*Ginkgo biloba* extract 761), includes 24% flavone glycosides (quercetin, kaempferol, and isorhamnetin), 6% terpene lactones (2.6–3.2% bilobalide, and 2.8–3.4% ginkgolides A, B, and C), 0.8% ginkgolide B, and 3% bilobalide [123]. Many of the substances present in the extract were associated with neuroprotective effects in disorders such as Parkinson's disease, Alzheimer's disease, and ischemic stroke [124]. In an observational study performed in individuals with ASD, 100mg/kg *Ginkgo biloba* extract taken twice a day improved autistic behaviors such as hyperactivity, irritability, and inappropriate speech [125]. Future study should further investigate the potential benefits of Ginkgo biloba extract on larger cohorts of autistic people.

7. Conclusions

It is now becoming evident how natural antioxidant and anti-inflammatory molecules may consistently help in counteracting symptoms in people with ASD (as summarized in Table 1). These effects can potentially be achieved by both the administration of selected antioxidants such as vitamin E, vitamin C, or NAC, or after the consumption of food rich in nutraceutical compounds, which may show additive or synergistic effects. In particular, nutraceutical compounds are present at very high concentrations in plants, fish, and crustaceans, which therefore can be considered important functional foods. Importantly, these molecules are extremely helpful for body health, as they can target inflammation and oxidative stress, and decrease damage within several organs, including the brain. Furthermore, as ASD individuals are characterized not only by high levels of oxidative stress and pro-inflammatory molecules but also by nutritional deficits, it is therefore important to perform a nutritional evaluation of every patient. In this way, the most appropriate strategy of intervention to counteract ASD-like behaviors can rapidly be selected.

Table 1. Summary of the studies describing the effects of natural antioxidants on autism spectrum disorder (ASD) animal models and humans with ASD. Dose, duration of the treatment, species, molecular effects, and behavioral improvements are reported in the table. IV: intravenously; IP: intraperitoneally; VPA: valproic acid.

Molecule/Formulation	Dose	Duration	Species	Molecular Effect	Behavioral Improvements	Reference
Glutathione	600 mg IV	once a week for 8 weeks	human	increased GSH/GSSG ratio	developmental skills and learning	70
Glutathione, vitamin C, NAC	600 mg, 2000 mg, 20 mg/kg(all IV)	once a week for 8 weeks	human	increased GSH/GSSG ratio	developmental skills and learning	70
Astaxanthin	2 mg/kg IP	once a day for 4 weeks	VPA-treated mouse	reduced oxidative stress (brain and liver)	sociability, social novelty and reduced anxiety	87
Capsule including: two flavonoids, luteolin, quercetin, rutin	in each capsule:>95% pure, 100 mg, 70 mg, 30 mg	1 capsule per 10 kg weight per day for 26 weeks	human	reduced IL-6 and TNF in the serum	communication, concentration, aberrant behavior	87,88
Palmitoylethanolamide and luteolin	700 mg orally	once a day for 1 year	human	-	stereotyped behaviors	100
Palmitoylethanolamide and luteolin	1 mg/kg orally	once a day for 3 months	VPA-treated mouse	reduced IL-6, IL-1β, Bax, and BCL-2 in the brain	social behaviors	100
DHA and EPA	800 mg, 700 mg orally	once a day for 6 weeks	human	-	reduced hyperactivity and stereotyped behaviors	105
DHA and EPA	1.5 g orally	once a day for 6 months	human	-	-	105
Green tea	300 mg/kg orally	once a day for 26 days	VPA-treated mouse	reduced lipid peroxidation and cerebellar damage	exploratory activity and spatial learning, reduced anxiety	113
Piperine	20 mg/kg IP	once a day for 26 days	VPA-treated mouse	increased GSH, decreased total nitrite and MDA	locomotor activity, social behaviors, spatial learning, reduced anxiety	119
Curcumin	1 g/kg IP	single dose	VPA-treated rat	reduced IL-6, IFNγ, glutamine and oxidative stress	-	121
Ginkgo biloba extract 761	100 mg/kg orally	twice a day for 4 weeks	human	-	aberrant behavior	125

Abbreviations

ALA	α-linolenic acid
ASD	Autism spectrum disorders
CRP	C-reactive protein
DHA	Dehidroascorbate
EPA	Eicosapentaenoic acid
GPx	Glutathione peroxidase
GR	Glutathione reductase
GSH	Glutathione
GSSG	Glutathione disulphide
IFN	Interferon
IL	Interleukin
NAC	N-Acetylcysteine
PUFAs	Polyunsaturated fatty acids
RNS	Reactive nitrogen species
ROS	Reactive oxygen species

References

1. American Psychiatric Association. *Diagnostic and Statistical Manual of Mental Disorders: DSM-5*; American Psychiatric Association: Arlington, VA, USA, 2013.
2. Hallmayer, J.; Cleveland, S.; Torres, A.; Phillips, J.; Cohen, B.; Torigoe, T.; Miller, J.; Fedele, A.; Collins, J.; Smith, K.; et al. Genetic heritability and shared environmental factors among twin pairs with autism. *Arch. Gen. Psychiatry* **2011**, *68*, 1095–1102. [CrossRef] [PubMed]
3. Belmonte, M.K.; Bourgeron, T. Fragile X syndrome and autism at the intersection of genetic and neural networks. *Nat. Neurosci* **2006**, *9*, 1221–1225. [CrossRef] [PubMed]
4. Wiznitzer, M. Autism and Tuberous Sclerosis. *J. Child Neurol.* **2004**, *19*, 675–679. [CrossRef] [PubMed]
5. Rademacher, S.; Eickholt, B.J. PTEN in autism and neurodevelopmental disorders. *Cold Spring Harb. Perspect. Med.* **2019**, *9*, a036780. [CrossRef] [PubMed]
6. Smith, S.E.P.; Zhou, Y.-D.; Zhang, G.; Jin, Z.; Stoppel, D.C.; Anderson, M.P. Increased gene dosage of Ube3a results in autism traits and decreased glutamate synaptic transmission in mice. *Sci. Transl. Med.* **2011**, *3*, 103ra97. [CrossRef]
7. Abrahams, B.S.; Geschwind, D.H. Advances in autism genetics: On the threshold of a new neurobiology. *Nat. Rev. Genet.* **2008**, *9*, 341–355. [CrossRef]
8. De la Torre-Ubieta, L.; Won, H.; Stein, J.L.; Geschwind, D.H. Advancing the understanding of autism disease mechanisms through genetics. *Nat. Med.* **2016**, *22*, 345–361. [CrossRef]
9. Satterstrom, F.K.; Kosmicki, J.A.; Wang, J.; Breen, M.S.; De Rubeis, S.; An, J.Y.; Peng, M.; Collins, R.; Grove, J.; Klei, L.; et al. Large-scale exome sequencing study implicates both developmental and functional changes in the neurobiology of autism. *Cell* **2020**, *180*, 568–584.e23. [CrossRef]
10. Thapar, A.; Rutter, M. Genetic advances in autism. *J. Autism Dev. Disord.* **2020**. [CrossRef]
11. Kazdoba, T.M.; Leach, P.T.; Yang, M.; Silverman, J.L.; Solomon, M.; Crawley, J.N. Translational mouse models of autism: Advancing toward pharmacological therapeutics. *Curr. Top. Behav. Neurosci.* **2016**, *28*, 1–52.
12. Won, H.; Mah, W.; Kim, E. Autism spectrum disorder causes, mechanisms, and treatments: Focus on neuronal synapses. *Front. Mol. Neurosci.* **2013**, *6*, 19. [CrossRef] [PubMed]
13. De Jong, M.; Punt, M.; De Groot, E.; Minderaa, R.B.; Hadders-Algra, M. Minor neurological dysfunction in children with autism spectrum disorder. *Dev. Med. Child Neurol.* **2011**, *53*, 641–646. [CrossRef] [PubMed]
14. Wang, T.T.; DU, L.; Shan, L.; Jia, F.Y. Research advances in immunological dysfunction in children with autism spectrum disorders (in Chinese). *Zhongguo Dang Dai Er Ke Za Zhi* **2014**, *16*, 1289–1293. [PubMed]
15. Young, A.M.; Chakrabarti, B.; Roberts, D.; Lai, M.C.; Suckling, J.; Baron-Cohen, S. From molecules to neural morphology: Understanding neuroinflammation in autism spectrum condition. *Mol. Autism* **2016**, *7*, 9. [CrossRef]

16. Hsiao, E.Y. Immune dysregulation in autism spectrum disorder. *Int. Rev. Neurobiol.* **2013**, *113*, 269–302.
17. Estes, M.L.; McAllister, A.K. Immune mediators in the brain and peripheral tissues in autism spectrum disorder. *Nat. Rev. Neurosci.* **2015**, *16*, 469–486. [CrossRef]
18. Masi, A.; Quintana, D.S.; Glozier, N.; Lloyd, A.R.; Hickie, I.B.; Guastella, A.J. Cytokine aberrations in autism spectrum disorder: A systematic review and meta-analysis. *Mol. Psychiatry* **2015**, *20*, 440–446. [CrossRef]
19. Pangrazzi, L.; Balasco, L.; Bozzi, Y. Oxidative stress and immune system dysfunction in autism spectrum disorders. *Int. J. Mol. Sci.* **2020**, *21*, 3293. [CrossRef]
20. Li, X.; Chauhan, A.; Sheikh, A.M.; Patil, S.; Chauhan, V.; Li, X.M.; Ji, L.; Brown, T.; Malik, M. Elevated immune response in the brain of autistic patients. *J. Neuroimmunol.* **2009**, *207*, 111–116. [CrossRef]
21. Morgan, J.T.; Chana, G.; Pardo, C.A.; Achim, C.; Semendeferi, K.; Buckwalter, J.; Courchesne, E.; Everall, I.P. Microglial activation and increased microglial density observed in the dorsolateral prefrontal cortex in autism. *Biol. Psychiatry* **2010**, *68*, 368–376. [CrossRef]
22. Edmonson, C.; Ziats, M.N.; Rennert, O.M. Altered glial marker expression in autistic post-mortem prefrontal cortex and cerebellum. *Mol. Autism* **2014**, *5*, 3. [CrossRef]
23. Crawley, J.N. Translational animal models of autism and neurodevelopmental disorders. *Dialogues Clin. Neurosci.* **2012**, *14*, 293–305. [PubMed]
24. Ergaz, Z.; Weinstein-Fudim, L.; Ornoy, A. Genetic and non-genetic animal models for autism spectrum disorders (ASD). *Reprod. Toxicol.* **2016**, *64*, 116–140. [CrossRef] [PubMed]
25. Balasco, L.; Provenzano, G.; Bozzi, Y. Sensory abnormalities in autism spectrum disorders: A focus on the tactile domain, from genetic mouse models to the clinic. *Front. Psychiatry* **2020**, *10*, 1016. [CrossRef] [PubMed]
26. Ronald, A.; Hoekstra, R.A. Autism spectrum disorders and autistic traits: A decade of new twin studies. *Am. J. Med. Genet. B Neuropsychiatr. Genet.* **2011**, *156*, 255–274. [CrossRef]
27. Gaugler, T.; Klei, L.; Sanders, S.J.; Bodea, C.A.; Goldberg, A.P.; Lee, A.B.; Mahajan, M.; Manaa, D.; Pawitan, Y.; Reichert, J.; et al. Most genetic risk for autism resides with common variation. *Nat. Genet.* **2014**, *46*, 881–885. [CrossRef]
28. Deng, W.; Zou, X.; Deng, H.; Li, J.; Tang, C.; Wang, X.; Guo, X. The relationship among genetic heritability, environmental effects, and autism spectrum disorders: 37 pairs of ascertained twin study. *J. Child Neurol.* **2015**, *30*, 1794–1799. [CrossRef]
29. Conway, F.; Brown, A.S. Maternal immune activation and related factors in the risk of offspring psychiatric disorders. *Front. Psychiatry* **2019**, *10*, 430. [CrossRef]
30. Christensen, J.; Gronborg, T.K.; Sorensen, M.J.; Schendel, D.; Partner, E.T.; Pedersen, L.H.; Vestergaard, M. Prenatal valproate exposure and risk of autism spectrum disorders and childhood autism. *JAMA* **2013**, *309*, 1696–1703. [CrossRef]
31. Patterson, P.H. Modeling autistic features in animals. *Pediatr. Res.* **2011**, *69 Pt 2*, 34R–40R. [CrossRef]
32. Brown, A.S.; Meyer, U. Maternal immune activation and neuropsychiatric illness: A translational research perspective. *Am. J. Psychiatry* **2018**, *175*, 1073–1083. [CrossRef] [PubMed]
33. Boksa, P. Effects of prenatal infection on brain development and behavior: A review of findings from animal models. *Brain Behav. Immun.* **2010**, *24*, 881–897. [CrossRef] [PubMed]
34. Nicolini, C.; Fahnestock, M. The valproic acid-induced rodent model of autism. *Exp. Neurol.* **2018**, *299*, 217–227. [CrossRef] [PubMed]
35. Schneider, T.; Roman, A.; Basta-Kaim, A.; Kubera, M.; Budziszewska, B.; Schneider, K. Gender-specific behavioral and immunological alterations in an animal model of autism induced by prenatal exposure to valproic acid. *Psychoneuroendocrinology* **2008**, *33*, 728–740. [CrossRef]
36. Silverman, J.L.; Yang, M.; Lord, C.; Crawley, J.N. Behavioural phenotyping assays for mouse models of autism. *Nat. Rev. Neurosci.* **2010**, *11*, 490–502. [CrossRef]
37. Meyza, K.Z.; Blanchard, D.C. The BTBR mouse model of idiopathic autism—Current view on mechanisms. *Neurosci. Biobehav. Rev.* **2017**, *76*, 99–110. [CrossRef]
38. Stubbs, E.G.; Crawford, M.L. Depressed lymphocyte responsiveness in autistic children. *J. Autism Child. Schizophr.* **1977**, *7*, 49–55. [CrossRef]
39. Siniscalco, D.; Schultz, S.; Brigida, A.; Antonucci, N. Inflammation and neuro-immune dysregulations in autism spectrum disorders. *Pharmaceuticals* **2018**, *11*, 56. [CrossRef]

40. Croonenberghs, J.; Bosmans, E.; Deboutte, D.; Kenis, G.; Maes, M. Activation of the inflammatory response system in autism. *Neuropsychobiology* **2002**, *45*, 1–6. [CrossRef]
41. Gottfried, C.; Bambini-Junior, V.; Francis, F.; Riesgo, R.; Savino, W. The impact of neuroimmune alterations in autism spectrum disorder. *Front. Psychol.* **2015**, *6*, 95. [CrossRef]
42. Hsiao, E.Y.; McBride, S.W.; Chow, J.; Mazmanian, S.K.; Patterson, P.H. Modeling an autism risk factor in mice leads to permanent immune dysregulation. *Proc. Natl. Acad. Sci. USA* **2012**, *109*, 12776–12781. [CrossRef] [PubMed]
43. Lucchina, L.; Depino, A.M. Altered peripheral and central inflammatory responses in a mouse model of autism. *Autism Res.* **2014**, *7*, 273–289. [CrossRef] [PubMed]
44. Codagnone, M.G.; Podestá, M.F.; Uccelli, N.A.; Reinés, A. Differential local connectivity and neuroinflammation profiles in the medial prefrontal cortex and hippocampus in the valproic acid rat model of autism. *Dev. Neurosci.* **2015**, *37*, 215–231. [CrossRef] [PubMed]
45. Matta, S.M.; Hill-Yardin, E.L.; Crack, P.J. The influence of neuroinflammation in Autism Spectrum Disorder. *Brain Behav. Immun.* **2019**, *79*, 75–90. [CrossRef]
46. Kazlauskas, N.; Robinson-Agramonte, M.; Depino, A. Neuroinflammation in animal models of autism. In *Translational Approaches to Autism Spectrum Disorder*; Robinson-Agramonte, M., Ed.; Springer: Cham, Switzerland, 2015.
47. Constantinescu, A.; Han, D.; Packer, L. Vitamin E recycling in human erythrocyte membranes. *J. Biol. Chem.* **1993**, *268*, 10906–10913.
48. Stewart, M.S.; Cameron, G.S.; Pence, B.C. Antioxidant nutrients protect against UVB-induced oxidative damage to DNA of mouse keratinocytes in culture. *J. Investig. Dermatol.* **1996**, *106*, 1086–1089. [CrossRef]
49. Figueroa-Méndez, R.; Rivas-Arancibia, S. Vitamin C in health and disease: Its role in the metabolism of cells and redox state in the brain. *Front. Physiol.* **2015**, *6*, 397. [CrossRef]
50. Rebouche, C.J. Ascorbic acid and carnitine biosynthesis. *Am. J. Clin. Nutr.* **1991**, *54*, 1147S–1152S. [CrossRef]
51. Cobley, J.N.; McHardy, H.; Morton, J.P.; Nikolaidis, M.G.; Close, G.L. Influence of vitamin C and vitamin E on redox signaling: Implications for exercise adaptations. *Free Radic Biol. Med.* **2015**, *84*, 65–76. [CrossRef]
52. Grosso, G.; Bei, R.; Mistretta, A.; Marventano, S.; Calabrese, G.; Masuelli, L.; Vestergaard, M.G.; Modesti, A.; Galvano, F.; Gazzolo, D. Effects of vitamin C on health: A review of evidence. *Front. Biosci.* **2013**, *18*, 1017–1029.
53. Qiu, S.; Li, L.; Weeber, E.J.; May, J.M. Ascorbate transport by primary cultured neurons and its role in neuronal function and protection against excitotoxicity. *J. Neurosci. Res.* **2007**, *85*, 1046–1056. [CrossRef] [PubMed]
54. Lasram, M.M.; Dhouib, I.B.; Annabi, A.; El Fazaa, S.; Gharbi, N. A review on the possible molecular mechanism of action of N-acetylcysteine against insulin resistance and type-2 diabetes development. *Clin. Biochem.* **2015**, *48*, 1200–1208. [CrossRef] [PubMed]
55. Rushworth, G.F.; Megson, I.L. Existing and potential therapeutic uses for N-acetylcysteine: The need for conversion to intracellular glutathione for antioxidant benefits. *Pharmacol. Ther.* **2014**, *141*, 150–159. [CrossRef] [PubMed]
56. James, S.J.; Melnyk, S.; Jernigan, S.; Cleves, M.A.; Halsted, C.H.; Wong, D.H.; Cutler, P.; Bock, K.; Boris, M.; Bradstreet, J.J.; et al. Metabolic endophenotype and related genotypes are associated with oxidative stress in children with autism. *Am. J. Med. Genet. B Neuropsychiatr. Genet.* **2006**, *141*, 947–956. [CrossRef] [PubMed]
57. Rose, S.; Melnyk, S.; Pavliv, O.; Bai, S.; Nick, T.G.; Frye, R.E.; James, S.J. Evidence of oxidative damage and inflammation associated with low glutathione redox status in the autism brain. *Transl. Psychiatry* **2012**, *2*, e134. [CrossRef]
58. James, S.J.; Melnyk, S.; Jernigan, S.; Pavliv, O.; Trusty, T.; Lehman, S.; Seidel, L.; Gaylor, D.W.; Cleves, M.A. A functional polymorphism in the reduced folate carrier gene and DNA hypomethylation in mothers of children with autism. *Am. J. Med. Genet. B Neuropsychiatr. Genet.* **2010**, *153*, 1209–1220. [CrossRef]
59. Al-Gadani, Y.; El-Ansary, A.; Attas, O.; El Ayadhi, L. Metabolic biomarkers related to oxidative stress and antioxidant status in Saudi autistic children. *Clin. Biochem.* **2009**, *42*, 1032–1040. [CrossRef]
60. González-Fraguela, M.E.; Diaz Hung, M.-L.; Vera, H.; Maragoto, C.; Noris, E.; Blanco, L.; Galvizu, R.; Robinson, M. Oxidative stress markers in children with autism spectrum disorders. *Br. J. Med. Med. Res.* **2013**, *3*, 307–317. [CrossRef]

61. Meguid, N.A.; Ghozlan, S.A.S.; Mohamed, M.F.; Ibrahim, M.K.; Dawood, R.M.; Din, N.G.B.E.; Abdelhafez, T.H.; Hemimi, M.; El Awady, M.K. Expression of reactive oxygen species-related transcripts in Egyptian children with autism. *Biomark Insights* **2017**, *12*, 1177271917691035. [CrossRef]
62. Krajcovicova-Kudlackova, M.; Valachovicova, M.; Mislanova, C.; Hudecova, Z.; Sustrova, M.; Ostatnikova, D. Plasma concentrations of selected antioxidants in autistic children and adolescents. *Bratisl. Lek. Listy* **2009**, *110*, 247–250.
63. Duconge, J.; Miranda-Massari, J.R.; Gonzalez, M.J.; Jackson, J.A.; Warnock, W.; Riordan, N.H. Pharmacokinetics of vitamin C: Insights into the oral and intravenous administration of ascorbate. *Puerto Rico Health Sci. J.* **2008**, *27*, 7–19.
64. Kothari, P.; Tate, A.; Adewumi, A.; Kinlin, L.M.; Ritwik, P. The risk for scurvy in children with neurodevelopmental disorders. *Spec. Care Dent.* **2020**, *40*, 251–259. [CrossRef] [PubMed]
65. Meguid, N.A.; Anwar, M.; Bjørklund, G.; Hashish, A.; Chirumbolo, S.; Hemimi, M.; Sultan, E. Dietary adequacy of Egyptian children with autism spectrum disorder compared to healthy developing children. *Metab. Brain Dis.* **2017**, *32*, 607–615. [CrossRef] [PubMed]
66. Marí-Bauset, S.; Llopis-González, A.; Zazpe-García, I.; Marí-Sanchis, A.; Morales-Suárez-Varela, M. Nutritional status of children with autism spectrum disorders (ASDs): A case-control study. *J. Autism Dev. Disord* **2015**, *45*, 203–212. [CrossRef] [PubMed]
67. Geier, D.A.; Kern, J.K.; Garver, C.R.; Adams, J.B.; Audhya, T.; Geier, M.R. A prospective study of transsulfuration biomarkers in autistic disorders. *Neurochem. Res.* **2009**, *34*, 386–393. [CrossRef]
68. Geier, D.A.; Kern, J.K.; Adams, J.B.; Geier, M.R. Biomarkers of environmental toxicity and susceptibility in autism. *J. Neurol. Sci.* **2009**, *280*, 101–108. [CrossRef]
69. James, S.J.; Cutler, P.; Melnyk, S.; Jernigan, S.; Janak, L.; Gaylor, D.W.; Neubrander, J.A. Metabolic biomarkers of oxidative stress and impaired methylation capacity in children with autism. *Am. J. Clin. Nutr.* **2004**, *80*, 1611–1617. [CrossRef]
70. ClinicalTrials.gov. Available online: https://clinicaltrials.gov/ct2/show/NCT00889538 (accessed on 25 November 2020).
71. De Felice, S. *The Nutraceutical Revolution: Fueling a Powerful, New International Market*; Havard University Advanced Management Program in Biomedical Research and Development: Como, Italy, 1989.
72. Onaolapo, A.Y.; Onaolapo, O.J. Nutraceuticals and Diet-based Phytochemicals in Type 2 Diabetes Mellitus: From Whole Food to Components with Defined Roles and Mechanisms. *Curr. Diabetes Rev.* **2019**, *16*, 12–25. [CrossRef]
73. Sosnowska, B.; Penson, P.; Banach, M. The role of nutraceuticals in the prevention of cardiovascular disease. *Cardiovasc. Diagn. Ther.* **2017**, *7* (Suppl. 1), S21–S31. [CrossRef]
74. Setorki, M.; Rafieian-Kopaei, M.; Merikhi, A.; Heidarian, E.; Shahinfard, N.; Ansari, R.; Nasri, H.; Esmael, N.; Baradaran, A. Suppressive impact of anethum graveolens consumption on biochemical risk factors of atherosclerosis in hypercholesterolemic rabbits. *Int. J. Prev. Med.* **2013**, *4*, 889–895.
75. Shirzad, M.; Kordyazdi, R.; Shahinfard, N.; Nikokar, M. Does Royal Jelly affect tumor cells? *J. HerbMed. Pharmacol.* **2013**, *2*, 45–48.
76. Rafieian-Kopaie, M.; Baradaran, A. Plants antioxidants: From laboratory to clinic. *J. Nephropathol.* **2013**, *2*, 152–153. [CrossRef]
77. Skibsted, L.H. Carotenoids in antioxidant networks. Colorants or radical scavengers. *J. Agric. Food Chem.* **2012**, *60*, 2409–2417. [CrossRef] [PubMed]
78. Mayne, S.T. Beta-carotene, carotenoids, and disease prevention in humans. *FASEB J.* **1996**, *10*, 690–701. [CrossRef] [PubMed]
79. Kesse-Guyot, E.; Andreeva, V.A.; Ducros, V.; Jeandel, C.; Julia, C.; Hercberg, S. Carotenoid-rich dietary patterns during midlife and subsequent cognitive function. *Br. J. Nutr.* **2014**, *111*, 915–923. [CrossRef]
80. Shimidzu, N.; Goto, M.; Miki, W. Carotenoids as singlet oxygen quenchers in marine organisms. *Fisheries Sci.* **1996**, *62*, 134–137. [CrossRef]
81. Igielska-Kalwat, J.; Gościańska, J.; Nowak, I. Karotenoidy jako naturalne antyoksydanty (Carotenoids as natural antioxidants). *Postepy Hig. Med. Dosw.* **2015**, *69*, 418–428. [CrossRef]
82. Ambati, R.R.; Phang, S.M.; Ravi, S.; Aswathanarayana, R.G. Astaxanthin: Sources, extraction, stability, biological activities and its commercial applications—A review. *Mar. Drugs* **2014**, *12*, 128–152. [CrossRef]

83. Grimmig, B.; Hudson, C.; Moss, L.; Peters, M.; Subbarayan, M.; Weeber, E.J.; Bickford, P.C. Astaxanthin supplementation modulates cognitive function and synaptic plasticity in young and aged mice. *Geroscience* **2019**, *41*, 77–87. [CrossRef]
84. Wibrand, K.; Berge, K.; Messaoudi, M.; Duffaud, A.; Panja, D.; Bramham, C.R.; Burri, L. Enhanced cognitive function and antidepressant-like effects after krill oil supplementation in rats. *Lipids Health Dis.* **2013**, *12*, 6. [CrossRef]
85. Wu, W.; Wang, X.; Xiang, Q.; Meng, X.; Peng, Y.; Du, N.; Liu, Z.; Sun, Q.; Wang, C.; Liu, X. Astaxanthin alleviates brain aging in rats by attenuating oxidative stress and increasing BDNF levels. *Food Funct.* **2014**, *5*, 158–166. [CrossRef] [PubMed]
86. Yook, J.S.; Okamoto, M.; Rakwal, R.; Shibato, J.; Lee, M.C.; Matsui, T.; Chang, H.; Chang, J.Y.; Soya, H. Astaxanthin supplementation enhances adult hippocampal neurogenesis and spatial memory in mice. *Mol. Nutr. Food Res.* **2016**, *60*, 589–599. [CrossRef] [PubMed]
87. Al-Amin, M.M.; Rahman, M.M.; Khan, F.R.; Zaman, F.; Mahmud Reza, H. Astaxanthin improves behavioral disorder and oxidative stress in prenatal valproic acid-induced mice model of autism. *Behav. Brain Res.* **2015**, *286*, 112–121. [CrossRef] [PubMed]
88. Ajami, M.; Pazoki-Toroudi, H.; Amani, H.; Nabavi, S.F.; Braidy, N.; Vacca, R.A.; Atanasov, A.G.; Mocan, A.; Nabavi, S.M. Therapeutic role of sirtuins in neurodegenerative disease and their modulation by polyphenols. *Neurosci. Biobehav. Rev.* **2017**, *73*, 39–47. [CrossRef] [PubMed]
89. Tewari, D.; Nabavi, S.F.; Nabavi, S.M.; Sureda, A.; Farooqi, A.A.; Atanasov, A.G.; Vacca, R.A.; Sethi, G.; Bishayee, A. Targeting activator protein 1 signaling pathway by bioactive natural agents: Possible therapeutic strategy for cancer prevention and intervention. *Pharmacol. Res.* **2018**, *128*, 366–375. [CrossRef]
90. Serra, D.; Paixão, J.; Nunes, C.; Dinis, T.C.; Almeida, L.M. Cyanidin-3-glucoside suppresses cytokine-induced inflammatory response in human intestinal cells: Comparison with 5-aminosalicylic acid. *PLoS ONE* **2013**, *8*, e73001. [CrossRef]
91. Li, Y.; Yao, J.; Han, C.; Yang, J.; Chaudhry, M.T.; Wang, S.; Liu, H.; Yin, Y. Quercetin, inflammation and immunity. *Nutrients* **2016**, *8*, 167. [CrossRef]
92. Nabavi, S.F.; Braidy, N.; Gortzi, O.; Sobarzo-Sanchez, E.; Daglia, M.; Skalicka-Woźniak, K.; Nabavi, S.M. Luteolin as an anti-inflammatory and neuroprotective agent: A brief review. *Brain Res. Bull.* **2015**, *119*, 1–11. [CrossRef]
93. Jardim, F.R.; De Rossi, F.T.; Nascimento, M.X.; Da Silva Barros, R.G.; Borges, P.A.; Prescilio, I.C.; Roberto de Oliveira, M. Resveratrol and brain mitochondria: A review. *Mol. Neurobiol.* **2018**, *55*, 2085–2101. [CrossRef]
94. Bellaver, B.; Bobermin, L.D.; Souza, D.G.; Rodrigues, M.D.; De Assis, A.M.; Wajner, M.; Gonçalves, C.-A.; OnofreSouza, D.; Quincozes-Santos, A. Signaling mechanisms underlying the glioprotective effects of resveratrol against mitochondrial dysfunction. *Biochim. Biophys. Acta* **2016**, *1862*, 1827–1838. [CrossRef]
95. Halliwell, B. Dietary polyphenols: Good, bad, or indifferent for your health? *Cardiovasc. Res.* **2007**, *73*, 341–347. [CrossRef] [PubMed]
96. Schaffer, S.; Halliwell, B. Do polyphenols enter the brain and does it matter? Some theoretical and practical considerations. *Genes Nutr.* **2012**, *7*, 99–109. [CrossRef] [PubMed]
97. Duda-Chodak, A.; Tarko, T.; Satora, P.; Sroka, P. Interaction of dietary compounds, especially polyphenols, with the intestinal microbiota: A review. *Eur. J. Nutr.* **2015**, *54*, 325–341. [CrossRef] [PubMed]
98. Taliou, A.; Zintzaras, E.; Lykouras, L.; Francis, K. An open-label pilot study of a formulation containing the anti-inflammatory flavonoid luteolin and its effects on behavior in children with autism spectrum disorders. *Clin. Ther.* **2013**, *35*, 592–602. [CrossRef]
99. Tsilioni, I.; Taliou, A.; Francis, K.; Theoharides, T.C. Children with autism spectrum disorders, who improved with a luteolin-containing dietary formulation, show reduced serum levels of TNF and IL-6. *Transl. Psychiatry* **2015**, *5*, e647. [CrossRef]
100. Bertolino, B.; Crupi, R.; Impellizzeri, D.; Bruschetta, G.; Cordaro, M.; Siracusa, R.; Esposito, E.; Cuzzocrea, S. Beneficial effects of co-ultramicronized palmitoylethanolamide/luteolin in a mouse model of autism and in a case report of autism. *CNS Neurosci. Ther.* **2017**, *23*, 87–98. [CrossRef]
101. Calder, P.C. Omega-3 fatty acids and inflammatory processes. *Nutrients* **2010**, *2*, 355–374. [CrossRef]
102. Van Elst, K.; Bruining, H.; Birtoli, B.; Terreaux, C.; Buitelaar, J.K.; Kas, M.J. Food for thought: Dietary changes in essential fatty acid ratios and the increase in autism spectrum disorders. *Neurosci. Biobehav. Rev.* **2014**, *45*, 369–378. [CrossRef]

103. Weiser, M.J.; Butt, C.M.; Mohajeri, M.H. Docosahexaenoic acid and cognition throughout the lifespan. *Nutrients* **2016**, *8*, 99. [CrossRef]
104. Chauhan, A.; Chauhan, V.; Brown, W.T.; Cohen, I. Oxidative stress in autism: Increased lipid peroxidation and reduced serum levels of ceruloplasmin and transferrin—The antioxidant proteins. *Life Sci.* **2004**, *75*, 2539–2549. [CrossRef]
105. Bozzatello, P.; Brignolo, E.; De Grandi, E.; Bellino, S. Supplementation with omega-3 fatty acids in psychiatric disorders: A review of literature data. *J. Clin. Med.* **2016**, *5*, 67. [CrossRef] [PubMed]
106. Mazahery, H.; Stonehouse, W.; Delshad, M.; Kruger, M.C.; Conlon, C.A.; Beck, K.L. Relationship between long chain n-3 polyunsaturated fatty acids and autism spectrum disorder: Systematic review and meta-analysis of case-control and randomised controlled trials. *Nutrients* **2017**, *9*, 155. [CrossRef] [PubMed]
107. Das, U.N. Nutritional factors in the pathobiology of autism. *Nutrition* **2013**, *29*, 1066–1069. [CrossRef]
108. Hall, B. The role of brain lipids in the causal model of autism: Re-interpretation of the existing data. *Hypothesis* **2016**, *14*, 1–6. [CrossRef]
109. Madore, C.; Leyrolle, Q.; Lacabanne, C.; Benmamar-Badel, A.; Joffre, C.; Nadjar, A.; Layé, S. Neuroinflammation in autism: Plausible role of maternal inflammation, Dietary omega 3, and microbiota. *Neural Plasticity* **2016**, *2016*, 1–15. [CrossRef]
110. Gibson, D.L.; Gill, S.K.; Brown, K.; Tasnim, N.; Ghosh, S.; Innis, S.; Jacobson, K. Maternal exposure to fish oil primes offspring to harbor intestinal pathobionts associated with altered immune cell balance. *Gut. Microbes* **2015**, *6*, 24–32. [CrossRef]
111. Bjorklund, G.; Saad, K.; Chirumbolo, S.; Kern, J.K.; Geier, D.A.; Geier, M.R.; Urbina, M.A. Immune dysfunction and neuroinflammation in autism spectrum disorder. *Acta Neurobiol. Exp.* **2016**, *76*, 257–268. [CrossRef]
112. Cabrera, C.; Artacho, R.; Gimenez, R. Beneficial effects of green tea. *J. Am. Coll Nutr.* **2006**, *25*, 79–99. [CrossRef]
113. Banji, D.; Banji, O.J.; Abbagoni, S.; Hayath, M.S.; Kambam, S.; Chiluka, V.L. Amelioration of behavioral aberrations and oxidative markers by green tea extract in valproate induced autism in animal. *Brain Res.* **2011**, *1410*, 141–151. [CrossRef]
114. Lardner, A.L. Neurobiological effects of the green tea constituent theanine and its potential role in the treatment of psychiatric and neurodegenerative disorders. *Nutr. Neurosci.* **2014**, *17*, 145–155. [CrossRef]
115. Sundberg, M.; Sahin, M. Cerebellar development and autism spectrum disorder in tuberous sclerosis complex. *J. Child Neurol.* **2015**, *30*, 1954–1962. [CrossRef] [PubMed]
116. Choi, B.M.; Kim, S.M.; Park, T.K.; Li, G.; Hong, S.J.; Park, R.; Chung, H.T.; Kim, B.R. Piperine protects cisplatin-induced apoptosis via heme oxygenase-1 induction in auditory cells. *J. Nutr. Biochem.* **2007**, *18*, 615–622. [CrossRef] [PubMed]
117. Fu, M.; Sun, Z.H.; Zuo, H.C. Neuroprotective effect of Piperine on pri-marily cultured hippocampal neurons. *Biol. Pharm. Bull.* **2010**, *33*, 598–603. [CrossRef] [PubMed]
118. Wattanathorn, J.; Chonpathompikunlert, P.; Muchimapura, S.; Priprem, A.; Tankamnerdthai, O. Piperine, the potential functional food for mood and cognitive disorders. *Food Chem. Toxicol.* **2008**, *46*, 3106–3110. [CrossRef] [PubMed]
119. Pragnya, B.; Kameshwari, J.S.L.; Veeresh, B. Ameliorating effect of piperine on behavioral abnormalities and oxidative markers in sodium valproate induced autism in BALB/C mice. *Behav. Brain Res.* **2014**, *270*, 86–94. [CrossRef] [PubMed]
120. Bhandari, R.; Kuhad, A. Neuropsychopharmacotherapeutic efficacy of curcumin in experimental paradigm of autism spectrum disorders. *J. Life Sci.* **2015**, *141*, 156–169. [CrossRef]
121. Al-Askar, M.; Bhat, R.S.; Selim, M.; Al-Ayadhi, L.; El-Ansary, A. Postnatal treatment using curcumin supplements to amend the damage in VPA-induced rodent models of autism. *BMC Chem. Biol.* **2017**, *17*, 259. [CrossRef]
122. Dong, S.; Zeng, Q.; Mitchell, E.S.; Xiu, J.; Duan, Y.; Li, C.; Tiwari, J.K.; Hu, Y.; Cao, X.; Zhao, Z. Curcumin enhances neurogenesis and cognition in aged rats: Implications for transcriptional interactions related to growth and synaptic plasticity. *PLoS ONE* **2012**, *7*, e31211. [CrossRef]
123. Uebel-von Sandersleben, H.; Rothenberger, A.; Albrecht, B.; Rothenberger, L.G.; Klement, S.; Bock, N. Ginkgo biloba extract EGb 761® in children with ADHD. *Z. Kinder Jugendpsychiatr. Psychother.* **2014**, *42*, 337–347. [CrossRef]

124. Ude, C.; Schubert-Zsilavecz, M.; Wurglics, M. Ginkgo biloba extracts: A review of the pharmacokinetics of the active ingredients. *Clin. Pharm.* **2013**, *52*, 727–749. [CrossRef]
125. Niederhofer, H. First preliminary results of an observation of Ginkgo Biloba treating patients with autistic disorder. *Phytother. Res.* **2009**, *23*, 1645–1646. [CrossRef] [PubMed]

3

Suicidal Ideation and Suicidal Attempts in Referred Adolescents with High Functioning Autism Spectrum Disorder and Comorbid Bipolar Disorder

Gabriele Masi [1,*], Silvia Scullin [1], Antonio Narzisi [1], Pietro Muratori [1], Marinella Paciello [2], Deborah Fabiani [1], Francesca Lenzi [1], Maria Mucci [1] and Giulia D'Acunto [1]

1 IRCCS Stella Maris, Scientific Institute of Child Neurology and Psychiatry, Calambrone, 56018 Pisa, Italy; silviascullin@gmail.com (S.S.); antonio.narzisi@fsm.unipi.it (A.N.); pmuratori@fsm.unipi.it (P.M.); deborah.fabiani@gmail.com (D.F.); flenzi@fsm.unipi.it (F.L.); mmucci@fsm.unipi.it (M.M.); gdacunto@fsm.unipi.it (G.D.)

2 Faculty of Psychology, Università Telematica Internazionale Uninettuno, 00186 Rome, Italy; m.paciello@uninettunouniversity.net

* Correspondence: gabriele.masi@fsm.unipi.it

Abstract: Suicidal ideation and attempts in adolescents are closely associated to bipolar disorders (BD). Growing evidence also suggests that high functioning autism spectrum disorders (HF-ASD) are at increased risk for suicidal ideation and behaviors. Although BD and HF-ASD are frequently comorbid, no studies explored suicidality in these individuals. This exploratory study addressed this issue in a clinical group of inpatient adolescents referred to a psychiatric emergency unit. Seventeen adolescents with BD and HF-ASD and severe suicidal ideation or attempts (BD-ASD-S), were compared to 17 adolescents with BD and HF-ASD without suicidal ideation or attempts (BD-ASD-noS), and to 18 adolescents with BD and suicidal ideation or attempts without ASD (BD-noASD-S), using a structured assessment methodology. Individuals with BD-ASD-S had a higher intelligence quotient, more severe clinical impairment, more lethality in suicide attempts, more internalizing symptoms, less impulsiveness, and lower social competence. Severity of ASD traits in individuals and parents did not correlate with suicidal risk. Some dimensions of resilience were protective in terms of repulsion by life and attraction to death. Main limitations are the small sample size, the lack of a control group of typically developing adolescents. However, a better understanding of the specificities of bipolar HF-ASD individuals with suicidality may improve prevention and treatment strategies.

Keywords: autism spectrum disorder; bipolar disorder; suicidal ideation; suicidal attempts; adolescence

1. Introduction

The concept of suicidality includes both suicidal ideation, with or without a plan, and with a wide range of severity, and suicidal attempts, that is self-injurious behaviors intended to kill oneself, with or without medical implications, but nonfatal, while completed suicides are fatal [1]. The term suicidality has long fallen out of favor with psychiatrists and psychologists, due to its imprecision, as it includes heterogeneous clinical conditions, not only in terms of presentation, but also in etiology, diagnosis, prognosis, and treatment. Disentangling this wide range of individuals in more specific subgroups, according to age and gender, psychiatric diagnoses, neurodevelopmental pathways, personality traits, psychiatric familial load, previous traumatic experiences, and social difficulties, may favor a more precise definition of risk factors, and more focused and appropriate prevention and treatment strategies [2,3].

There is growing evidence that a diagnosis of Autism Spectrum Disorders (ASD) is one of the risk factors for suicide [4,5]. In a population-based cohort of ASD probands ($n = 27{,}122$, all diagnosed between 1987 and 2009) compared with gender-, age-, and county of residence-matched controls ($n = 2{,}672{,}185$), Hirvikoski et al. [6] reported a probability for ASD to die by suicide 10 times greater than in the general population. In a clinical cohort study, including 367 high functioning individuals with ASD, 243 (66%) presented self-reported suicidal ideation, and 127 (35%) self-reported plans or attempts at suicide. They more likely reported lifetime experience of suicidal ideation than the UK population sample (odds ratio 9.6 (95% CI 7.6–11.9), $p < 0.0001$), than people with one, two, or more medical illnesses ($p < 0.0001$), or with psychotic illness ($p = 0.019$) [7].

Suicidality in high functioning (HF)-ASD can present with specific features [4]. Thoughts can become easily ruminative, not only in terms of triggering situations for suicidal ideation (i.e., impaired interpretation of social relationships), but also in methods of searching information aimed at planning a suicide attempt [8]. Furthermore, the high lethality and violence of the suicidal methods in ASD individuals (such as hanging, gunshot, railway hitting, or jumping off a bridge) increases the risk of a completed suicide during an attempt, compared to other psychiatric populations [9]. This evidence suggests that ASD should be considered a specific and independent risk factor for suicide [10,11].

Studies specifically addressing suicidal risk factors in youth with ASD have underlined the role of extreme loneliness [12,13], social adverse experiences [14,15], previous traumas [16], internalizing symptoms (anxiety/mood disorders), low emotional regulation, and ADHD [16,17], particularly in HF-ASD individuals [18–20]. Some cognitive features, such as decreased cognitive flexibility, insight of disease, and communication skills may flatten the expression of subjective suffering [21,22]. This is particularly true in adolescence, the age range with the highest suicidal risk [4]. HF-ASD adolescents are mostly exposed to increased social pressure, they can become more acutely aware of their disability, and they have to face the unbridgeable gap between themselves and neurotypical peers [22].

Among the factor increasing suicide risk, mood disorders, have been shown to be strongly related to suicidal outcomes [23]. Even if depressive disorders have been traditionally linked to the concept of suicidality [24], bipolar disorder (BD) has increasingly become, in the last decades, even more closely related to suicidal risk [25]. A systematic review (1970–2017) including articles on completed suicide in individuals with BD showed that suicide rates in BD are approximately 20- to 30-fold greater than in general population, with higher risk in BD-II individuals, and with a heritability of completed suicide of about 40%. Factors related to completed suicide are early onset, family history of suicide among first-degree relatives, previous attempted suicides, type of treatment, somatic, and psychiatric comorbidities [25].

Psychiatric comorbidity in ASD is still under-investigated, even if nearly 70% of people with ASD, including children and adolescents, experience at least one comorbid psychiatric disorder, and around 40% may have two or more psychiatric disorders [9,26,27]. Regarding the different comorbidities in ASD, the prevalence of mood disorder among 21,797 participants with ASD has been reported as 18.8% (95% CI: 10.6–31.1) [28]. The prevalence of depressive disorders has been reported by Lai and colleagues as 11% (95% CI: 9–13) in children and adults [29], and by Hudson and colleagues (meta-analysis including 66 studies) as 12.3% (95% CI: 9.7–15.5) and 14.4% (95% CI: 10.3–19.8) (current and lifetime prevalence, respectively) [30].

The BD-ASD association has been more recently highlighted, along with its important clinical and therapeutic implications [31]. Two reviews assessed the co-occurrence of bipolar disorders in ASD [29,32]. Vannucchi and colleagues found that the prevalence of bipolar disorders ranged from 6% to 21.4% across studies [32], whereas Lai and colleagues reported a prevalence of 5% (95% CI: 3–6) among 153,192 ASD individuals [29]. Regarding only children and adolescents, Joshi and colleagues [31] found that 30% (47/155) of bipolar I probands met criteria for ASD (diagnosis based on DSM-III-R criteria).

While both BD and HF-ASD represent independent risk factors for suicidal ideation and behavior, their association in terms of increased suicidal risk is strongly under-explored in clinical samples. Dell'Osso and colleagues [33] investigated the prevalence of suicidal ideation in 34 adult individuals with ASD without intellectual disability, 68 with subthreshold ASD ("autistic traits"), and 160 healthy controls. Individuals with ASD reported significantly higher scores than the other two groups in mood disorders and depression, while the subthreshold autistic individuals presented higher scores than the heathy control group. Of note, both individuals with ASD and subthreshold ASD scored higher in suicidality, compared to healthy controls, without significant differences between clinical and subthreshold ASD individuals. The depressive score and the restricted interests and rumination domain score were the strongest predictors of suicidality. These results underline the association between mood spectrum and suicidality in adult individuals with ASD, including those with subthreshold forms. These correlations have not been explored in adolescents with ASD, albeit the high rates of suicidal ideation and attempts in this age range.

Among the different personality features possibly related to suicidal risk in adolescents, three domains were considered as particularly significant, according to the available literature, the attitude to life and death, the impulsivity, and the resilience to life stressors. The repulsion by life and the attraction (or low fearlessness) about death have been proved to be related to suicidality in adolescents with psychiatric diagnoses [34,35]. Highly impulsive adolescents tend to act rashly in the context of negative emotions, because long-term benefits are less important than the immediate short-term gains of emotion regulation [36]. Finally, life adversities or stressful life events increase the risk of suicidal ideation and behaviors) [3], and low adaptive resilience abilities after stressful life events are a further vulnerability factor and a possible target for interventions [37].

The aim of our study is to explore if within the bipolar spectrum, adolescents with ASD and suicidality may present specificities in three personality dimensions usually related to suicidality in adolescence (resilience, impulsivity, and attitude to life and death). We compared subjects with BD, ASD, and suicidality (Group 1), with BD; and suicidality, but without ASD (Group 2); and BD and ASD, but without suicidality (Group 3), in order to possibly disentangle the role of autism and suicidality in bipolarity. We hypothesized that bipolar adolescents with HF-ASD could present specific clinical characteristics in their suicidal manifestations, including clinical severity, cognitive abilities, psychiatric comorbidities, and personality features, compared to those without suicidality or without ASD, which may represent possible targets for the diagnostic procedures and treatment plans. Given the exploratory design of the study, we investigated these psychological features without a-priori hypotheses.

2. Materials and Methods

2.1. Sample

This was a naturalistic study based on a clinical database of 52 adolescents (age range 11 to 18 years) with BD, all referred as individuals to our psychiatric emergency unit between January 2018 and July 2019. Seventeen individuals (age range 11 to 18 years) had a comorbid HF-ASD and severe suicidal ideation or suicide attempt(s) (BD-ASD-S group), 17 (age range 11 to 18 years) a comorbid HF-ASD, but without suicidal ideation or suicidal attempt(s) (BD-ASD-noS group), and 18 (age range 11 to 18 years) with severe suicidal ideation or suicide attempts, but not ASD (BD-NoASD-S). The diagnosis of BD was based on DSM 5 criteria, and a diagnostic interview, the Kiddie Schedule for Affective Disorders and Schizophrenia for School-Aged Children-Present and Lifetime Version (K-SADS-PL) [38], administered to the patient and at least one parent.

The diagnosis of ASD was based on the DSM 5 diagnostic criteria [39], and confirmed with the module 3 of Autism Diagnostic Observation Schedule—Second Version (ADOS-2) [40]. Only a minority of individuals' caregivers were interviewed with the Autism Diagnostic Interview-Revised (ADI-R) [41]. The ADI-R is less effective in the diagnosis of HF-ASDA and it may not recognize more subtle forms of ASD [42]. It is therefore possible that, in these individuals with HF-ASD, the symptoms may not be evident at 4 to 5 years of age (developmental period investigated in the ADI-R), but could emerge only when social demands exceed these individuals' limited capacities [39].

The diagnosis of severe suicidal ideation or suicide attempt was based on a score 3 or above at the Columbia–Suicide Severity Rating Scale [CSSRS] [43]. All the individuals presented normal intelligence (Full scale IQ above 85), based on the Wechsler Intelligence Scale for Children—Fourth Edition (WISC-IV) [44].

2.2. Measures

All the individuals received a diagnostic assessment with the K-SADS-PL, a semi-structured interview to diagnose childhood mental disorders in children aged 6 to 18, administered by trained child psychiatrists, in order to diagnose BD (including Type I, Type II, and type NOS), ASD, and comorbidities. All the individuals were assessed with the WISC-IV, to exclude an Intellectual Disability.

The ADOS-2 was administered to support the diagnosis of ASD to all the individuals with first diagnosis of ASD based on historical information and the diagnostic interview K-SADS-PL. The ADOS-2 is a semi-structured interaction that measures symptoms of autism through a standard set of probes. It provides an empirically derived algorithm that differentiates children with ASDs from those with other delays or with typical development. The ADOS-Calibrated Severity Score was used to assess the severity of autistic symptoms [45].

The global clinical severity was assessed with the Clinical Global Impression Severity (CGI-S) [46], while the functional impairment with the Child Global Assessment Scale (C-GAS) [47].

For a dimensional assessment of psychopathology, all individuals were assessed with the Child Behavior Checklist (CBCL) [42,48], a 118-item scale, completed by parents, assessing how often a certain behavior applies to their offspring, on a three-point scale (0 = absent, 1 = occurs sometimes, 2 = occurs often), clustered in two broad-band scores, designated as Internalizing Problems and Externalizing Problems, a Total Problem Score, and with 8 different syndromes scales (Withdrawal, Somatic complaints, Anxiety/depression, Social problems, Thought problems, Attention, Rule-breaking behavior, Aggressive behavior). In the current study, we assessed the presence of Emotional Dysregulation using the CBCL Dysregulation Profile (CBCL-DP), based on the sum of t-scores of the three CBCL subscales, Anxious/depression, Attention problems, and Aggressive behaviors [43,49]. The reliability coefficients (Cronbach) of CBCL Attention Problems, Aggression, and Anxious/Depressed subscales were 0.82, 0.81, and 0.82, respectively.

Type of suicidality and severity of suicidal ideation and behavior were assessed using the Columbia–Suicide Severity Rating Scale (CSSRS), (score 3 or higher), recommended by the Center for Disease Control and Prevention and Food and Drug Administration for the assessment of adolescents at high suicidal risk.

In order to explore further psychological features possibly related to suicidal risk, that is attitude to life and death, impulsivity, and resilience abilities facing life adversities, three specific measures were included in the assessment for all the individuals included in the study.

The Multi-Attitude Suicide Tendency Scale (MAST) [50] was used to assess attitude for life and death, related to the fearlessness about death, and to the capability for suicide. This measure, designed to assess suicidal tendencies in youth, is a 30-item scale exploring four types of attitudes: attraction to life, repulsion by life, attraction to death, and repulsion by death. All four factor scales showed good reliability estimates, as well as relationships with measures of suicidal behavior and ideation and general psychopathology [50,51].

Impulsivity was assessed with the Barratt Impulsiveness Scale-11 (BIS-11) [52,53], including 30 items that are scored to yield second-order factors, Attentional, Motor, and Non-planning impulsiveness.

Resilience was explored with the Resilience scale for Adolescent (READ) [54–56], a self-administered 28-item questionnaire, with a score for each item ranging from 1 (totally disagree) to 5 (totally agree), which incorporates intrapersonal and interpersonal protective factors mapping onto the three salient domains of resilience, including individual, family, and external environment. Confirmatory factor analysis validated the original five-factor structure of the READ, including Personal Competence,

Social Competence, Structured Style, Family Cohesion, and Social Resources. The measures showed good reliability and validity in adolescents [57].

All participants and parents were informed about the assessment instruments. Written informed consent was obtained from participants and parents. The study conformed to Declaration of Helsinki; the Ethics Committee of the Hospital approved the methodology of the study (Identification Code 2014/0001507).

2.3. Statistical Analyses

Descriptive analyses were used to describe demographic and clinical characteristics of the whole sample. Chi-square analyses were performed on categorical variables, and a t-test or one-way ANOVA on continuous variables, with statistical significance set at 0.05. The Bonferroni–Holm method was used for multiple comparisons. The Student's t-test, with Bonferroni correction, was used in order to compare the calibrated severity score of ADOS-2 between BD-ASD-S and BD-ASD-noS.

A structural equation modeling (SEM) was conducted to examine the association between resilience protective factors measured by READ scales and suicide tendency measured by the MAST (attraction and/or repulsion to life and/or death) in all individuals. The SEM model has been tested using the maximum likelihood (ML) method since none of the variables exceed the value of |1| for univariate skewness and kurtosis. To examine model fit, several goodness-of-fit indices were used: the comparative fit index (CFI), the Tucker and Lewis index (TLI), the standardized root mean square residual (SRMR), and the root mean square error of approximation (RMSEA).

3. Results

The three groups BD-ASD-S, BD-noASD—S, and BD-ASD-noS did not differ according to mean age (14.53 ± 2.03 years, 14.78 ± 1.86 years and 14.94 ± 2.22 years, respectively, $F = 0.175$, $df = 51$, $p = 0.840$), while gender ratio was uneven, as in the BD-ASD-S the male/female was 14/3, in BD-noASD-S 6/12, and in BD-ASD-noS 10/7, ($\chi^2 = 8.62$, $df = 2$, $p = 0.013$). Regarding the frequency of the BD types (BD I, BD II, and BD Not Otherwise Specified) in the three groups, they were respectively, six, seven, and five in the BD-ASD-S; six, eight, and three in the BD-noASD—S; and seven, five, and five in the BD-ASD-noS. Differences among groups were not statistically significant ($\chi^2 = 0.92$, $df = 4$, $p = 0.921$, ns).

The intellectual quotient, measured with the WISC-IV, was significantly higher in the BD-ASD-S group than in the other two groups for the full scale IQ and for the verbal comprehension index, while for the perceptual reasoning and working memory indices, BD-ASD-S scored significantly higher than BD-ASD-NoS. The processing speed index did not differ among groups (Table 1).

Regarding clinical severity, assessed with the CGI-S, the BD-ASD-S group was the most severely impaired (6.41 ± 0.71), compared to the BD-noASD-S (6.00 ± 0.68), and BD-ASD-noS (4.82 ± 0.95) ($F = 18.5$, $p < 0.001$). Similarly, the BD-ASD-S group presented the greatest functional impairment, assessed with the C-GAS (28.76 ± 7.35), compared to the BD-noASD-S (35.06 ± 7.11), and the BD-ASD-noS (41.47 ± 7.97) ($F = 12.25$, $p < 0.001$).

According to the type of suicidality, assessed with the CSSI-R, types of suicidal ideation, frequency of ideation, control over ideation, deterrents from suicide behavior, and reasons for ideation did not differ among groups. Preparatory acts did not differ, but potential lethality higher than 1 was more frequent in the BD-ASD-S group (41.2%), compared to the BD-noASD-S group (11.1%) ($p = 0.042$).

Regarding psychiatric diagnoses, according the K-SADS-PL, only obsessive compulsive disorder was more frequently reported in individuals with BD-ASD-S (70.6%), and with BD-ASD-noS (41.2%), compared to those with BD-noASD-S (5.6%) ($\chi^2 = 15.70$, $df = 2$, $p < 0.001$ for both BD- ASD-S and BD-ASD-noS after Bonferroni–Helm method). All the other categorical diagnoses (ADHD, anxiety disorders, depression, and disruptive behavior disorders) did not differ among groups.

Regarding the comparison among groups according to the CBCL, individuals with BD-ASD-S presented higher scores in the internalizing problems, and, among the syndrome scales, in the thought disorders scale, while the anxiety-depressed and the withdrawal scales only approached statistical significance, and the three groups did not differ according to the dysregulation profile score (Table 2).

Table 1. Wechsler Intelligence Scale for Children—Fourth Edition (WISC-IV) (Wechsler, 2003). Comparisons among groups. Legenda; BD-ASD-S = Bipolar Disorder + High Functioning Autism Spectrum Disorder + Severe Suicide Ideation or Attempt; BD-noASD-S = Bipolar Disorder + Severe Suicide Ideation or Attempt, without High Functioning Autism Spectrum Disorder; BD-ASD-noS = Bipolar Disorder + High Functioning Autism Spectrum Disorder, without Severe Suicide Ideation or Attempt; SD: Standard Deviations; FSIQ: Total Intellectual Quotient; VCI: Verbal Comprehension Index; PRI: Perceptual Reasoning Index; WMI: Working Memory Index; PSI: Processing Speed Index. Statistical significance at $p < 0.05$.

	Group 1 BD-ASD-S Mean; SD	Group 2 BD-no ASD-S Mean; SD	Group 3 BD-ASD-NoS Mean; SD	One-Way ANOVA (F); *p*	Bonferroni–Holm Gr1 vs. Gr.2 *p*	 Gr.1 vs. Gr.3 *p*	 Gr.2 vs. Gr.3 *p*
FSIQ	112.9; 16.2	97.3; 13.2	84.8; 18.8	(9.43); 0.001	0.041	0.000	ns
VCI	116.6; 18.4	99.8; 15.1	91.0; 17.1	(7.67); 0.002	0.029	0.002	ns
PRI	115.5; 16.9	104.2; 13.2	96.9; 19.8	(4.12); 0.024	Ns	0.023	ns
WMI	102.4; 14.1	91.4; 11.7	80.0; 12.1	(7.59); 0.002	Ns	0.001	ns
PSI	92.3; 10.7	94.94; 18.4	80.0; 18.4	(2.43); ns	Ns	ns	ns

Table 2. Child Behavior Checklist (CBCL): Comparisons among groups. Legenda: BD-ASD-S = Bipolar Disorder + High Functioning Autism Spectrum Disorder + Severe Suicide Ideation or Attempt; BD-noASD-S = Bipolar Disorder + Severe Suicide Ideation or Attempt, without High Functioning Autism Spectrum Disorder; BD-ASD-noS = Bipolar Disorder + High Functioning Autism Spectrum Disorder, without Severe Suicide Ideation or Attempt. Statistical significance at $p < 0.05$.

	Group 1 BD-ASD-S Mean; SD	Group 2 BD-no ASD-S Mean; SD	Group 3 BD-ASD-NoS Mean; SD	One-Way ANOVA (F); *p*	Gr1 vs. Gr.2 *p*	Gr.1 vs. Gr.3 *p*	Gr.2 vs. Gr.3 *p*
Internalizing	72.7; 7.6	69.9; 4.8	66.4;9.1	(3.1); ns	ns	0.049	ns
Externalizing	60.8; 7.9	63.2; 9.1	60.7; 6.4	(0.57); ns	ns	ns	ns
Total	68.1; 6.2	67.6; 5.6	65.6; 6.7	(0.79); ns	ns	ns	ns
Anxious/Depressed	75.1; 9.8	72.9; 9.2	66.9; 10.8	(3.1); ns	ns	ns	ns
Withdrawn	75.7; 9.3	73.2; 11.3	67.3; 9,9	(3.0); ns	ns	ns	ns
Somatic Complaints	62.8; 9.9	59.3; 7.0	59.2; 9.3	(0.93); ns	ns	ns	ns
Social Problems	65.9; 8.2	64.9; 7.6	67.4; 7.4	(0.46); ns	ns	ns	ns
Thought Problems	70.9; 9.3	70.2; 5.3	63.28: 9.2	(4.7); 0.013	ns	0.023	0.042
Attention	59.4.; 4.9	62.9; 8.9	64.2; 7.9	(1.9); ns	ns	ns	ns
Rule Breaking Problems	59.5; 6.2	627; 8.8	58,8; 5.83	(1.5); ns	ns	ns	ns
Aggressive behavior	61.9; 9.4	64.8; 9.5	60.9; 6.1	(1.0); ns	ns	ns	ns
Dysregulation Profile	196.4; 16.0	200.7; 19.1	192.1; 19.7	(0 96); ns	ns	ns	ns

Autism severity according to ADOS-Calibrated Severity Score, did not differ significantly between suicidal and non-suicidal individuals with ASD (BD-ASD-S: M = 5.85, SD = 1.15 versus BD-ASD-noS: M = 5.59, SD = 0.76 t = 0.701, $p = 0.243$).

All the four scales of the prevalent attitude (repulsion or attraction) for life and death (attraction to life, repulsion by life, attraction to death, and repulsion by death) failed to reach statistical difference among groups.

Similarly, the attentional and motor impulsivity, as well as the total score of the BIS, did not differ in the three groups. On the contrary, the non-planned impulsivity was higher in the BD-noASD-S group, compared to BD-ASD-S and BD-ASD-noS groups (F = 3.85, $p = 0.028$). More specifically, in multiple comparisons, ASD suicidal individuals presented less non planned impulsivity than individuals without ASD ($p = 0.040$).

On the Resilience test (READ), only Personal Competence differed among groups (F = 6.85, $p = 0.004$), as, after multiple comparisons, individuals with BD-ASD-noS significantly outscored those with BD-noASD-S ($p = 0.003$). All the other four dimensions of the scale (Social Competence, Structured Style, Family Cohesion, and Social Resources), as well as total score, were similar among groups.

Results of the path analysis (χ^2 (7) = 6.232, p = ns, CFI = 1, TLI = 1; SRMR = 0.057, RMSEA = 0.000 (0.000–0.164), p = ns) attest that some resilience dimensions were significantly associated with suicide tendency. In particular, personal competences (unstandardized coefficient: −0.19, S.E. = 0.09) and structured style (unstandardized coefficient: −0.29, S.E. = 0.10) were negatively associated with repulsion by life, and social resource (unstandardized coefficient: −0.24, S.E. = 0.12) was negatively associated with attraction to death. The model explained the 25% of repulsion by life variance, and 0.05% of attraction to death variance (Figure 1).

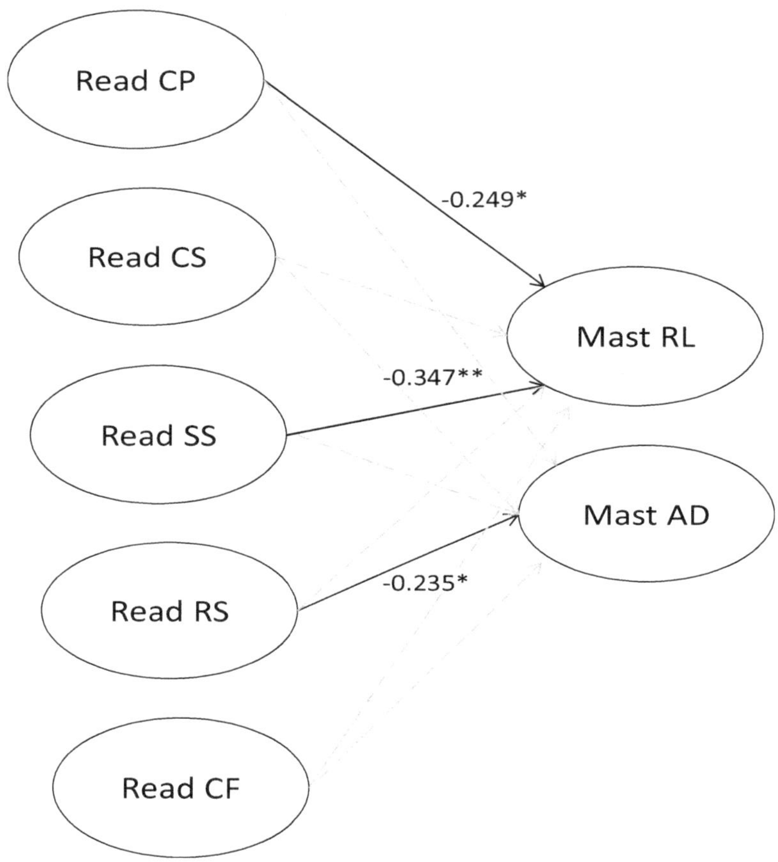

Figure 1. Relationships between Resiliency and Suicide Tendency. Note: READ CP = Personal Competence, READ CS = Social Competence, READ SS = Structured Style, READ RS = Social Resources, READ CF = Family Cohesion, Mast RL = repulsion by life, Mast AD = attraction to death. *: $p < 0.05$, **: $p < 0.01$.

4. Discussion

If BD is a well-known risk factor for suicide ideation and behavior, this risk may be markedly increased in bipolar individuals with HF-ASD. In fact, persons with HF-ASD experience the world in a specific way, compared with typically developing individuals, from basic information processing and attribution processing patterns, to social perspectives, such as the difficulties in expressing feelings and communicating with others [4,8,32,53,54,58]. A better comprehension of possible peculiarities in a very special population with both BD and HF-ASD may improve our understanding on how suicidal behaviors may be recognized, managed and treated. In our study, suicidal bipolar individuals with ASD were more frequently males, and presented greater clinical severity and functional impairment. Furthermore, they presented higher potential lethality of their suicidality, compared to the group without ASD, consistently with literature findings [17,32,55,56,59,60]. These differences were not accounted for by the type of BD, which did not differ among groups.

The suicidal individuals with ASD presented also a higher IQ, suggesting that the psychopathological severity has a greater impact on global functioning than their cognitive functioning [57,61]. Consistently, studies on populations with neurodevelopmental disorders reported that individuals with intellectual disabilities show a lower suicide rate than general population [57,58,61,62]. A high IQ may represent a specific risk factor [59,60,63,64], as it may imply an increased self-consciousness of one's own disability, leading to painful feelings of inadequacy, guilt, and exclusion from peer groups. Such aspects may be more evident during adolescence, when heightened social requests can easily go beyond the individual's coping abilities, further worsening the social withdrawal [58,61–63,65–68].

Regarding psychiatric diagnoses, only OCD differed among groups, and was more frequently reported in ASD individuals, irrespective of the presence of suicidality. However, a recent study showed that rumination was significantly associated with a history of attempted suicide in a sample of 75 adults with ASD [8,16].

Suicidal individuals with BD-ASD individuals presented at the CBCL (completed by parents) significantly more internalizing problems and thought problems. Internalized symptoms can represent a risk factor for suicide in individuals with ASD [16,24]. Hence, investigating symptoms with standardized scales with both individuals and caregivers, including direct psychiatric interviews, is crucial, given that many individuals with HF-ASD are able to "camouflage" internalized symptoms.

The severity of autistic traits in individuals with or without suicidality, according to ADOS-2, did not differ between the two groups, suggesting that this feature does not affect the suicidal risk. Available evidence on this topic is inconsistent. While a number of studies on "Asperger syndrome" populations have shown a negative correlation between suicidal ideation and autistic traits [15,23,67,69], on the contrary Cassidy et al. [7,15] reported that persons diagnosed with Asperger syndrome with previous suicide attempts showed significantly higher autistic traits than individuals with this diagnosis without a history of attempted suicide.

In our study, the three groups did not differ according to repulsion or attraction for life and death. On the contrary, non-planned impulsivity was highest in the BD-noASD-S group, compared to both the ASD groups (with or without suicidality), suggesting that in individuals with ASD the suicidality may be less impulsive than in individuals without ASD, although both the groups have a diagnosis of BD This could imply a "colder" transition from ideation to suicide attempt, leading to more lethal strategies [68,70].

Regarding resilience, personal competence was lowest in individuals with BD-noASD-S individuals, and highest in those with BD-non suicidal ASD, with intermediate scores in the BD-ASD-S group, suggesting that the feeling of a low personal competence is more urgent in non-autistic individuals, and namely in those who present suicidal ideation or behavior, in whom it may have a triggering role in their suicidality.

A structural equation modeling was applied to examine the influences among variables that may interact, namely, between resilience protective factors, and suicide tendency, in terms of attraction and/or repulsion to life and/or death. Some dimensions of resilience, particularly personal competences and structured style were protective in terms of repulsion by life, while social resource was protective in terms of attraction to death. This information may guide possible therapeutic interventions aimed at reinforcing specific areas of resilience in order to improve some risk factors related to suicide vulnerability in adolescence.

Our study shows a number of limitations that could limit the generalization of the results. Major limitations of the study are the small sample size, and the lack of a control group of typically developing adolescents. Furthermore, these groups were not recruited through an age- and gender-matching protocol design, although no statistically significant age difference emerged, and the female component was only scarcely represented. Finally, only a selected number of features were considered as relevant, and the diagnostic exploration did not include other potentially important elements.

Our study provides a first, exploratory contribution for better understanding the peculiarities of adolescents with BD and ASD and severe suicide ideation or suicide attempts, helpful for subsequent targeted examination of suicidality in autism/bipolar disorder. These specificities may help clinicians not only in the diagnostic process, focusing investigations on specific areas, but also in the prevention and treatment strategies, for planning timely and finely customized educational and therapeutic approaches, at the individual level, contributing to a precision medicine even in these complex and often misunderstood individuals.

Author Contributions: Conceptualization: G.M., S.S., M.M., G.D.; Methodology: G.M., G.D., A.N., P.M., M.P.; Data collection: S.S, D.F., F.L., G.D.; Statistical analyses: P.M. and M.P.; Writing first draft: G.M.; Discussion on the first draft and conclusions: S.S., A.N., P.M., M.P., D.F., F.L., M.M., G.D.; All authors have read and agreed to the published version of the manuscript.

Acknowledgments: The authors wish to thank all the participants, the adolescent and their parents

References

1. Nock, M.W.; Green, J.G.; Hwang, I.; Mclaughlin, K.A.; Sampson, M.A.; Zaslavsky, A.M.; Kessler, R.C. Prevalence, correlates and treatment of lifetime suicidal behavior among adolescents: Results from the National Comorbidity Survey Replication –Adolescent Supplement (NCSA). *JAMA Psychiatry* **2013**, *70*, 300–310. [CrossRef] [PubMed]
2. Glenn, C.R.; Kleiman, E.M.; Kellerman, J.; Pollak, O.; Cha, C.B.; Esposito, E.C.; Porter, A.C.; Wyman, P.A.; Boatman, A.E. Annual Research Review: A meta-analytic review of worldwide suicide rates in adolescents. *J. Child Psychol. Psychiatry* **2020**, *61*, 294–308. [CrossRef] [PubMed]
3. Hawton, K.; Saunders, K.E.; O'Connor, R.C. Self-harm and suicide in adolescents. *Lancet* **2012**, *379*, 2373–2382. [CrossRef]
4. Oliphant, R.Y.K.; Smith, E.M.; Grahame, V. What is the Prevalence of Self-harming and Suicidal Behaviour in Under 18s with ASD, with or Without an Intellectual Disability? *J. Autism. Dev. Disord.* **2020**. [CrossRef] [PubMed]
5. Wijnhoven, L.A.; Niels-Kessels, H.; Creemers, D.H.; Verhulst, A.A.; Otten, R.; Engels, R.C. Prevalence of comorbid depressive symptoms and suicidal ideation in children with autism spectrum disorder and elevated anxiety symptoms. *J. Child Adolesc. Mental Health* **2019**, *31*, 77–84. [CrossRef]
6. Hirvikoski, T.; Mittendorfer-Rutz, E.; Boman, M.; Larsson, H.; Lichtenstein, P.; Bölte, S. Premature mortality in autism spectrum disorder. *Br. J. Psychiatry* **2016**, *208*, 232–238. [CrossRef]
7. Cassidy, S.; Bradley, P.; Robinson, J.; Allison, C.; McHugh, M.; Baron-Cohen, S. Suicidal ideation and suicide plans or attempts in adults with Asperger's syndrome attending a specialist diagnostic clinic: A clinical cohort study. *Lancet Psychiatry* **2014**, *1*, 142–147. [CrossRef]
8. Arwert, T.G.; Sizoo, B.B. Self-reported Suicidality in Male and Female Adults with Autism Spectrum Disorders: Rumination and Self-esteem. *J. Autism Dev. Disord.* **2020**. [CrossRef]
9. Fitzgerald, M. Suicide and Asperger's syndrome. *Crisis* **2007**, *28*, 1–3. [CrossRef]
10. Cassidy, S.; Bradley, L.; Shaw, R. Baron-Cohen, S. Risk markers for suicidality in autistic adults. *Mol. Autism.* **2018**, *31*, 9–42.
11. Chen, M.H.; Pan, T.L.; Lan, W.H.; Hsu, J.W.; Huang, K.L.; Su, T.P.; Li, C.T.; Lin, W.C.; Wei, H.T.; Chen, T.J.; et al. Risk of Suicide Attempts among Adolescents and Young Adults with Autism Spectrum Disorder: A Nationwide Longitudinal Follow-Up Study. *J. Clin. Psychiatry* **2017**, *78*, e1174–e1179. [CrossRef] [PubMed]
12. Culpin, I.; Mars, B.; Pearson, R.M.; Golding, J.; Heron, J.; Bubak, I.; Carpenter, P.; Magnusson, C.; Gunnell, D.; Rai, D. Autistic Traits and Suicidal Thoughts, Plans, and Self-Harm in Late Adolescence: Population-Based Cohort Study. *J. Am. Acad. Child Adolesc. Psychiatry* **2018**, *57*, 313–320. [CrossRef]
13. Veenstra-VanderWeele, J. Recognizing the Problem of Suicidality in Autism Spectrum Disorder. *J. Am. Acad. Child Adolesc. Psychiatry* **2018**, *57*, 302–303. [CrossRef] [PubMed]
14. Cappadocia, M.C.; Weiss, J.A.; Pepler, D. Bullying experiences among children and youth with autism spectrum disorders. *J. Autism Dev. Disord.* **2012**, *42*, 266–277. [CrossRef] [PubMed]
15. Shtayermman, O. Peer victimization in adolescents and young adults diagnosed with Asperger's Syndrome: A link to depressive symptomatology, anxiety symptomatology and suicidal ideation. *Issues Compr. Pediatr. Nurs.* **2007**, *30*, 87–107. [CrossRef]

16. Storch, E.A.; Sulkowski, M.L.; Nadeau, J.; Lewin, A.B.; Arnold, E.B.; Mutch, P.J.; Jones, A.M.; Murphy, T.K. The phenomenology and clinical correlates of suicidal thoughts and behaviors in youth with autism spectrum disorders. *J. Autism. Dev. Disord.* **2013**, *43*, 2450–2459. [CrossRef] [PubMed]
17. Hedley, D.; Uljarević, M.; Foley, K.R.; Richdale, A.; Trollor, J. Risk and protective factors underlying depression and suicidal ideation in Autism Spectrum Disorder. *Depress. Anxiety* **2018**, *35*, 648–657. [CrossRef]
18. Leyfer, O.T.; Folstein, S.E.; Bacalman, S.; Davis, N.O.; Dinh, E.; Morgan, J.; Tager-Flusberg, H.; Lainhart, J.E. Comorbid psychiatric disorders in children with autism: Interview development and rates of disorders. *J. Autism Dev. Disord.* **2006**, *36*, 849–861. [CrossRef]
19. van Steensel, F.J.; Bögels, S.M.; Perrin, S. Anxiety disorders in children and adolescents with autistic spectrum disorders: A meta-analysis. *Clin. Child Fam. Psychol. Rev.* **2011**, *14*, 302–317. [CrossRef] [PubMed]
20. Ben-Sasson, A.; Hen, L.; Fluss, R.; Cermak, S.A.; Engel-Yeger, B.; Gal, E. A meta-analysis of sensory modulation symptoms in individuals with autism spectrum disorders. *J. Autism Dev. Disord.* **2009**, *39*, 1–11. [CrossRef]
21. Foley Nicpon, M.; Doobay, A.F.; Assouline, S.G. Parent, teacher, and self-perceptions of psychosocial functioning in intellectually gifted children and adolescents with autism spectrum disorder. *J. Autism Dev. Disord.* **2010**, *40*, 1028–1038. [CrossRef] [PubMed]
22. Meyer, J.A.; Mundy, P.C.; Vaughan Van Hecke, A.; Durocher, J.S. Social attribution processes and comorbid psychiatric symptoms in children with Asperger syndrome. *Autism* **2006**, *10*, 383–402. [CrossRef]
23. Twenge, J.M.; Cooper, A.B.; Joiner, T.E.; Duffy, M.E.; Binau, S.G. Age, period, and cohort trends in mood disorder indicators and suicide-related outcomes in a nationally representative dataset, 2005–2017. *J. Abnorm. Psychol.* **2019**, *128*, 185–199. [CrossRef] [PubMed]
24. Rao, U.; Weissman, M.M.; Martin, J.A.; Hammond, R.W. Childhood depression and risk of suicide: A preliminary report of a longitudinal study. *J. Am. Acad. Child Adolesc. Psychiatry* **1993**, *32*, 21–27. [CrossRef] [PubMed]
25. Plans, L.; Barrot, C.; Nieto, E.; Rios, J.; Schulze, T.G.; Papiol, S.; Mitjians, M.; Vieta, E.; Benabarre, A. Association between completed suicide and bipolar disorder: A systematic review of the literature. *J. Affect. Disord.* **2019**, *242*, 111–122. [CrossRef] [PubMed]
26. Hossain, M.M.; Khan, N.; Sultana, A.; Ma, P.; McKyer, E.L.J.; Ahmed, H.U.; Purohit, N. Prevalence of comorbid psychiatric disorders among people with autism spectrum disorder: An umbrella review of systematic reviews and meta-analyses. *Psychiat. Res.* **2020**, *18*, 112922. [CrossRef]
27. Simonoff, E.; Pickels, A.; Charman, T.; Chandler, S.; Loucas, T.; Baird, G. Psychiatric disorders in children and adolescents with autism spectrum disorders: Prevalence, comorbidity, and associated factors in a population-derived sample. *J. Am. Acad. Child Adolesc. Psychiatry* **2008**, *47*, 921–929. [CrossRef]
28. Lugo Marín, J.; Alviani Rodríguez-Franco, M.; Mahtani Chugani, V.; Magán Maganto, M.; Díez Villoria, E.; Canal Bedia, R. Prevalence of schizophrenia spectrum disorders in average-iq adults with autism spectrum disorders: A meta-analysis. *J. Autism Dev. Disord.* **2018**, *48*, 239–250. [CrossRef]
29. Lai, M.-C.; Kassee, C.; Besney, R.; Bonato, S.; Hull, L.; Mandy, W.; Szatmari, P.; Ameis, S.H. Prevalence of co-occurring mental health diagnoses in the autism population: A systematic review and meta-analysis. *Lancet Psychiatry* **2019**. [CrossRef]
30. Hudson, C.C.; Hall, L.; Harkness, K.L. Prevalence of depressive disorders in individuals with autism spectrum disorder: A meta-analysis. *J. Abnorm. Child Psychol.* **2019**, *47*, 165–175. [CrossRef]
31. Joshi, G.; Biederman, J.; Petty, C.; Goldin, R.I.; Eurtak, S.L.; Wozniak, J. Examining the comorbidity of bipolar disorder and autism spectrum disorders: A large controlled analysis of phenotypic and familial correlates in a referred population of youth with bipolar I disorder with and without autism spectrum disorders. *J. Clin. Psychiatry* **2013**, *74*, 578–586. [CrossRef] [PubMed]
32. Vannucchi, G.; Masi, G.; Toni, C.; Dell'Osso, L.; Erfurth, A.; Perugi, G. Bipolar disorder in adults with Asperger's Syndrome: A systematic review. *J. Affect. Disord.* **2014**, *168*, 151–160. [CrossRef] [PubMed]
33. Dell'Osso, L.; Carpita, B.; Muti, D.; Morelli, V.; Salarpi, G.; Salerni, A.; Scotto, J.; Massimetti, C.; Gesi, C.; Ballerio, M.; et al. Mood symptoms and suicidality across the autism spectrum. *Compr. Psychiatry* **2019**, *91*, 34–38. [CrossRef]
34. Osman, A.; Gilpin, A.R.; Kopper, B.A.; Barrios, F.X.; Gutierrez, P.M.; Chiros, C.E. The Multi Attitude Suicide Tendency Scale: Further Validation with Adolescent Psychiatric Inpatients. *Suicide Life Threat Behav.* **2000**, *30*, 377–385. [PubMed]

35. Klomek, A.B.; Orbach, I.; Sher, L.; Sommerfeld, E.; Diller, R.; Apter, A.; Shahar, G.; Zalsman, G. Quality of depression among suicidal inpatient youth. *Arch. Suicide Res.* **2008**, *12*, 133–140. [CrossRef]
36. Park, C.H.K.; Lee, J.W.; Lee, S.Y.; Shim, S.H.; Moon, J.J.; Paik, J.W.; Cho, S.J.; Kim, S.G.; Kim, M.H.; Kim, S.; et al. Implications of Increased Trait Impulsivity on Psychopathology and Experienced Stress in the Victims of Early Trauma With Suicidality. *J. Nerv. Ment. Dis.* **2018**, *206*, 840–849. [CrossRef]
37. Jakobsen, I.S.; Larsen, K.J.; Horwood, J.L. Suicide Risk Assessment in Adolescents -C-SSRS, K10, and READ. *Crisis* **2017**, *38*, 247–254. [CrossRef]
38. Kaufman, J.; Birmaher, B.; Brent, D.; Rao, U.; Flynn, C.; Moreci, P.; Williamson, D.; Ryan, N. Schedule for Affective Disorders and Schizophrenia for School-Age Children-Present and Lifetime Version (K-SADS-PL): Initial reliability and validity data. *J. Am. Acad. Child Adolesc. Psychiatry* **1997**, *36*, 980–988. [CrossRef]
39. American Psychiatric Association. *Diagnostic and Statistical Manual for Mental Disorders – Fifth Edition (DSM 5)*; American Psychiatric Association: Arlington, VA, USA, 2013.
40. Lord, C.; Rutter, M.; DiLavore, P.C.; Risi, S.; Gotham, K.; Bishop, S. *Autism Diagnostic Observation Schedule*, 2nd ed.; Western Psychological Services: Torrance, CA, USA, 2012.
41. Rutter, M.; Le Couteur, A.; Lord, C. *Autism Diagnostic Interview – Revised*; Western Psychological Services: Torrance, CA, USA, 2003.
42. Saemundsen, E.; Magnússon, P.; Smári, J.; Sigurdardóttir, S. Autism Diagnostic Interview-Revised and the Childhood Autism Rating Scale: Convergence and discrepancy in diagnosing autism. *J. Autism Dev. Disord.* **2003**, *33*, 319–328. [CrossRef]
43. Posner, K.; Brown, G.K.; Stanley, B.; Brent, D.A.; Yershova, K.V.; Oquendo, M.A.; Currier, G.W.; Melvin, G.A.; Greenhill, L.; Shen, S.; et al. The Columbia-Suicide Severity Rating Scale: Initial validity and internal consistency findings from three multisite studies with adolescents and adults. *Am. J. Psychiatry* **2011**, *168*, 1266–1277. [CrossRef]
44. Wechsler, D. *The Wechsler Intelligence Scale for Children*, 4th ed.; Pearson: London, UK, 2003.
45. Gotham, K.; Pickles, A.; Lord, C. Standardizing ADOS scores for a measure of severity in autism spectrum disorders. *J. Autism Dev. Disord.* **2009**, *39*, 693–705. [CrossRef] [PubMed]
46. Guy, W. *ECDEU Assessment Manual for Psychopharmacology, Revised*; US Department of Health, Education and Welfare: Rockville, MD, USA, 1976.
47. Shaffer, D.; Gould, M.S.; Brasic, J.; Ambrosini, P.; Fisher, P.; Bird, H.; Aluwahlia, S.A. Children's Global Assessment Scale (CGAS). *Arch. Gen. Psychiatry* **1983**, *40*, 1228–1231. [CrossRef] [PubMed]
48. Achenbach, T.M.; Rescorla, L.A. *Manual for the ASEBA School-Age Forms and Profiles. Burlington, VT: University of Vermont Research Center for Children, Youth, & Families*; University of Vermont: Burlington, VT, USA, 2001.
49. Deutz, M.H.; Geeraerts, S.B.; van Baar, A.L.; Deković, M.; Prinzie, P. The Dysregulation Profile in middle childhood and adolescence across reporters: Factor structure, measurement invariance, and links with self-harm and suicidal ideation. *Eur. Child Adolesc. Psychiatry* **2016**, *25*, 431–442. [CrossRef] [PubMed]
50. Orbach, I.; Milstein, I.; Har-Even, D.; Apter, A.; Tiano, S.; Elizur, A. A Multi-Attitude Suicide Tendency Scale for adolescents. *J. Consult. Clin. Psychol.* **1991**, *3*, 398–404. [CrossRef]
51. Osman, A.; Barrios, F.X.; Panak, W.F.; Osman, J.R.; Hoffman, J.; Hammer, R. Validation of the Multi-Attitude Suicide Tendency scale in adolescent samples. *J. Clin. Psychol.* **1994**, *50*, 847–855. [CrossRef]
52. Patton, J.H.; Stanford, M.S.; Barratt, E.S. Factor structure of the Barratt impulsiveness scale. *J. Clin. Psychol.* **1995**, *51*, 768–774. [CrossRef]
53. Fossati, A.; Di Ceglie, A.; Acquarini, E.; Barratt, E.S. Psychometric properties of an Italian version of the Barratt Impulsiveness Scale-11 (BIS-11) in nonclinical subjects. *J. Clin. Psychol.* **2001**, *57*, 815–828. [CrossRef] [PubMed]
54. Hjemdal, O.; Friborg, O.; Stiles, T.C.; Martinussen, M.; Rosenvinge, J. A new scale for adolescent resilience: Grasping the central protective resources behind healthy development. *Measur. Eval. Couns. Dev.* **2006**, *39*, 84–96. [CrossRef]
55. Stratta, P.; Riccardi, I.; Di Cosimo, A.; Rossi, A.; Rossi, A. A validation study of the italian version of the resilience scale for adolescents (READ). *J. Commun. Psychol.* **2012**, *40*. [CrossRef]
56. von Soest, T.; Mossige, S.; Stefansen, K.; Hjemdal, O.A. Validation Study of the Resilience Scale for Adolescents (READ). *J. Psychopathol. Behav. Assess.* **2010**, *32*, 215–225. [CrossRef]

57. Hjemdal, O.; Vogel, P.A.; Solem, S.; Hagan, K.; Stiles, T.C. The relationship between resilience and levels of anxiety, depression and obsessive-compulsive symptoms in adolescents. *Clin. Psychol. Psychother.* **2011**, *18*, 314–321. [CrossRef] [PubMed]
58. Lai, M.C.; Anagnostou, E.; Wiznitzer, M.; Allison, C.; Baron-Cohen, S. Evidence-based support for autistic people across the lifespan: Maximising potential, minimising barriers, and optimising the person-environment fit. *Lancet Neurol.* **2020**. [CrossRef]
59. Kato, K.; Mikami, K.; Akama, F.; Yamada, K.; Maehara, M.; Kimoto, K.; Kimoto, K.; Sato, R.; Takahashi, Y.; Fukushima, R.; et al. Clinical features of suicide attempts in adults with autism spectrum disorders. *Gen. Hosp. Psychiatry* **2013**, *35*, 50–53. [CrossRef] [PubMed]
60. Hannon, G.; Taylor, E.P. Suicidal behaviour in adolescents and young adults with ASD: Findings from a systematic review. *Clin. Psychol. Rev.* **2013**, *33*, 1197–1204. [CrossRef]
61. Howlin, P.; Asgharian, A. The diagnosis of autism and Asperger syndrome: Findings from a survey of 770 families. *Dev. Med. Child Neurol.* **1999**, *41*, 834–839. [CrossRef]
62. Huband, N.; Tantam, D. Attitudes to self-injury within a group of mental health staff. *Br. J. Med. Psychol.* **2000**, *73*, 495–504. [CrossRef]
63. Myriam De-la-Iglesia, M.; Olivar, J.S. Risk factors for depression in children and adolescents with high functioning autosm spectrum disorders. *Sci. World J.* **2015**, 127853. [CrossRef]
64. Balfe, M.; Tantam, D. A descriptive social and health profile of a community sample of adults and adolescents with Asperger syndrome. *BMC Res. Notes* **2010**, *3*, 300. [CrossRef]
65. Gotham, K.; Bishop, S.L.; Brunwasser, S.; Lord, C. Rumination and perceived impairment associated with depressive symptoms in a verbal adolescent-adult ASD sample. *Autism Res.* **2014**, *7*, 381–391. [CrossRef]
66. Hedley, D.; Young, R. Social comparison processes and depressive symptoms in children and adolescents with Asperger syndrome. *Autism* **2006**, *10*, 139–153. [CrossRef]
67. Turecki, G. Preventing suicide: Where are we? *Lancet Psychiatry* **2016**, *3*, 597–598. [CrossRef]
68. Brent, D.A.; Perper, J.; Goldstein, C.; Kolko, D.J.; Allan, M.J.; Allman, C.J.; Zelenak, J.P. Risk factor for adolescent suicide. A comparison of adolescent suicide victims with suicidal in patients. *Arch. Gen. Psychiatry.* **1988**, *45*, 581–588. [CrossRef] [PubMed]
69. Demirkaya Karakoç, S.; Tutkunkardaş, M.D.; Mukaddes, N.M. Assessment of suicidality in children and adolescents with diagnosis of high functioning autism spectrum disorder in a Turkish clinical sample. *Neuropsychiatr. Dis. Treat.* **2016**, *11*, 2921–2926. [CrossRef] [PubMed]
70. McDonnell, C.G.; Bradley, C.C.; Kanne, S.M.; Lajonchere, C.; Warren, Z.; Carpenter, L.A. When Are We Sure? Predictors of Clinician Certainty in the Diagnosis of Autism Spectrum Disorder. *J. Autism Dev. Disord.* **2019**, *49*, 1391–1401. [CrossRef]

4

Broader Autism Phenotype in Siblings of Children with ASD

Ewa Pisula [†,*] **and Karolina Ziegart-Sadowska** [†]

Faculty of Psychology, University of Warsaw, Stawki 5/7, 00-183 Warsaw, Poland; karolinaziegart@gmail.com
* Author to whom correspondence should be addressed; ewa.pisula@psych.uw.edu.pl

† These authors contributed equally to this work.

Academic Editor: Merlin G. Butler

Abstract: Although less pronounced, social, cognitive, and personality characteristics associated with autism spectrum disorders (ASD) may be present in people who do not meet ASD diagnostic criteria, especially in first-degree relatives of individuals with ASD. Research on these characteristics, referred to as broader autism phenotype (BAP), provides valuable data on potential expressions of autism-specific deficits in the context of family relations. This paper offers a review of research on BAP in siblings of individuals with ASD, focusing on reports regarding social, communication, and cognitive deficits, published from 1993 to 2014. The studies are divided into two groups based on participants' age: papers on preschool and older siblings of individuals with ASD; and publications on infants at risk for ASD. On the basis of this review, suggestions are offered for further research and its significance for our understanding of the genetic determinants of autism.

Keywords: broad autism phenotype; siblings; review; at-risk infants

1. Introduction

Autism spectrum disorders (ASD) are neurodevelopmental disorders characterized by deficits in social communication and the presence of repetitive patterns of behavior, activity, and interests [1,2]. An important contributing factor in ASD etiology could be genetic liability, since the occurrence rate for ASD in siblings is on average 20- or 25-fold higher than in the general population [3–5].

The genetic mechanisms involved in the development of ASD are complex and heterogeneous [4,6,7]. This complexity is reflected by the variety of clinical characteristics of ASD, involving differences in the combination and expression of symptoms and severity of disorders in affected individuals. The heterogeneous, multifaceted nature of ASD is what drives research into the many possible expressions of autism that incorporate its typical deficits. The data obtained in that research may help us understand the genetic mechanisms that contribute to the development of autism-specific functional traits and atypical developmental trajectories. Moreover, this data may be useful in identifying genetic factors specific for various autism phenotypes, both in subjects with ASD and individuals from the general population.

A clear diagnostic conceptualization of autism still has yet to be established. It has been proposed that behavioral and cognitive characteristics of ASD, which include social, communication, and cognitive processes, rigid and persistent interests, and rigid and aloof personality traits, are continuously distributed throughout the general population [8]. These characteristics are likely to be more prevalent in first-degree relatives of individuals with ASD than in other groups [6,9–15]. Frazier and colleagues [16] studied how caregivers reported autism symptoms among children in their charge diagnosed with ASD and their unaffected siblings. They obtained data supporting the view that ASD is best characterized as a category. However, they note that "these data do not discount the possibility of endophenotypes or subthreshold ASD symptoms in unaffected family members" [16]. Wheelwright and colleagues [17] point out that studying ASD in nonclinical samples may be valuable in the context of the variety of genetic factors that seem to be connected to ASD. The genetic research on autism may benefit from a more inclusive concept of genetic expression that comprises cognitive, social, and communication deficits, as well as personality traits [18,19]. Characteristics similar to autism but less severe are referred to as broader autism phenotype (BAP) [20]. The notion of BAP facilitated involvement in studies on ASD and related phenomena of a large number of individuals without a clinical diagnosis of ASD. Consequently, it became possible to apply methods of the quantitative genetics typically used in the studies of normally distributed characteristics [21]. Research on BAP may help identify more functionally homogeneous subgroups of affected individuals and pinpoint the genetic factors that contribute to the development of ASD symptoms or traits [22]. The identification of phenotype may, therefore, open up the possibility of hypothetically assigning responsibility to a candidate gene or chromosome region. It therefore seems that data obtained in studies on BAP may provide promising cues for more detailed hypotheses on the genetic background of ASD. These studies may also contribute to a better understanding of the lesser variants of autism [23]. Since the data collected to date are not uniform, their applicability to genetic studies remains limited, and indicating the phenotypes with a clear genetic connection is still a difficult question. This may be due to the fact that the BAP concept covers a range of cognitive and social abilities and personality traits. Precisely establishing which characteristics should be included in BAP is a somewhat controversial undertaking. The lack of standardized criteria for BAP complicates attempts to engage in a comparative review of research on the topic. The features generally recognized as the most typical are deficits in social functioning, pragmatic language difficulties, restricted, repetitive behaviors and interests, as well as cognitive deficits (with respect to theory of mind in particular and social cognition in general, executive function, weak central coherence) and rigid personality [23]. Therefore, this paper focuses on the phenotypic characteristics of the individuals, observed from the perspective of clinical and experimental psychology. It seems that the concise summary of studies on BAP proposed here may provide some assistance in designing more advanced future studies aimed at identifying specific genetic mechanisms. Moreover, this paper will also demonstrate the methodological diversity in this field of study, which might help us in understanding the inconsistency of results across papers being published.

Gottesman and Gould [24] pointed out that phenotypes, understood as measurable characteristics, are heritable traits that are located in the path of pathogenesis from genetic predisposition to psychopathology. These traits are found at a higher rate in unaffected relatives of diagnosed family members than in the general population. The search for phenotypes may be conducted in specific populations that carry risk genes, but remain unaffected. Therefore unaffected relatives of individuals with the diagnosis, like healthy siblings, fulfill both criteria: they are enriched in risk genes and are healthy [25].

Therefore, a number of studies on BAP have been conducted on siblings of individuals with ASD. Initial findings have already indicated a significantly higher risk of autism in siblings than in the general population. Autism was initially reported to occur in approximately 2%–3% of siblings of affected children [26,27]. Folstein and Rutter [19], studying 21 pairs of same-sex siblings of whom one of the pairs was diagnosed with autism, found a concordance for autism in 4 of 11 sets of monozygotic twins, while in 10 dizygotic twin pairs they found no coexistence of autism in both children. Bolton and colleagues [28] analyzed family histories of autism in 137 individuals whose siblings had been diagnosed with the disorder, and found that 5.8% of siblings were diagnosed with autism, atypical autism, or Asperger syndrome, while no ASD diagnoses were reported among the siblings of individuals with Down syndrome. In a study by Ghaziuddin [29], 4.3% of siblings of 114 children with Asperger syndrome or autism were also diagnosed with Asperger syndrome or autism disorder.

Rates of BAP among siblings of individuals with ASD are much higher. August, Stewart, and Tsai [18] found cognitive disabilities in 15.5% of 71 siblings of probands with autism (compared to less than 3% in the control group). Folstein and Rutter [19] put forward a hypothesis that it is not autism as such that is inherited, but rather a pervasive cognitive deficit present both in individuals with autism and their immediate family. Currently, it is estimated that characteristics typical for ASD are present in at least 10%–20% of siblings of children diagnosed with ASD [28,30]. Ozonoff and colleagues [31], whose study involved a sample of 600 children in the USA and Canada, reported that autism-characteristic symptoms developed in nearly 19% of children whose older siblings had ASD. Boys are particularly at risk, with the correlation three times higher than in girls. At least one BAP trait is found in approximately 50% of family members of individuals with ASD when parents are included [32]. Biological siblings are attracting the attention of researchers studying BAP due to the large percentage of shared genes and environmental factors affecting their development.

Over the past few decades the corpus of data on BAP in siblings of individuals with ASD has expanded significantly. However, the studies in this area are highly diverse in terms of aspects such as design, instruments used, participant groups, as well as number of participants, their ages, and functions of interest, which lead to their findings being particularly difficult to integrate. Some help in overcoming that difficulty is offered by review papers that pool information on various aspects of studies and their results [23,33–37]. These reviews, especially those on preschool or older siblings, rarely provide information on participants' age. Due to the neurodevelopmental nature of ASD and the specifics of the processes involved, the inclusion of that information would seem reasonable. In the light of increasing interest in studying infant siblings of children with ASD among researchers seeking early predictors of ASD, summarizing the data collected from siblings could provide valuable information. Moreover, the methods for collecting data from children, adolescents, and adults are different, which provides even greater encouragement to have a closer look at the studies on BAP in different groups of siblings of individuals with ASD. The present paper provides a review of research on BAP traits in siblings of individuals with ASD, wherein the body of research will be divided into two groups: preschool or older siblings, and at-risk infants. The two will be treated as distinct due to the different nature of studies on infant siblings of children with ASD compared to research on older siblings. The studies on infants and toddlers are quite often prospective, enrolling both healthy children and children later diagnosed with ASD. With repeated measures it is possible to follow the siblings' developmental trajectories, unlike in most available studies on children over three or four years of age. Studies on at-risk infants have only emerged in the last decade; earlier research focused on older children, and as such these studies will be discussed first. For the reasons mentioned above, we have not attempted to propose a systematic review as defined in the PRISMA statement [38]. The present paper rather involves the subjective perspective of the authors reflected by the choice of the reviewed papers.

2. Research on Preschool-Age or Older Siblings

Table 1 presents a list of studies on broader autism phenotype in preschool or older siblings of individuals with ASD, published in the years 1993–2014. The list includes mainly studies that enrolled healthy siblings not affected by autism, although in a handful of them some participants were diagnosed with ASD or another disorder (*i.e.*, delayed language development) during the course of the study [28,39,40]. We have rejected studies in which the results of siblings were pooled in statistical analysis with the results of parents or other relatives *i.e.*, [41,42], which was sometimes a consequence of very small sibling subgroup size (like in [43]—only four siblings). Furthermore, publications included in the list meet the following criteria: (a) Peer-reviewed articles published in English; (b) Original studies; (c) Containing a control group; and (d) The social communication, language, and cognitive characteristics of autism in siblings of individuals with autism were the objects of study.

As shown in Table 1, studies that involve healthy siblings of individuals with ASD vary in design. They differ in terms of compared groups, sibling ages, sample sizes, analyzed aspects of functioning, as well as instruments and methods.

Table 1. Social communication, language, and cognitive BAP characteristics in siblings of individuals with ASD.

Study	Journal & Year	Characteristics	Sample	Age of Siblings of Individuals with ASD	Control Group, Matching Criteria	Measures/Instruments (Samples)	Main Findings
Ozonoff, Rogers, Farnham, & Pennington [45]	*J. Autism Dev. Disord.*, 1993	Executive function, theory of mind	18 Siblings of high functioning autism (HFA) children	8–18 years	18 siblings of children with learning disability, 18 HFA individuals, 18 learning-disabled children, matched on the basis of IQ, gender, socioeconomic status (SES), and ethnic background	Wechsler Intelligence Scale for Children–Revised (WISC-R), Wechsler Adults Intelligence Scale–Revised (WAIS-R), Wisconsin Card Sorting Test (WCST), Tower of Hanoi, Second-Order Belief Atribution Task, Fox and Grapes Task, Apple-Dog Task	HFA siblings performed worse than controls in the measure of planning (Tower of Hanoi). No differences between siblings groups in: set-shifting, working memory, and inhibitory control, theory-of-mind, Verbal IQ, Performance IQ, and Full Scale IQ
Szatmari *et al.* [45]	*J. Am. Acad. Child Adolesc. Psychiatry*, 1993	Cognitive impairments, adaptive behavior, developmental history	Siblings (and parents) of 52 pervasive developmental disorders (PDD) probands	6–18 years	Siblings (and parents) of 33 Down syndrome and low birth weight controls, matching criteria: IQ, family size, SES	Vineland Adaptive Behavior Scales (VABS), the Revised Stanford-Binet, Wide Range Achievement Test-Revised (WRAT-R), WCST	No differences between ASD siblings compared to control siblings on the social and communication domains of the VABS. No group differences in developmental history of language delays
Bolton *et al.* [28]	*J. Child Psychol. Psychiatry*, 1994	Social and communication impairments	137 Siblings (and 198 parents) of ASD individuals	Younger than 8 years	Down syndrome probands relatives (64 siblings, 72 parents); matching for age, sex, social class, birth order, and maternal age	Family History Interview, Autism Diagnostic Interview	20.4% of ASD siblings (and 3.1% of control siblings) demonstrated communication atypicalities, social impairments, or restricted behaviors; 4 out of 137 siblings met ICD-10 criteria for autism (two of them were mentally retarded), a further three were classified as having atypical autism and one was diagnosed with Asperger syndrome
Fombonne *et al.* [46]	*J. Child Psychol. Psychiatry*, 1997	General intellectual functioning, reading and spelling skills	Siblings (and parents) of 99 autism probands	Children and adults, lack of precise data	Siblings (and parents) of 36 Down syndrome individuals, matched for age, sex, social class, birth order, and maternal age with the autism probands	Family History Schedule, WAIS-R, WISC-R, Gray Oral Reading Test (GORT), Edinburgh Reading Tests, National Adult Reading Test, The Schonell Graded Word Spelling Test-B	Slightly higher mean verbal IQ scores in siblings of ASD individuals. Only the group of siblings of ASD individuals identified as affected with the BAP had significantly lower IQ scores and poorer reading and spelling abilities than unaffected siblings
Piven, Palmer, Jacobi, Childress, and Arndt [14]	*Am. J. Psychiatry*, 1997	Social and communication deficits	12 siblings from multiple incidence autism families	4–30 years	53 siblings of Down syndrome individuals; matched by probands age; no differences in parental education level and age	Family History Interview for Developmental Disorders of Cognition and Social Functioning	Higher rates of social deficits in siblings from families with multiple incidence autism. No differences in the rates of communication deficits or stereotyped behaviors in siblings
Folstein *et al.* [47]	*J. Child Psychol. Psychiatry*, 1999	Pragmatic language, verbal IQ, reading and spelling skills	87 siblings (and 166 parents) of individuals with autism	5–46 years	64 siblings (and 75 parents) of individuals with Down syndrome; very similar age of siblings and parental education	WISC-R, WAIS-R, GORT, Kaufman Battery	No differences in verbal IQ scores, reading and spelling skills
Hughes, Hughes, Plumet, & Leboyer [48]	*J. Child Psychol. Psychiatry*, 1999	Executive function: verbal fluency, planning, flexibility	31 siblings of children with autism	5 years 8 months–19 years 11 months	32 siblings of children with developmental delay, 32 children from unaffected families (with no family history of ASD); similar family backgrounds (living in a low-income area)	Cambridge Neuropsychological Test Automated Battery, Multistage set-shifting task, akin to the WCST, Corsi Block Tapping task, Tower of London, Verbal Fluency task	Superior verbal and spatial span in siblings of children with autism; higher number of autism siblings than controls performed poorly on the verbal fluency tasks, planning, and set-shifting
Briskman, Happé, and Frith [49]	*J. Child Psychol. Psychiatry*, 2001	Everyday-life preferences and activities	19 siblings of children with autism	8–18 years	13 dyslexic siblings, 11 controls; matched on the basis of SES, parental education	Parental report	No differences between ASD siblings and other groups in everyday skills and preferences (parent-rated) with the exception of two boys subsequently diagnosed on the Autism Spectrum

Table 1. *Cont.*

Study	Journal & Year	Characteristics	Sample	Age of Siblings of Individuals with ASD	Control Group, Matching Criteria	Measures/Instruments (Samples)	Main Findings
Happé, Briskman and Frith [50]	*J. Child Psychol. Psychiatry*, 2001	Information processing, "Central coherence"	19 siblings of children with autism	8–18 years	14 dyslexia siblings, 17 controls; matched on the basis of SES, parental education; no difference in chronological age between autism group probands, dyslexia group probands, or normal controls	WISC-R, WISC-III, phonological measures (*i.e.*, the Reading tests); Experimental measures (*i.e.*, the Embedded Figures Test, Block Design Task, Titchener Circles Illusion Task)	Intact central coherence in siblings
Pilowsky, Yirmiya, Shalev, & Gross-Tsur [51]	*J. Child Psychol. Psychiatry*, 2003	Language abilities	27 siblings of children with autism	6 years–15 years 1 month	23 siblings of children with mental retardation of unknown etiology, 22 siblings of children with developmental language disorders; groups matched by siblings' age, gender, birth order, family size, ethnicity, and family income and by probands' gender and mental age	Children's Evaluation of Language Fundamentals (CELF)	Higher scores in siblings of children with autism on receptive, expressive, and total language scales and on verbal IQ compared to siblings of children with developmental language disorders
Dorris, Espie, Knott, & Salt [52]	*J. Child Psychol. Psychiatry*, 2004	Mind-reading	27 siblings of children with Asperger syndrome (AS)	7 years 6 months–17 years	27 control children matched for age, sex, and a measure of verbal comprehension	"Eyes Test", British Picture Vocabulary Scale II	Poorer performance of AS siblings in the "Eyes Test"
Bishop, Maybery, Wong, Maley, & Hallmayer [11]	*Am. J. Med. Genet. B: Neuropsychiatr. Genet.*, 2006	Communication deficits	43 ASD siblings	4–16 years	46 control children; matching criteria: age, sex	Parent' report on Children's Communication Checklist-2 (CCC-2)	The only difference between groups was syntax; 23.8% of ASD siblings scored 2 SD below the control mean on CCC-2, compared to 2.2% of controls. Some differences in structural language skills
Constantino *et al.* [6]	*Am. J. Psychiatry*, 2006	Subsyndromal autistic impairments	49 siblings of children with autism from multiple-incidence families, 100 siblings of children with any PDD	4–18 years	45 siblings of children with psychopathology unrelated to autism, no matching criteria discussed	Social Responsiveness Scale (SRS)	Siblings of children with autism from multiple-incidence families—the highest scores in the SRS; followed by siblings of probands with any PDD, and then siblings of the probands with psychopathology unrelated to autism
Shaked, Gamliel, & Yirmiya [53]	*Autism*, 2006	Theory of mind	24 siblings of children with ASD (SIBS-A)	54–57 months	24 typically developing siblings (SIBS-TD), matched by siblings' age, gender, birth order, parents' age, and education	The false belief and the strange stories tasks	No differences on both theory of mind tasks
Christ, Holt, White, & Green [54]	*J. Autism Dev. Disord.*, 2007	Executive function: inhibitory control, processing speed	21 siblings of children with ASD	6–15 years	18 children with ASD, 25 typically developing (TD) controls, matched on age, overall IQ, and processing speed	Stroop Card Task, Stroop Computer Task, Flanker Task, Go/No-go Task	No differences between ASD siblings and controls in processing speed and inhibitory control
Chuthapisith, Ruangdaraganon, Sombuntham, & Roongpraiwan [39]	*Autism*, 2007	Language development	32 preschool siblings of children with autism	2–6 years	28 control children, matched by siblings' age, gender, maternal educational level and family income	The Stanford-Binet IV	Delayed language development in eight of the autism siblings. Following exclusion of siblings with ASD and developmental language disorder (DLD) diagnosis, the remaining 29 siblings' verbal IQs were not significantly different from the control group
Dalton, Nacewicz, Alexander, & Davidson [55]	*Biol. Psychiatry*, 2007	Face processing	12 ASD siblings	8–18 years	21 individuals with autism, 19 TD controls, matched for age and intelligence quotient (IQ)	Facial Recognition Task, eye tracking, brain functional magnetic resonance imaging	Decreased gaze fixation and brain function in response to images of human faces in ASD siblings; less time than the control group fixating the eye region in response to naturalistic photographs of both familiar and unfamiliar human faces

Table 1. *Cont.*

Study	Journal & Year	Characteristics	Sample	Age of Siblings of Individuals with ASD	Control Group, Matching Criteria	Measures/Instruments (Samples)	Main Findings
Gamliel, Yirmiya, & Sigman [56]	*J. Autism Dev. Disord.*, 2007	Cognitive and language development—a prospective study	39 ASD siblings (SIBS-A)	4–54 months	39 siblings of TD children (SIBS-TD); matched at 4 months according to chronological age, sex, birth order, number of children in the family, sex of the older proband, temperament profile, and mental and motor scores	Bayley Scales of Infant Development—2nd Edition (BSID-II), Reynell Developmental Language Scales (RDLS), Kaufman Assessment Battery for Children (K-ABC), Clinical Evaluation of Language Fundamentals-Preschool (CELF-P)	A delay in cognition and/or language in 12 of the SIBS-A and only two SIBS-TD; one child subsequently diagnosed with autism. Cognitive differences disappeared by age 54 months, while some differences in receptive and expressive language abilities remained. Most SIBS-A were well-functioning
Pilowsky, Yirmiya, Gross-Tsur, & Shalev [40]	*J. Autism Dev. Disord.*, 2007	Neurocognitive functioning (*i.e.*, intellectual abilities, acquired knowledge and achievement, executive function, attention and distractibility, sequential and simultaneous processing), behavior problems, developmental history, language abilities	30 siblings of children with autism	6–16 years	28 siblings of children with mental retardation, 30 siblings of children with developmental language delay; matched by siblings' chronological age, gender, birth order, probands' gender, and family income	WISC-III, WRAT-III, Tower of Hanoi, CELF-III (Word Associations Test), Rapid Automatic Naming test, Attention Deficit and Hyperactivity Questionnaire, Sequences Test, Visual Perception Test, Child Behavior Checklist, Family History Questionnaire	After excluding from ASD sibling group two siblings diagnosed with PDD, there were no differences between siblings of children with autism and the other groups
Gamliel, Yirmiya, Jaffe, Manor, & Sigman [57]	*J. Autism Dev. Disord.*, 2009	Cognitive and language development–a prospective study	37 siblings of children with ASD (SIBS-A)	4 months–7 years	47 siblings of TD children (SIBS-TD); matched at 4 months on the basis of age, sex, birth order, number of children in the family, sex of the older proband, and temperament profile	BSID-II, K-ABC, RDLS, CELF-P, WISC-III, WRAT-III, CELF-III	At 7 years, 40% of the SIBS-A (and 16% of SIBS-TD) showed cognitive, language and/or academic difficulties (this sub-group was named SIBS-A-BP). Early language scores (14–54 months) were significantly lower in SIBS-A-BP compared to the language scores of SIBS-TD. Language as a major area of difficulty for SIBS-A during the preschool years
Kawakubo *et al.* [58]	*PLoS ONE*, 2009	Verbal fluency	24 siblings of children with ASD	Children (n = 12; M age = 11.1; SD = 3); Adults (n = 12)	27 high functioning individuals with ASD, 27 unrelated healthy controls with no family history of ASD, matched for age and IQ	Letter fluency task	No differences between either the child or the adult group
Koh, Milne, & Dobkins [59]	*Neuropsychologia*, 2010	Motor perception	13 adolescents with siblings diagnosed with ASD	13 years–17 years 11 months	23 adolescents with ASD, 42 TD adolescents, matched for age and gender	Two experiments: "detection task", and the "motion task"	SIBS showed higher chromatic contrast sensitivity than both participants with ASD and TD participants, what authors interpreted as the possible existence of a protective factor in these individuals against developing ASD
Ben-Yizhak *et al.* [60]	*J. Autism Dev. Disord.*, 2011	Pragmatic language, school related linguistic abilities	35 siblings of children with autism (SIBS-A)	9–12 years	42 siblings of TD children; matching criteria at age 4 months: chronological age, sex, birth order, number of children in the family, sex of the older proband, temperament profile, and mental and motor scores	ADOS, SCQ, WISC-III, CELF-III, WRAT-III) Diagnostic Battery for Reading Processes in Hebrew	Lower pragmatic language abilities in a subgroup of SIBS-A identified with BAP-related difficulties. No differences between groups in general linguistic measures, school achievements, and reading processes
Levy and Bar-Yuda [61]	*Autism*, 2011	Language performance	28 siblings of nonverbal children with autism SIBS-ANV	4–9 years	27 controls matched for age, family background, socioeconomic status, and type of school they attended	CELF, spontaneous speech samples	SIBS-ANV achieved lower scores on the Receptive Scale, Expressive Scale and the Total Language Scale of the CELF; differences in the language scores were associated with IQ. No differences between groups in the results of grammatical analysis of spontaneous speech samples

Table 1. *Cont.*

Study	Journal & Year	Characteristics	Sample	Age of Siblings of Individuals with ASD	Control Group, Matching Criteria	Measures/Instruments (Samples)	Main Findings
Sumiyoshi, Kawakubo, Suga, Sumiyoshi, & Kasai [62]	*Neurosci. Res.*, 2011	Ability to organize information, executive function	14 siblings of individuals with ASD	Adults: M age = 24.5; SD = 4.0	22 individuals with ASD, 15 age-matched control subjects	WCST, Verbal Learning Task (VLT), AQ, CARS	No differences between siblings and controls in the WCST and VLT results. Authors noticed that a linear increase of the memory organization score in the VLT was absent in siblings as well as the ASD group. More autistic traits measured by AQ and CARS in siblings than in controls
Fiorentini *et al.* [63]	*Neuropsychologia*, 2012	Face identity	8 siblings (and 20 parents) of ASD children	7 years 11 months–16 years 3 months	10 TD children, (and 20 parents of TD children); matched for age, IQ	Face identity after effect task	Face-coding mechanisms in relatives of ASD individuals similar but less efficient compared to the relatives of typical children
Warren *et al.* [64]	*J. Autism Dev. Disord.*, 2012	Neurocognitive, language, and behavior measures—a prospective study	39 younger siblings of children with ASD (SIBS-ASD)	4 years 2 months–7 years 4 months	22 younger siblings of TD children; matching criteria: gender, chronological age, and SES	Differential Ability Scales—Second Edition, NEPSY-II, CELF-P, Children's Communication Checklist-2 for Parents, ADOS, SRS, CBCL, Social Skills Rating System	Executive functioning composite, Auditory attention, Inhibition–naming–worse in SIBS-ASD compared to controls. No differences in CBCL results
Gerdts, Bernier, Dawson, & Estes [65]	*J. Autism Dev. Disord.*, 2013	Broader autism phenotype traits as measured by Broader Phenotype Autism Symptom Scale	Siblings and parents from 87 multiplex and 41 simplex ASD families	Simplex families: M age = 11.51 (SD = 3.59); Multiplex families: M age = 10.20 (SD = 4.20)	Only members of ASD families	Broader Phenotype Autism Symptom Scale	Siblings from multiplex ASD families revealed less social interest, poorer conversational skills, higher rigidity, and intense interests and were less expressive in the use of nonverbal communication than siblings from simplex ASD families
Malesa *et al.* [66]	*Autism*, 2013	Prospective study–follow-up evaluation at age 5 years	38 from 54 later-born SIBS-ASD, participating in the original study by Yoder *et al.* [67] (see: Table 2)	4–7 years	23 from 31 later-born SIBS-TD, participating in the original study; matching criteria: chronological age, race, and gender	ADOS, ADI-R, CELF-P, CELF-4, Differential Ability Scales-Second Edition (DAS-II), Social Skills Rating System (SSRS)	Two SIBS-ASD received a diagnosis of ASD at follow-up; none of the SIBS-TD received a clinical diagnosis. At age five there were no differences between SIBS-ASD and SIBS-TD in performance on most social and language domains assessed with standardized measures
Oerlemans *et al.* [68]	*J. Autism Dev. Disord.*, 2013	Executive function, social cognition, local processing style	172 siblings of children with ASD	6–21 years	140 Children with ASD, 127 controls; matched on the basis of age and ethnic background	Face recognition task, the Identification of Facial Emotions task, the Prosody task, Go/No-Go task, The Response Organization Objects task, Digit Span task (from Wechsler Scale)	ASD siblings performed worse than controls in face recognition task and inhibition task (but the differences referred only to processing speed)
Pickles, St Clair, & Conti-Ramsden [69]	*J. Autism Dev. Disord.*, 2013	Communication and social deficits	134 siblings (and 193 parents) of probands with ASD	8–42 years	Specific Language Impairment (SLI-only, 79 siblings, 103 parents), SLI + ASD (43 siblings, 30 parents), Down syndrome (DS, 63 siblings, 70 parents), matched on the basis of age and other criteria (not listed precisely)	Family History Information (with modifications)	ASD and SLI siblings had higher levels of communication deficits in relation to DS siblings (especially in the rate of language delay, level of spelling difficulties). More social deficits in ASD relatives in comparison to DS and SLI-only relatives
Robel *et al.* [70]	*Eur. Child Adolesc. Psychiatry*, 2013	Autistic traits	24 siblings of children with autism	M age = 9.4 (SD = 1.82)	96 siblings of TD children, aged three or older, from different socioeconomic backgrounds	French Autism Quotient (two main factors: F1 corresponding to socialization and communication, F2 to imagination and rigidity)	F1 and total AQ score higher in siblings of children with autism and global scores; no differences in F2 scores

Table 1. *Cont.*

Study	Journal & Year	Characteristics	Sample	Age of Siblings of Individuals with ASD	Control Group, Matching Criteria	Measures/Instruments (Samples)	Main Findings
Gizzonio *et al.* [71]	*Exp. Brain Res.*, 2014	Cognitive profile	21 siblings of children with ASD	6–16 years	32 Affected with ASD brothers of participating siblings, 43 TD children; matching criteria not listed precisely	WISC-III, SRS	No significant differences between Verbal Intelligence Quotient and Performance Intelligent Quotient scores among groups. Not significant, predominance of performance over verbal abilities observed in siblings group. Common cognitive profile in ASD group and ASD siblings
Holt *et al.* [22]	*Psychol. Med.*, 2014	Theory of mind	40 full siblings of individuals with autism or AS	12–18 years	50 adolescents with HFA or AS, 40 TD controls; matching criteria: age, full scale IQ above 70	"Reading the Mind in the Eyes" task	No differences between siblings and controls
Oerlemans *et al.* [72]	*Eur. Child Adolesc. Psychiatry*, 2014	Recognition of facial emotion and affective prosody; verbal attention	79 siblings of children with ASD	6–13 years	90 children with ASD (43 with and 47 without ADHD), 139 controls; matched on the basis of age and ethnic background	Facial emotion and affective prosody experimental tasks	Poorer performance of unaffected siblings than controls and better than the ASD probands in recognition of facial emotion and affective prosody tasks

2.1. Comparison Groups

All papers listed in Table 1 included one or more comparison groups. One exception is the paper by Gerdts *et al.* [65], which is listed despite the fact that only ASD families were included in that study. However, the inclusion of multiplex and simplex ASD families provides valuable insight into the severity of BAP traits in families with more than one child with autism.

Analysis of the groups used in comparisons with siblings of individuals with ASD reveals several strategies adopted by researchers. The most commonly-used comparison group consists of healthy siblings of typically developing individuals, or simply typically developing individuals themselves with no family history of autism [48,54,60,63,64,70]. This strategy allows for a comparison of the development of ASD siblings with their typically developing peers from families with no autism.

In many studies, one of the comparison groups was composed of individuals diagnosed with ASD, usually high-functioning autism or Asperger syndrome [22,44,54,55,58,59,62,68,72]. This way, the results of siblings could be compared with those obtained from individuals with ASD, and it was possible to determine whether the instruments used actually identified these deficits. In some of these studies, the results achieved by siblings of individuals with ASD landed in the middle, between the scores of individuals with ASD and those achieved by typically developing controls *i.e.*, [62,71]. This could indicate qualitatively similar traits or behavioral profiles of siblings and individuals with ASD, although the results of siblings are closer to the developmental norm. Some studies evaluated affected and unaffected siblings from the same family, *i.e.*, [71]. This empirical approach has particular merit in light of the fact that siblings share on average 50% of genes with their affected brother or sister [68]. Verifying similarities between siblings in terms of autistic traits may offer new insights into genetic susceptibility to autism.

In several studies, typically older ones, the comparison group for siblings of individuals with ASD was composed of siblings of individuals with Down syndrome, *i.e.*, [14,45–47,69]. This was to control for the effects of a family member with a hereditary disability not associated with ASD on the development and functioning of siblings. Recently, however, the focus has been on the comorbidity of Autism Spectrum Disorders and Down syndrome. Lowenthal *et al.* [73] showed that the frequency of Pervasive Developmental Disorders in individuals with Down syndrome was 15.6%, including 5.58% for autism. These findings must be taken into account in the selection of siblings of individuals with Down syndrome for the group compared with the siblings of ASD individuals. The presence and severity of autistic traits and symptoms in probands with Down syndrome must also be controlled for. With the high incidence of ASD (see [74]), this should be a universally-observed principle applied in the selection of comparison groups in studies on BAP, not limited to Down syndrome participants.

In some research projects, comparison groups consisted of siblings of individuals with developmental delay [48], mental retardation of unknown etiology [40,51], or psychopathology unrelated to autism, such as ADHD, affective disorders, and anxiety disorders [6]. There is also an interesting group of studies that included siblings of children with such developmental problems as dyslexia [49,50] and specific language impairment [69]. Extensive research has recently been done on potential associations between these complex developmental disorders and autism as, similarly to autism, their incidence is greater in males, they involve a number of neurophysiological and neuroanatomical abnormalities, they are likely to have strong genetic components, and they encompass language and communication deficits [75,76].

There is no question that the type of comparison groups should be taken into consideration when interpreting results and forming generalizations regarding the presence or absence of specificity in the functioning of siblings of individuals with ASD. In the case of heritable conditions that share features with ASD (e.g., SLI), it is possible that the first-degree relatives of probands will present some characteristics that overlap with the BAP [23]. This may cause additional difficulties in comparisons and the isolation of the autism phenotype.

2.2. Participants' Age and Sample Size

In the majority of studies listed in Table 1, the participants' functioning was measured only once. The exceptions are two longitudinal studies by Gamliel and colleagues [56,57] that include children aged 4 months to 4.6 and 7 years, and studies by Warren *et al.* [64] and Malesa *et al.* [66], which were a continuation of a study by Yoder *et al.* [67]. As these studies provide information about preschool and school-age children, we decided to include them in Table 1. There is only one other study [39] in which participants were under 4 years of age. In all other works the siblings of individuals with ASD were aged 4 or older, and in a number of them the age range was quite large. In some papers it exceeded 10 years, *i.e.*, [44,49,55], and could be as high as 40 years, *i.e.*, [47,69].

The age of siblings at the time of the study is not always crucial; in designs where caregivers were asked to provide information on the child's development history, that variable is less significant *i.e.*, [46,69]. However, in those studies that measure developmental levels across various domains or mastery of specific functions, a wide age range of participants may compromise the precision of inferences. It also cannot capture any developmental delays or irregularities that may be present during a certain period. However, knowledge of the specifics of that aspect of development could help in planning support for children in ASD families. A wide sibling age range makes it difficult to determine the level of that group's functioning, especially when coupled with a small sample size, which precludes statistical analysis on subgroups more homogenous in terms of age. In some studies the ASD siblings group counted under 20 participants *i.e.*, [14,44,49,50,55,59,62,63]. There is, however, a clear trend towards increased sample size in more recent studies, *i.e.*, [68,69]. In turn, small groups tend to be more homogenous, including in respect of participants' age. One illustration is the study by Warren *et al.* [64], which enrolled 40 siblings aged 4 to 7; another comes from research on preschool and early school children aged 2 to 9 years *i.e.*, [39,61]. Ben-Yizhak *et al.* [60] assessed older children in a narrow age range from 9 to 12 years, while Koh *et al.* [59] and Holt *et al.* [22] evaluated adolescents aged 12–18. Nevertheless, the majority of studies are conducted on children and adolescents with wider age ranges: from 6–8 to 16–18 years, *i.e.*, [6,40,54,71].

As we have previously mentioned, research on siblings who are of preschool age, or on older children and adolescents, suffers from a lack of longitudinal studies. In one of a handful of reports that provide such information, Gamliel *et al.* [56] stated that cognitive deficits originally present in siblings of children with ASD disappeared during the preschool period (age: 54 months), but—compared to controls—some differences in terms of receptive and expressive language abilities remained. The results indicating differences in language development were confirmed in the next phase of the study, conducted when the children reached 7 years of age. Data of that sort is particularly relevant for understanding the specifics of developmental processes in children from ASD-affected families. While not meeting the diagnostic criteria for the disorder, these children may experience difficulties due to atypical development. Some of these difficulties are resolved, but there are some that may compromise their adjustment at a given moment in life. Thus, longitudinal studies that enable us to follow developmental processes, as well as to identify their determinants and effective methods of developmental support, are particularly valuable.

2.3. Functioning Characteristics of Interest

The studies listed in Table 1 cover a wide variety of characteristics. In some, non-affected siblings were assessed for autism symptomatology with instruments used in diagnosis (Autism Diagnostic Observation Schedule, ADOS [77] or Autism Diagnostic Interview-Revised, ADI-R [78]) or based on developmental history established from medical history or interviews other than ADI-R *i.e.*, [14,28,69]. The results of these studies suggest a greater incidence of deficits in at least one domain typical for ASD. However, their results are not fully consistent in terms of the domains affected by the deficits and the depth of the deficits in question.

Greater severity of autistic traits in the siblings of individuals with ASD compared to controls was shown in those studies that measured such traits using the Social Communication Questionnaire (SCQ [79]), Childhood Autism Rating Scale (CARS [80]), Autism Spectrum Quotient (AQ [8]) and Broader Phenotype Autism Symptom Scale (BPASS [32]) [6,62,65,79]. Another finding was that autistic traits, including less social interest, poorer conversational skills, higher rigidity, and intense interests, as well as less expressiveness in the use of nonverbal communication, are more pronounced in siblings from multiplex ASD families than in children from simplex ASD families [65]. Based on similar results obtained for social and communication domains of BAP in parents, Bernier *et al.* [81] concluded that different genetic transfer mechanisms may operate in families with one and families with several children with autism displaying many of these characteristics. It has been suggested that *de novo* mutations and non-inherited copy number variants may be particularly important risk factors in simplex ASD families, while in multiplex ASD families they are present to a much lesser degree [82]. However, this finding was not confirmed in all studies [83]. As noted by Spiker and colleagues [84], the variability of autistic phenotype expressed in multiplex families is relatively low. In their study on families with two or more children with autism, in 37 out of 44 participating families at least two children met the ADI diagnostic criteria. Out of all the children in these families, 71% met all of the criteria for autism diagnosis in ADI, 22% failed to meet any of the criteria, and 7% met one or more criteria without reaching all of the ADI cutpoints. The number of items classified as "uncertain" was small, and there was a clear-cut distinction between children affected and unaffected by autism. It should also be noted that studies involving siblings from simplex ASD families, siblings from multiplex ASD families, and controls are scarce. This reduces the possibility of identifying the scope of the differences between the three groups with respect to the BAP.

A substantial body of research into the functioning of ASD siblings concerns language and communication as part of the phenotype(s) of ASD. Findings vary, as do methods and instruments. In their grammatical analysis of spontaneous speech samples, Levy and Bar-Yuda [61] found no significant differences between ASD siblings and preschool controls. In some studies ASD siblings were found to be more likely to have language delays relative to their comparison groups [39,56,57], while in other papers such differences were not stated, *i.e.*, [45]. A frequently encountered pattern of results is one in which the group of ASD siblings as a whole does not differ from controls, but a subgroup may be distinguished that demonstrates more pronounced BAP traits, including inferior language development, *i.e.*, [39,60]. Interesting data comes from comparisons of ASD siblings with siblings of individuals with language disorders. Some researchers found less severe difficulties in language and communication in siblings of individuals with ASD than siblings of people with language disorders, *i.e.*, [51], while others demonstrated that ASD siblings, similar to specific language impairment siblings, demonstrate higher levels of communication deficits in relation to siblings of individuals with Down syndrome [69].

A number of studies analyzed siblings' intellectual abilities [44,46,47,51,71]. This is an important issue since intellectual disability (ID) and autism are highly co-morbid [85]. It is estimated that ID is present in 50%–70% of all ASD cases [85]. Precise estimation of the co-morbidity of ASD and ID is complicated due to changing criteria, diagnostic procedures, and educational policy (e.g., providing more support to certain groups of pupils) as well as the methodological problems (screening tools properties) [86]. Nevertheless, it has been shown that the number of high-functioning individuals with ASD diagnosis has increased in recent years (see [74]). It is also noteworthy that IQ may be underestimated in people with high levels of autistic traits [87]. However, the interrelationships among the level of autistic traits and intellectual abilities are still far from being fully recognized, and the results of studies on IQ in siblings of individuals with ASD are equally difficult to generalize. In some of them, no differences were found between ASD siblings and controls in terms of IQ levels (e.g., [40,44,47]), while Fombonne *et al.* [46] and Pilowsky *et al.* [51] reported even higher verbal IQ in ASD siblings. Gizzonio *et al.* [71] found no differences between ASD siblings and controls in terms of Verbal IQ and Performance IQ, but reported a slight (non-significant) predominance of performance over verbal abilities. As the authors have suggested, this could indicate the presence of a certain cognitive profile common for individuals with ASD and their siblings, but statistically non-significant differences make this a very tentative conclusion. Fombonne *et al.* [46] identified a subgroup of participants who demonstrated BAP traits (referred to as BAP+) and had significantly lower IQ scores than the group of siblings non-affected with BAP. Similar results were reported by Chuthapisith *et al.* [39].

There have been numerous studies on autism-specific cognitive deficits: in theory of mind, central coherence, and executive function. Research on theory of mind, recognition of facial emotions, and face processing indicate that they are less developed in siblings of individuals with ASD compared to controls, *i.e.*, [55,63,68,72]. By contrast, the results of a study using the "Reading the Mind in the Eyes" task were inconclusive. Dorris *et al.* [52] showed that siblings scored lower than controls, but Holt *et al.* [22] found no differences between adolescent ASD siblings and typically developing control adolescents. Similarly, no differences in theory of mind between siblings and controls were reported by Ozonoff [44]. The key in studies of this type is to take into account the age of participating siblings, which is often overlooked. It is also noteworthy that this area of study is still strongly affected by a lack of precise conceptual definitions and methodological scrutiny, which makes the discussion even more complex. It must be noted that the results of studies on deficits discussed above in individuals with ASD are mixed, and are far from conclusive. A detailed discussion of the definitional controversies relating to particular aspects of cognitive deficits typical for ASD, as well as a presentation of current opinion concerning theory of mind, emotion recognition, central coherence, and executive function in people with ASD, remain outside the scope of this paper.

A complex picture also emerges from research on executive function. Siblings of individuals with ASD were found to be no different from controls in terms of inhibitory control and processing speed [54], but performed worse in planning tasks [44,48]. Ozonoff and colleagues [44] found no differences in working memory and set-shifting, while Hughes *et al.* [48] concluded that a larger than expected proportion of siblings of individuals with autism demonstrated difficulties in set-shifting. In the study conducted by Pilowsky *et al.* [40], differences in executive function between ASD siblings and controls disappeared once two participants diagnosed with Pervasive Developmental Disorders were removed from the former group. It should be also mentioned that Happe, Briskman, and Frith [50] reported no differences in terms of weak central coherence. In recent years the field of research on siblings of individuals diagnosed with ASD has been dominated by studies focused on infants at high familial risk for ASD (see [35]). It is estimated that about 10%–20% of high-risk infants can be affected with subclinical ASD traits or other developmental problems [88]. It should be emphasized that the analyses in some of the studies on infants also included children who later received an ASD diagnosis, which is why these results should be approached with caution. Nevertheless, research on infant siblings of children with ASD can not only provide us with valuable information on early signs of autism, but also pave the way for investigation of BAP traits [35].

3. Research on High-Risk Infants

Most studies focus on infant siblings of older children diagnosed with ASD, aged from 4 to 24 or 36 months. Diagnosis of the ASD proband is usually confirmed with ADOS and ADI-R outcomes, and the age of the proband is not relevant. Infant siblings are usually participants in long-lasting longitudinal studies in which different aspects of infants' functioning are assessed, *i.e.*, [56,77,89]. The control groups mainly consist of typically developing infants without familial risk for ASD. Some research projects perform comparison analyses between high-risk infants (HR, siblings of older children diagnosed with ASD) and low-risk infants (LR, infants without familial risk for ASD) [90–94], while others strive for interpretation of infants' functioning and test performance in the context of later ASD diagnoses or BAP characteristics [30,95–98]. Many studies differ in the sizes of HR and LR infant samples involved in analysis (*i.e.*, nine HR infants in [99] to 507 HR infants in [88]), making interpretation and comparison of results problematic.

A number of research projects on infant siblings are focused on early characteristics of ASD core symptoms, as well as overall risk for developing ASD, *i.e.*, [88,94,100–102]. Macari *et al.* [101] suggest that two thirds of infants at high risk for ASD experience some kind of developmental difficulties in the second year of life. A large study conducted by Messinger *et al.* [88] indicated elevated levels of autistic traits (higher mean ADOS severity scores) in HR infants compared to LR infants. Georgiades *et al.* [100] suggested that significantly more HR infants had exhibited higher levels of autistic-like traits than LR children, and at the age of three years these children had more social communication impairments, lower cognitive abilities, and more internalizing problems than typically developing children.

As shown in Table 2, many authors report early communication and language deficits [56,89,90,94, 96,102–104], social interaction impairments [91,94,97,98,105–107], and increased levels of stereotyped behaviors [108–110] in HR infant siblings.

It should be noted that the emergence of some of the highlighted differences are probably caused by inclusion in analyses of high-risk infant siblings who later developed ASD. For instance, Rozga *et al.* [97] ascertained that high-risk infant siblings who later developed ASD exhibited lower rates of joint attention and requesting behavior than typically developing children. However, HR infant siblings without ASD outcomes did not differ in these characteristics from the control infants. Similarly, Bedford *et al.* [111] indicated that only the high-risk infants with later emerging socio-communication difficulties (ASD and atypical development) differed significantly from the control group in the gaze following task. What is more, high-risk infants without ASD outcome performed similarly to typically developing infants. Hutman *et al.* [95] also suggest social impairments only in the high-risk infants with later ASD diagnosis. Hudry *et al.* [104] observed reduced receptive vocabulary advantage in all HR infants by 14 months, but this difference was maintained through 24 months only in children with ASD outcome, while typically developing HR infants regained a more normative profile.

Some empirical data suggest the presence of deficits in quality of mother–infant interaction and differences in responses to separation events in high-risk infant siblings. For instance, Esposito *et al.* [112] found differences in cry sample patterns in HR toddlers compared to LR toddlers in expression of distress during the separation phase. However, Haltigan *et al.* [113] concluded that HR infants are not less likely to form secure affectional bonds with their caregivers than LR infants, but also mentioned that infant siblings of children with ASD are less distressed during separation and more reserved after reunion with a caregiver compared to typically developing children. Finally, a study conducted by Wan *et al.* [114] indicated that infant attentiveness to parent and positive affect were lower in the high-risk group later diagnosed with ASD. These characteristics, as well as dyadic mutuality, predicted a three-year ASD outcome.

A number of studies analyzed face processing and social visual fixation patterns as predictors of autistic traits in infants. Some HR siblings demonstrated diminished gaze to the mother's eyes relative to her mouth in the Still Face episode [93]. During the face processing task, LR infants demonstrated a preference for looking at the left side of the face (characteristic left visual field bias) that emerged by 11 months of age and was absent in HR infants at any age [115]. Hutman *et al.* [95] observed no difference in the proportion of attention to social stimuli or attention shifting during the play condition between HR and LR infants. However, children later diagnosed with ASD tended to continue looking at a toy during the distress condition despite the salience of social information. Overall, no group differences between HR and LR infants in gaze following behavior at either age was observed in the study by Bedford *et al.* [111]. Nevertheless, it should be noted that HR infants with later emerging socio-communication difficulties (ASD and atypical development) allocated less attention to a congruent object compared to typically developing HR siblings and LR controls.

Table 2. Studies on infants and toddlers at risk for ASD.

Study	Journal & Year	Characteristics	Sample	Age of Siblings of Individuals with ASD	Control Group, Matching Criteria	Measures/Instruments (Samples)	Main Findings
Goldberg *et al.* [105]	*J. Autism Dev. Disord.*, 2005	Social communication behaviors	8 children diagnosed with ASD; 8 younger siblings of children with ASD	Below 3 years old	9 TD children, age and IQ controlled	ADI-R, ADOS-G, CARS, Early Social Communication Scales (ESCS)	On three of four of the ESCS subscales (Responds to Social Interaction, Initiates of Joint Attention, and Requesting Behaviors) social communicative behaviors of younger siblings differed from those of typically developing children but not from the behaviors displayed by ASD group
Zwaigenbaum *et al.* [102]	*Int. J. Dev. Neurosci.*, 2005	Autistic traits, autism-specific behavior	65 siblings of children with ASD	6 to 24 months	75 low risk infants, gender-, birth-order, and age-matched to high-risk infants	Novel observational scale a computerized visual orienting task, and standardized measures of temperament, cognitive and language development	Lower receptive language scores and use of fewer gestures and phrases at 24 months in non-autistic siblings. By 12 months of age, siblings who are later diagnosed with autism may be distinguished from other siblings and low-risk controls on the basis of: (1) behavioral markers, including atypicalities in eye contact or visual tracking; (2) prolonged latency to disengage visual attention; (3) a characteristic pattern of early temperament, with marked passivity and decreased activity level at six months; and (4) delayed expressive and receptive language
Landa and Garrett-Mayer [30]	*J. Child Psychol. Psychiatry*, 2006	Autistic traits, autism-specific behavior	60 HR infants (siblings of children with autism, SIBS-A) and 27 LR infants (no family history of autism), at 24 months of age categorized as: unaffected, ASD, or language delayed (LD)	6–24 months	27 low risk infants (no family history of autism), age, ethnic group, and SES were controlled	Language test scores, ADOS, MSEL	Lower scores on all MSEL scales in SIB-A at 14 months, compared to LD and TD children. By 14 months of age, the ASD group performed significantly worse than the unaffected group on all scales except Visual Reception. By 24 months of age, the ASD group performed significantly worse than the unaffected group in all domains, and worse than the language delayed group in Gross Motor, Fine Motor, and Receptive Language
Mitchell *et al.* [96]	*J. Dev. Behav. Pediatr.*, 2006	Early language and communication development	97 SIBS-A (then part of them diagnosed with ASD)	12 to 24 months	49 control children, recruited from three regions in numbers roughly proportionate to each region's high-risk siblings	MacArthur Communicative Development Inventory (CDI), Preschool Language Scale—Third Edition, MSEL	Children with ASD showed delays in early language and communication compared with non-ASD siblings and controls. At 12 months, the ASD group was reported to understand significantly fewer phrases and to produce fewer gestures. At 18 months, they showed delays in their understanding of phrases, comprehension and production of single words, and use of gestures. Siblings not diagnosed with ASD also used fewer play-related gestures at 18 months than low-risk controls, even when children with identified language delays were excluded
Yirmiya *et al.* [90]	*J. Child Psychol. Psychiatry*, 2006	Social engagement, communication, and cognition	21 SIBS-A	4–14 months	21 TD infants, age-matched	Bayley Scales of Infant Development–2nd edition, Infant Characteristics Questionnaire (ICQ), Still-face paradigm, Name-calling responsiveness, Early Social Communication Scales (ESCS), Checklist for Autism in Toddlers (CHAT)	At 14 months, SIBS-A made fewer nonverbal requesting gestures and achieved lower language scores on the Bayley Scale. Infant SIBS-A, who showed more neutral affect to the still face and were less able to respond to their name being called by their mothers, initiated fewer nonverbal joint attention and requesting behaviors at 14 months, respectively

Table 2. *Cont.*

Study	Journal &Year	Characteristics	Sample	Age of Siblings of Individuals with ASD	Control Group, Matching Criteria	Measures/Instruments (Samples)	Main Findings
Bryson *et al.* [99]	*J. Autism Dev. Disord.*, 2007	Autistic traits, IQ	9 HR infants with older siblings with ASD, all of them diagnosed with ASD at 36 months	6–24 months, assessment every 6 months	Developmental study, no control group	ADOS, Bayley Scales of Infant Development, 2nd ed. or MSEL, CDI-Words and Gestures, Infant Temperament Scale or Toddler Behavior Assessment Questionnaire	Two groups were identified: 1st subgroup ($n = 6$) showed a decrease in IQ between 12 and 24 or 36 months; 2nd subgroup ($n = 3$) continued to obtain average IQs. Signs of autism emerged and/or were more striking earlier in the 1st group ($n = 6$). In all children early impairment in social-communicative development coexisted with atypical sensory and/or motor behaviors and temperamental profile marked by irritability/distress and dysregulated state
Cassel *et al.* [91]	*J. Autism Dev. Disord.*, 2007	Social and emotional communication	12 infant siblings of children with autism	6–18 months	19 age-matched TD control children	Face-to-face/still-face (FFSF), Early Social Communication Scale (ESCS)	Siblings smiled for a lower proportion of the FFSF than TD and lacked emotional continuity between episodes. Siblings engaged in lower rates of initiating joint attention at 15 months, lower rates of higher-level behavioral requests at 12 months, and responded to fewer joint attention bids at 18 months. Infant siblings experience subtle, inconsistent, but multi-faceted deficits in emotional expression and referential communication
Iverson *et al.* [92]	*J. Autism Dev. Disord.*, 2007	Vocal-motor development	21 infant siblings of children with autism	5–18 months	18 TD control children, maternal and parental age and levels of parental education comparable in sample and control group	Videotaping: naturalistic observation, semi-structured play, play in a Johnny Jump-Up, face-to-face interaction, and play with toys; MacArthur–Bates Communicative Development Inventory; Pervasive Developmental Disorder Screening Test-II	Infant siblings were delayed in the onset of early developmental milestones and spent significantly less time in a greater number of postures, suggestive of relative postural instability. Infant siblings demonstrated attenuated patterns of change in rhythmic arm activity around the time of reduplicated babble onset; and were highly likely to exhibit delayed language development at 18 months
Loh *et al.* [108]	*J. Autism Dev. Disord.*, 2007	Stereotyped motor behaviors	8 infant siblings of children with autism later diagnosed with ASD, 9 infant siblings of children with autism not diagnosed with ASD	12 and 18 months	15 TD control children, same geographic area as the sibling sample and age-matched to the high-risk infants	Measurement of Repetitive Motor Behaviors, videotaping	At 12 and 18 months the ASD group "arm waved" more frequently and at 18 months, one posture ("hands to ears") was more frequently observed in the ASD and non-diagnosed group compared to the TD
Merin *et al.* [93]	*J. Autism Dev. Disord.*, 2007	Visual fixation patterns during reciprocal social interaction	31 infant siblings of children with autism	6 months	24 Comparison infants with no autism family history, age and gender controlled	Modified Still Face paradigm, Eye tracking	Eleven infants demonstrated diminished gaze to the mother's eyes relative to her mouth during the Still Face episode; 10 of them had an older sibling with ASD
Stone *et al.* [103]	*Arch. Pediatr. Adolesc. Med.*, 2007	Communicative and cognitive development	64 siblings of children with ASD (SIBS-A)	12–23 months	42 control children with no autism family history, no matching criteria except for age range	MSEL, CARS, Screening Tool for Autism in Two-Year-Olds (STAT), MacArthur Communicative Development Inventories, Detection of Autism by Infant Sociability Interview	Younger siblings of children with ASD demonstrated poorer performance in nonverbal problem solving, directing attention, understanding words, understanding phrases, gesture use, and social-communicative interactions with parents, and had increased autism symptoms relative to control siblings

Table 2. *Cont.*

Study	Journal & Year	Characteristics	Sample	Age of Siblings of Individuals with ASD	Control Group, Matching Criteria	Measures/Instruments (Samples)	Main Findings
Sullivan *et al.* [98]	*J. Autism Dev. Disord.*, 2007	Response to joint attention	51 infant siblings of children with autism; Outcome groups at age 3 years: 16 ASD, 8 broader autism phenotype, and 27 non-broader autism phenotype	14 and 24 months	Developmental study, no control group	Adaptation of a task described by Butterworth and Jarrett (1991) to assess response to joint attention; the Communication and Symbolic Behavior Scales Developmental Profile, MSEL, ADOS	Lower response to joint attention was observed for the ASD group at 24 months. Response to joint attention performance at 14 months predicted ASD outcome. The ASD group made minimal improvement in response to joint attention between 14 and 24 months
Toth *et al.* [94]	*J. Autism Dev. Disord.*, 2007	Social, imitation, play and language abilities	42 non-autistic siblings of children with autism 20 toddlers with no family history of autism	18–27 months	20 toddlers with no family history of autism, controlled for age and ethnic group	MSEL, The Vineland Social-Emotional Early Childhood Scales, The Communication and Symbolic Behavior Scale-Developmental Profile, Imitation battery developed by Meltzoff, The Play Assessment Scale, The Early Development Interview	Siblings scored poorer in Receptive language scale (MSEL), Daily living skills, Motor and Composite (Vineland)
Yirmiya *et al.* [89]	*J. Autism Dev. Disord.*, 2007	Cognitive and language profile —a prospective study	30 siblings of children with autism (SIBS-A)	24–36 months	30 siblings of typically developing children (SIBS-TD); matched on the basis of chronological age, gender, birth order, scores on mental and psychomotor indices, temperamental characteristics and number of children in the family	BSID-II, RDLS, CHAT, K-ABC, CELF-P, The Social and Communication Questionnaire (SCQ)	At 24 months: more SIBS-A demonstrated language scores one or two standard deviations below the mean compared to SIBS-TD. At 36 months: more SIBS-A displayed receptive and expressive difficulties compared to SIBS-TD. Six SIBS-A (including one diagnosed with autism) revealed language scores more than two standard deviations below the mean at both ages, a pattern not seen in the SIBS-TD
Garon *et al.* [116]	*J. Abnorm. Child Psychol.*, 2009	Temperamental traits	138 HR infants with an older sibling with autistic spectrum disorder	6–36 months	73 low risk infants with no family history of ASD, no matching criteria listed except for age range	Toddler Behavior Assessment Questionnaire-Revised, MSEL, ADOS, ADI R	HR children, who were diagnosed with ASD at 36 months, had temperament profile marked by lower positive affect, higher negative affect, and difficulty controlling attention and behavior (labelled as Effortful Emotion Regulation). This temperamental profile distinguished also HR children without ASD diagnosis at 36 months from LR children
Yoder *et al.* [67]	*J. Autism Dev. Disord.*, 2009	Social impairment and ASD diagnosis	43 siblings of children with autism (SIBS-ASD)	15–34 months	24 SIBS-TD, matched on the basis of child's age and maternal education	MSEL, STAT, Responding to Joint Attention (RJA), Social Behavior Checklist (SBC), ADOS, ADI-R	Initial level of responding to joint attention and growth rate of weighted triadic communication predicted the degree of social impairment at the final measurement period of SIBS-ASD. Both predictors were associated with later ASD diagnosis, contrary to unweighted triadic communication, age of entry into the study, and initial language level, which did not predict later social impairment
Christensen *et al.* [117]	*J. Autism Dev. Disord.*, 2010	Play behaviors	17 ASD siblings later diagnosed with ASD, infant siblings of children with autism with and without other delays (Other Delays and No Delays siblings; $n = 12$ and $n = 19$, respectively)	18 months	19 TD children, no matching criteria listed except for age range	Free-play task: functional, symbolic, and repeated play actions	ASD siblings showed fewer functional and more non-functional repeated play behaviors than TD children. Other Delays siblings showed more non-functional repeated play than TD controls. Group differences disappeared with the inclusion of verbal mental age

Table 2. *Cont.*

Study	Journal &Year	Characteristics	Sample	Age of Siblings of Individuals with ASD	Control Group, Matching Criteria	Measures/Instruments (Samples)	Main Findings
Holmboe *et al.* [109]	*Infant Behav. Dev.*, 2010	Executive functions, attention and inhibition, frontal cortex functioning	31 SIBS-ASD	9–10 months	33 typically developing children with no family history of autism, no matching criteria listed except for age range	Freeze-Frame task	SIBS-ASD had difficulty disengaging attention and showed less selective inhibition than controls (less difference between interesting and boring trials); however, they demonstrated selective inhibitory learning (tendency to show a larger decrease in looks to the distractors in the interesting trials than in the boring trials, whereas controls showed a similar decrease in the two trial type)
Haltigan *et al.* [113]	*J. Autism Dev. Disord.*, 2011	Attachment security	51 infant siblings of older children with ASD (SIBS-ASD)	15 months	34 typically developing children with no family history of autism (SIBS-COMP); no matching criteria listed except for age range	Strange Situation Procedure (SSP)	SIBS-ASD are not less likely to form secure affectional bonds with their caregivers than SIBS-COMP. Larger rate of B1–B2 secure subclassifications in SIBS-ASD than controls (B1–B2 infants are less distressed during separation and are more reserved after reunion with caregiver)
Ozonoff *et al.* [31]	*Pediatrics*, 2011	Recurrence risk for ASD	664 infants with an older sibling with ASD	18–36 months	No control group, developmental study	ADOS, MSEL	18.7% of the infants developed ASD. Infant gender (threefold increase in risk for male subjects) and the presence of 1 affected older sibling (twofold increase in risk) were significant predictors of ASD outcome
Paul *et al.* [118]	*J. Child Psychol. Psychiatry*, 2011	Vocal production	At 6 months: 28 high-risk (HR) infants; at 9 months: 37 HR infants; at 12 months: 38 HR infants; at 24 months: 24 HR infants	6–24 months	At 6 months: 20 low-risk (LR) infants; at 9 months: 29 LR infants; at 12 months: 31 LR infants; at 24 months: 21 LR infants; no matching criteria listed except for age range	ADOS, MSEL, Vocalization Sample Collection	Differences were seen between risk groups for certain vocal behaviors. Differences in vocal production in the first year of life were associated with outcomes in terms of autistic symptomatology in the second year
Rozga *et al.* [97]	*J. Autism Dev. Disord.*, 2011	Mother–infant interaction and nonverbal communication, social gaze, affect, and joint attention behaviors	17 infant siblings of older children with ASD, later diagnosed with autism; 84 infant siblings of older children with ASD without ASD diagnosis (NoASD-sib)	6–36 months	66 TD children, no matching criteria listed except for age range	Free Play Mother–Infant Interaction, Still Face Procedure, ESCS	The ASD group did not differ from the other two groups at six months in the frequency of gaze, smiles and vocalizations directed toward the caregiver, nor in their sensitivity to her withdrawal from interaction. By 12 months, infants in the ASD group exhibited lower rates of joint attention and requesting behaviors. NoASD-sibs did not differ from comparison infants on any variables of interest at 6 and 12 months
Bedford *et al.* [111]	*J. Autism Dev. Disord.*, 2012	Social gaze, communication and attentional engagement	54 HR infants	7 and 13 months	50 LR infants, no matching criteria listed except for age range	Eye-tracking	No group difference between high-risk and low-risk infants in gaze-following behavior at either age. At-risk infants with later emerging socio- communication difficulties (ASD and atypical development) allocated less attention to the congruent object compared to typically developing high-risk siblings and low-risk controls

Table 2. *Cont.*

Study	Journal & Year	Characteristics	Sample	Age of Siblings of Individuals with ASD	Control Group, Matching Criteria	Measures/Instruments (Samples)	Main Findings
Cornew *et al.* [119]	*J. Autism Dev. Disord.*, 2012	Social referencing	38 HR infants	17.7–20.6 months	44 LR infants; LR and HR groups controlled for equality of mean age and infants' maturity at birth	Social referencing procedure	Compared to both typically developing infants and high-risk infants without ASD, infants later diagnosed with ASD engaged in slower information seeking. High-risk infants, both those who were and those who were not later diagnosed with ASD, exhibited impairments in regulating their behavior based on the adults' emotional signals
Dundas *et al.* [115]	*J. Autism Dev. Disord.*, 2012	Face processing	43 HR infants	6 and 11 months	31 LR infants; gender, ethnicity, and age of infants in LR and HR groups described	Eye-tracking	Low-risk infants demonstrated a preference for looking at the left side of the face, which emerged by 11 months of age. High-risk infants did not demonstrate a left visual field bias at either age
Hutman *et al.* [95]	*J. Autism Dev. Disord.*, 2012	Social interactions, selective visual attention	81 HR infants; Outcome groups: 15 ASD; 12 Other Concerns; 59 High-Risk Typical; and 43 Low-Risk Typical	12 months	48 LR infants, no matching criteria listed except for age range	Examiner–Child Interaction, play, and distress condition	No difference in proportion of attention to social stimuli or attention shifting during the play condition between groups. Infants later diagnosed with ASD tended to continue looking at a toy during the distress condition despite the salience of social information. Emotion recognition is intact in infants who later develop autism, but the emotional value of the information appears to be less salient
Macari *et al.* [101]	*J. Autism Dev. Disord.*, 2012	Risk for ASD	53 HR infants	12, 18 and 24 months	31 LR infants; no matching criteria listed except for age range	MSEL, ADOS-Toddler	About 2/3 of infants at high risk for ASD experience some kind of developmental difficulties in the second year of life
Curtin &Vouloumanos [120]	*J. Autism Dev. Disord.*, 2013	Speech preference	31 HR infants	12–18 months	31 LR infants; no matching criteria listed except for age range	Speech/Non-Speech task, MSEL, MacArthur–Bates Communicative Development Inventories	Only low-risk infants listened significantly longer to speech than to non-speech at 12 months. In both groups, relative preference for speech correlated positively with general cognitive ability at 12 months. However, in high-risk infants only, preference for speech was associated with autistic-like behavior at 18 months, while in low-risk infants, preference for speech correlated with language abilities
Damiano *et al.* [110]	*J. Autism Dev. Disord.*, 2013	Repetitive and stereotyped movements	20 HR infants (SIBS-ASD)	15–24 months	20 typically developing siblings (SIBS-TD), differences in maternal educational between HR and LR groups were noted	STAT, Repetitive and Stereotyped Movement Scales (RSMS)	SIBS-ASD displayed higher rates of repetitive and stereotyped movements (RSM) relative to SIBS-TD; SIBS-ASD as a group demonstrated a significantly higher inventory of RSMs than controls, but this difference was no longer significant after excluding subgroup of ASD diagnosed SIBS-ASD. Different patterns for Object vs. Body RSM inventory for the high-risk groups with different diagnostic outcomes (Sibs-ASD/+ *vs.* Sibs-ASD/−)

Table 2. *Cont.*

Study	Journal & Year	Characteristics	Sample	Age of Siblings of Individuals with ASD	Control Group, Matching Criteria	Measures/Instruments (Samples)	Main Findings
Georgiades *et al.* [100]	*JAMA Psychiatry*, 2013	Autistic-like traits	170 HR infants	12 months	90 LR control subjects with no family history of ASD; no matching criteria listed except for age range	The Autism Observation Scale for Infants	Cluster 1 (*n* = 37), having significantly higher levels of autistic-like traits, consisted of 33 children from the siblings and only four from the control subjects. At the age of three, children from cluster 1 had more social-communication impairments, lower cognitive abilities, and more internalizing problems. Nineteen percent of HR siblings who did not meet ASD diagnostic criteria at the age of three showed autistic-like traits resembling a BAP by 12 months
Messinger *et al.* [88]	*J. Am. Acad. Child Adolesc. Psychiatry*, 2013	ASD risk, autistic traits	507 HR siblings	8–36 months	324 LR control subjects, no matching criteria listed except for age range	ADOS calibrated severity scores, and Mullen Verbal and Non-Verbal Developmental Quotients (DQ)	At three years, HR siblings without an ASD outcome exhibited higher mean ADOS severity scores and lower verbal and non-verbal DQs than LR controls. HR siblings were over-represented (21% HR vs. 7% LR) in latent classes characterized by elevated ADOS severity and/or low to low-average DQs. The remaining HR siblings without ASD outcomes (79%) belonged to classes in which they were not differentially represented with respect to LR siblings
Wan *et al.* [114]	*J. Child Psychol. Psychiatry*, 2013	Quality of interaction	At 6–10 months: 45 HR infants; at 12–15 months: 43 HR siblings	6–10 and 12–15 months	At 6–10 months: 47 LR siblings; at 12–15 months: 48 LR siblings; no matching criteria listed except for age range	Six-min videotaped episodes of parent-infant free play; Manchester Assessment of Caregiver-Infant Interaction (MACI)	At six months, infant liveliness was lower in the at-risk groups; at 12 months, infant attentiveness to parent and positive affect were lower in the at-risk group later diagnosed with ASD. Dyadic mutuality, infant positive affect and infant attentiveness to parent at 12 months predicted three-year ASD outcome, whereas infant ASD-related behavioral atypicality did not
Del Rosario *et al.* [121]	*J. Autism Dev. Disord.*, 2014	Temperament trajectories	16 HR infants who were later diagnosed with ASD (SIBS-ASD), 27 HR infants who demonstrated typical patterns of development (SIBS-HR-TD)	6–36 months	No control group	Carey Temperament Scales completed by parents, MSEL	Temperament trajectories of children with ASD reflected increases over time in activity level, and decreasing adaptability and approach behaviors relative to high-risk typically developing (HR-TD) children
Esposito *et al.* [112]	*J. Autism Dev. Disord.*, 2014	Expression of distress during the separation phase	13 HR infants	15 months	14 LR infants; LR and HR groups were controlled for the age of infants and the age of older siblings	Cry samples derived from vocal recordings	HR toddlers, compared to those with LR, produced cries that were shorter and had a higher fundamental frequency (F0). Three HR toddlers later classified with an ASD at 36 months produced cries that had among the highest F0 and shortest durations
Gangi *et al.* [106]	*J. Autism Dev. Disord.*, 2014	Joint attention initiation, social communication	56 HR siblings	8–12 months	26 LR siblings; LR and HR groups were controlled for age and ethnicity	Initiating joint attention (IJA) smiling patterns (*i.e.*, anticipatory smiling, reactive smiling, and no smiling) assessed with Early Social Communication Scales	High-risk siblings produced less anticipatory smiling than low-risk siblings, suggesting early differences in communicating pre-existing positive affect. Among high-risk siblings, only IJA without smiling was associated with later ASD severity scores

Table 2. *Cont.*

Study	Journal &Year	Characteristics	Sample	Age of Siblings of Individuals with ASD	Control Group, Matching Criteria	Measures/Instruments (Samples)	Main Findings
Gliga *et al.* [122]	*Dev. Psychol.*, 2014	Spontaneous belief attribution, mental state understanding for action prediction	47 siblings of children with ASD	36 months	39 typically developing children; no matching criteria listed except for age range	Eye-tracking	In tasks demanding mental state understanding for action prediction, at-risk siblings performed at chance (contrary to control children, who performed above the chance), independently of their later clinical outcome (ASD, broader autism phenotype, or typically developing). Performance was not related to children's verbal or general IQ, nor was it explained by children "missing out" on crucial information, as shown by an analysis of visual scanning during the task
Hudry *et al.* [104]	*J. Autism Dev. Disord.*, 2014	Early language profiles, communication	54 HR infants	7–38 months	50 LR controls, no matching criteria listed except for the age range	MCDI: Words and Gestures (WG) and Words and Sentences (WS), VABS—2nd edition and MSEL	Reduced receptive vocabulary advantage was observed in HR infants by 14 months, but was maintained to 24 months only in children with ASD outcome, while typically-developing HR infants regained a more normative profile
Nichols *et al.* [107]	*J. Autism Dev. Disord.*, 2014	Social communication, social smiling	15 SIBS-ASD/AS (siblings of children with ASD, who demonstrated later ASD symptomatology), 27 SIBS-ASD/NS (siblings of children with ASD, who did not demonstrate ASD symptoms)	15 months	25 siblings of children with no family history of ASD, SIBS-TD; no matching criteria listed except for the age range	MSEL, STAT, ADOS	Both SIBS-ASD subgroups demonstrated lower levels of social smiling than SIBS-TD. Only the SIBS-ASD/AS demonstrated less eye contact and non-social smiling than SIBS-TD
Patten *et al.* [123]	*J. Autism Dev. Disord.*, 2014	Vocal patterns, vocalization frequency	37 HR infants (23 obtained the ASD diagnosis later)	9–12 and 15–18 months	14 typically developing infants with no autism family history (LR); HR and LR groups did not differ in terms of age, gender or SES	Video records	Infants later diagnosed with ASD produced low rates of canonical babbling and low volubility by comparison with the typically developing infants

Some authors have posited alternative temperament development trajectories in HR infants, characteristic for early ASD symptoms or broader autism phenotype condition. HR children who were diagnosed with ASD at 36 months had a temperament profile marked by lower positive affect, higher negative affect, and difficulty controlling attention and behavior. This temperamental profile also distinguished HR children without ASD diagnosis at 36 months from LR children [116]. Rosario *et al.* [121] compared HR infants who were or were not later diagnosed with ASD and discovered that the temperament trajectories of children with ASD reflected increases over time in activity levels and decreasing adaptability and approach behaviors relative to high-risk typically developing (TD) children.

It is also predicted that HR infants will exhibit problems with executive functions, especially attention and inhibition deficits, which are considered to be associated with frontal cortex functioning impairments [109]. HR infants had difficulty disengaging attention and showed less selective inhibition than controls (less difference between interesting and boring trials); however, they demonstrated a larger decrease in looks to the distractors in the interesting trials than in the boring trials, whereas controls showed a similar decrease in the two trial types.

Studies investigating vocalization patterns in HR infants suggest that infants later diagnosed with ASD produce low rates of canonical babbling and low volubility in comparison with typically developing infants [123]. Iverson *et al.* [92] also found impaired vocal-motor developmental behaviors in HR infants. Infant siblings demonstrated attenuated patterns of change in rhythmic arm activity around the time of reduplicated babble onset, and were highly likely to exhibit delayed language development at 18 months.

It should be stressed that the analyzed studies have many limitations. As previously mentioned, some authors include in the analysis high-risk infant siblings who later developed ASD, which can lead to overestimation of the differences between high-risk and low-risk children, *i.e.*, [95,97,111]. Furthermore, some studies do not report any clear matching criteria of the control group participants during the recruitment procedure—there is only a description provided of recruited participants in terms of different parameters (such as gender, age, ethnicity, *etc.*), *i.e.*, [110,115,119]. It should be noted that these features often vary across studies, which can raise questions about the comparability and recurrence of obtained results with other research projects. There are also studies that do not have any control group at all, because of the aim of the study, *i.e.*, comparing HR siblings who later developed ASD or did not [107,121]. These research projects provide information about differences within the HR group, but lack data from comparisons of these HR infants with typically developing children that do not have an ASD family background. There are also discrepancies between infants' age ranges in different studies. Some papers focus on describing the features of children at exactly the same age (*i.e.*, 6, 12, or 24 months [102], or other time points [30,90,96]), while others collect data covering a fixed age range (18–27 months [94], below 3 years old [105], 12–23 months [103]). These distinct approaches produce different types of data and therefore variable quality of comparisons, which should be considered during an analysis of studies.

In summary, there are many studies suggesting the existence of a broad range of impairments in infant siblings of children with ASD. Some of the differences are probably characteristic for later ASD diagnosis, but it should be noted that infant siblings are also at a high risk of developing broader autism phenotype-like traits.

4. Summary and Conclusions

The review of studies on BAP traits in siblings of individuals with ASD shows that the issue has been extensively explored. This goes hand in hand with investigation of hereditary mechanisms involved in the etiology of autism spectrum disorders. Research on BAP provides important information about the varied expressions of autism-specific traits. Integration of the results of these studies presents a challenge due to differences in methods, control groups, age of participants, and other aspects of research protocols. Since the relationships between autistic traits and other individual characteristics in a general population, including first-degree relatives of individuals with ASD, have not yet been fully elaborated, this paper focuses on the phenotypic characteristics of individuals observed mainly in psychological studies.

A number of investigators reported cognitive deficits in siblings of children with ASD, which can be a part of ASD phenotype(s). These include emotion recognition tasks [52], lower levels of efficiency in planning, attention shifting, and verbal fluency [44,48]. Some studies indicated differences in social skills development [6,14,28,69]. Difficulties for siblings of children with ASD were also found with respect to communication and language. There are reports of histories of language delay and pragmatic language deficits in this group compared with the siblings of children with Down syndrome and typically developing children, *i.e.*, [28,60,61,94,102].

Researchers have posited various BAP traits in siblings of individuals with autism as important components of the neurocognitive endophenotype for autism. For instance, Dalton *et al.* [55] suggested that social and emotional processing along with underlying neural circuitry constitute an important element of the endophenotype. Fiorentini and colleagues [63] point to face-coding mechanisms, emphasizing their role in the impairment of adaptive mechanisms, while Holt and colleagues [22] highlight the role of mentalizing deficits and atypical social cognition. The inclusion of language deficits in BAP remains controversial. Based on their findings from research on children aged 4–9 years, Levy and Bar-Yuda [61] question whether these deficits should indeed be included in BAP, while Gamliel *et al.* [56,57] consider them to be the key component in the difficulties encountered by preschool and early school individuals with ASD.

It should also be noted that some researchers found no differences between siblings of people with ASD and comparison groups with respect to BAP characteristics [40,45]. Importantly, in a number of studies subgroups demonstrating developmental deficits were distinguished from the group of healthy siblings of people with autism [39,65]. The clear distinction between ASD symptoms and BAP traits is difficult in studies involving siblings of individuals with ASD. This is especially true in studies on infant siblings, in which the risk of ASD rather than the BAP characteristics is the main concern. Prospective studies in this group of children should be continued, in order to track the developmental trajectories in these children at subsequent stages of their development.

It should be stressed that in the light of BAP research, the majority of brothers and sisters of individuals with ASD develop typically, without displaying autistic traits to a greater extent than the relevant control groups. However, traits in the siblings group are often widely dispersed, suggesting that there is much variation among these children in the course of developmental processes and their outcomes.

Some data suggest that genetic susceptibility to autism may differ among families. It is likely to be higher in families with two or more children diagnosed with ASD. Other siblings in these families demonstrate more pronounced BAP traits [65,124]. Research on these families could provide valuable insights on genetic involvement in the development of autistic traits.

Longitudinal studies are especially useful, as they enable researchers to trace developmental dynamics of ASD siblings. Despite achieving the status of the gold standard in research on infants, more longitudinal studies on children over 36 months of age are needed.

The information available at present is insufficient to formulate final conclusions regarding BAP characteristics in siblings of people with ASD. There is no doubt, however, that current research is bringing us closer to an understanding of the genetic factors involved in the etiology of this group of disorders. The studies are also of fundamental importance due to the rising numbers of ASD diagnoses and the presence of autistic characteristics in the general population.

Acknowledgments: This paper was funded by the project of the National Science Center of Poland, #UMO-2011/03/B/HS6/03326 and by the University of Warsaw.

Author Contributions: Ewa Pisula: Study design, Literature search, Manuscript preparation, Funds collection; Karolina Ziegart-Sadowska: Literature search, Manuscript preparation.

References

1. American Psychiatric Association. *Diagnostic and Statistical Manual of Mental Disorders*, 5th ed.; American Psychiatric Association: Arlington, VA, USA, 2013.
2. World Health Organization. *Manual of the International Statistical Classification of the Diseases, and Related Health Problems*, 10th ed.; World Health Organization: Geneva, Switzerland, 2002; Volume 1.
3. Lauritsen, M.B.; Pedersen, C.B.; Mortensen, P.B. Effects of familial risk factors and place of birth on the risk of autism: A nationwide register-based study. *J. Child Psychol. Psychiatry* **2005**, *46*, 963–971. [CrossRef] [PubMed]
4. Persico, A.M.; Sacco, R. Endophenotypes in autism spectrum disorders. In *Comprehensive Guide to Autism*; Patel, V.B., Preedy, V.R., Martin, C.R., Eds.; Springer: New York, NY, USA, 2014; pp. 77–95.
5. Rogers, S.J. What are infant siblings teaching us about autism in infancy? *Autism Res.* **2009**, *2*, 125–137. [CrossRef] [PubMed]
6. Constantino, J.N.; Lajonchere, C.; Lutz, M.; Gray, T.; Abbacchi, A.; McKenna, K.; Singh, D.; Todd, R.D. Autistic social impairment in the siblings of children with pervasive developmental disorders. *Am. J. Psychiatry* **2006**, *163*, 294–296. [CrossRef] [PubMed]
7. Rutter, M.; Thapar, A. Genetics of autism spectrum disorders. In *Handbook of Autism and Pervasive Developmental Disorders*, 4th ed.; Volkmar, R., Rogers, S.J., Paul, R., Pelphrey, K.A., Eds.; Wiley & Sons: New Jersey, NJ, USA, 2014; Volume 1, pp. 411–423.
8. Baron-Cohen, S.; Wheelwright, S.; Skinner, R.; Martin, J.; Clubley, E. The autism-spectrum quotient (AQ): Evidence from Asperger syndrome/high-functioning autism, males and females, scientists and mathematicians. *J. Autism Dev. Disord.* **2001**, *31*, 5–17. [CrossRef] [PubMed]
9. Bailey, A.; Palferman, S.; Heavey, L.; Couteur, A.L. Autism: The phenotype in relatives. *J. Autism Dev. Disord.* **1998**, *28*, 369–392. [CrossRef] [PubMed]
10. Bishop, D.V.M.; Maybery, M.; Maley, A.; Wong, D.; Hill, W.; Hallmayer, J. Using self-report to identify the broad phenotype in parents of children with autistic spectrum disorders: A study using the Autism-Spectrum Quotient. *J. Child Psychol. Psychiatry* **2004**, *45*, 1431–1436. [CrossRef] [PubMed]
11. Bishop, D.V.M.; Maybery, M.; Wong, D.; Maley, A.; Hallmayer, J. Characteristics of the broader phenotype in autism: A study of siblings using the children's communication checklist-2. *Am. J. Med. Genet. Part B* **2006**, *141B*, 117–122. [CrossRef] [PubMed]
12. Losh, M.; Childress, D.; Lam, K.; Piven, J. Defining key features of the broad autism phenotype. *Am. J. Med. Genet. Part B* **2008**, *147B*, 424–433. [CrossRef] [PubMed]
13. Losh, M.; Piven, J. Social-cognition and the broad autism phenotype: Identifying genetically meaningful phenotypes. *J. Child Psychol. Psychiatry* **2007**, *48*, 105–112. [CrossRef] [PubMed]
14. Piven, J.; Palmer, P.; Jacobi, D.; Childress, D.; Arndt, S. Broader autism phenotype: Evidence from a family history study of multiple-incidence autism families. *Am. J. Psychiatry* **1997**, *154*, 185–190. [PubMed]
15. Piven, J.; Palmer, P.; Landa, R.; Santangelo, S.; Jacobi, D.; Childress, D. Personality and language characteristics in parents from multiple-incidence autism families. *Am. J. Med. Genet.* **1997**, *74*, 398–411. [CrossRef] [PubMed]
16. Frazier, T.W.; Youngstrom, E.A.; Sinclair, L.; Kubu, C.S.; Law, P.; Rezai, A.; Constantino, J.N.; Eng, C. Autism spectrum disorders as a qualitatively distinct category from typical behavior in a large, clinically ascertained sample. *Assessment* **2010**, *17*, 308–320. [CrossRef] [PubMed]
17. Wheelwright, S.; Auyeung, B.; Allison, C.; Baron-Cohen, S. Defining the broader, medium and narrow autism phenotype among parents using the Autism Spectrum Quotient (AQ). *Mol. Autism* **2010**, *1*. [CrossRef] [PubMed]
18. August, G.J.; Stewart, M.A.; Tsai, L. The incidence of cognitive disabilities in the siblings of autistic children. *Br. J. Psychiatry* **1981**, *138*, 416–422. [CrossRef] [PubMed]
19. Folstein, S.; Rutter, M. Infantile autism: A genetic study of 21 twin pairs. *J. Child Psychol. Psychiatry* **1977**, *18*, 297–321. [CrossRef] [PubMed]
20. Piven, J. The broad autism phenotype: A complementary strategy for molecular genetic studies of autism. *Am. J. Med. Genet.* **2001**, *105*, 34–35. [CrossRef]
21. Schlichting, C.D.; Pigliucci, M. Gene regulation, quantitative genetics and the evolution of reaction norms. *Evol. Ecol.* **1995**, *9*, 154–168. [CrossRef]

22. Holt, R.J.; Chura, L.R.; Lai, M.-C.; Suckling, J.; von dem Hagen, E.; Calder, A.J.; Bullmore, E.T.; Baron-Cohen, S.; Spencer, M.D. "Reading the Mind in the Eyes": An fMRI study of adolescents with autism and their siblings. *Psychol. Med.* **2014**, *44*, 3215–3227. [CrossRef] [PubMed]
23. Ingersoll, B.; Wainer, A. The broader autism phenotype. In *Handbook of Autism and Pervasive Developmental Disorders*, 4th ed.; Volkmar, F.R., Rogers, S.J., Paul, R., Pelphrey, K.A., Eds.; Wiley & Sons: New Jersey, NJ, USA, 2014; Volume 1, pp. 28–56.
24. Gottesman, I.I.; Gould, T.D. The endophenotype concept in psychiatry: Etymology and strategic intentions. *Am. J. Psychiatry* **2003**, *160*, 636–645. [CrossRef] [PubMed]
25. Rasetti, R.; Weinberger, D.R. Intermediate phenotypes in psychiatric disorders. *Curr. Opin. Genet. Dev.* **2011**, *21*, 340–348. [CrossRef] [PubMed]
26. Rutter, M. Concepts of autism: A review of research. *J. Child Psychol. Psychiatry* **1968**, *9*, 1–25. [CrossRef] [PubMed]
27. Smalley, S.L.; Asarnow, R.F.; Spence, M.A. Autism and genetics. A decade of research. *Arch. Gen. Psychiatry* **1988**, *45*, 953–961. [CrossRef] [PubMed]
28. Bolton, P.; Macdonald, H.; Pickles, A.; Rios, P.; Goode, S.; Crowson, M.; Bailey, A.; Rutter, M. A case-control family history study of autism. *J. Child Psychol. Psychiatry* **1994**, *35*, 877–900. [CrossRef] [PubMed]
29. Ghaziuddin, M. A family history study of Asperger syndrome. *J. Autism Dev. Disord.* **2005**, *35*, 177–182. [CrossRef] [PubMed]
30. Landa, R.; Garrett-Mayer, E. Development in infants with autism spectrum disorders: A prospective study. *J. Child Psychol. Psychiatry* **2006**, *47*, 629–638. [CrossRef] [PubMed]
31. Ozonoff, S.; Young, G.S.; Carter, A.; Messinger, D.; Yirmiya, N.; Zwaigenbaum, L.; Bryson, S.; Carver, L.J.; Constantino, J.N.; Dobkins, K.; *et al.* Recurrence risk for autism spectrum disorders: A Baby Siblings Research Consortium study. *Pediatrics* **2011**, *128*, e488–e495. [PubMed]
32. Dawson, G.; Estes, A.; Munson, J.; Schellenberg, G.; Bernier, R.; Abbott, R. Quantitative assessment of autism symptom-related traits in probands and parents: Broader Phenotype Autism Symptom Scale. *J. Autism Dev. Disord.* **2007**, *37*, 523–536. [CrossRef] [PubMed]
33. Bauminger, N.; Yirmiya, N. The functioning and well-being of SIBS-A: Behavioral-genetic and familial contributions. In *The Development of Autism: Perspectives from Theory and Research*; Burack, J.A., Charman, T., Yirmiya, N., Zelazo, P.R., Eds.; Erlbaum: Hillsdale, NJ, USA, 2001; pp. 61–80.
34. Gerdts, J.; Bernier, R. The broader autism phenotype and its implications on the etiology and treatment of autism spectrum disorders. *Autism Res. Treat.* **2011**, *2011*, e545901. [CrossRef] [PubMed]
35. Jones, E.J.H.; Gliga, T.; Bedford, R.; Charman, T.; Johnson, M.H. Developmental pathways to autism: A review of prospective studies of infants at risk. *Neurosci. Biobehav. Rev.* **2014**, *39*, 1–33. [CrossRef] [PubMed]
36. Losh, M.; Adolphs, R.; Piven, J. The broad autism phenotype. In *Autism Spectrum Disorders*; Dawson, G., Amaral, D., Geschwind, D., Eds.; Oxford University Press: Oxford, UK, 2011; pp. 457–476.
37. Sucksmith, E.; Roth, I.; Hoekstra, R.A. Autistic traits below the clinical threshold: Re-examining the broader autism phenotype in the 21st century. *Neuropsychol. Rev.* **2011**, *21*, 360–389. [CrossRef] [PubMed]
38. Moher, D.; Liberati, A.; Tetzlaff, J.; Altman, D.G. Preferred reporting items for systematic reviews and meta-analyses: The PRISMA statement. *PLoS Med.* **2009**, *6*, e1000097. [CrossRef] [PubMed]
39. Chuthapisith, J.; Ruangdaraganon, N.; Sombuntham, T.; Roongpraiwan, R. Language development among the siblings of children with autistic spectrum disorder. *Autism* **2007**, *11*, 149–160. [CrossRef] [PubMed]
40. Pilowsky, T.; Yirmiya, N.; Gross-Tsur, V.; Shalev, R.S. Neuropsychological functioning of siblings of children with autism, siblings of children with developmental language delay, and siblings of children with mental retardation of unknown genetic etiology. *J. Autism Dev. Disord.* **2007**, *37*, 537–552. [CrossRef] [PubMed]
41. Delorme, R.; Goussé, V.; Roy, I.; Trandafir, A.; Mathieu, F.; Mouren-Siméoni, M.-C.; Betancur, C.; Leboyer, M. Shared executive dysfunctions in unaffected relatives of patients with autism and obsessive-compulsive disorder. *Eur. Psychiatry* **2007**, *22*, 32–38. [CrossRef] [PubMed]
42. Pickles, A.; Starr, E.; Kazak, S.; Bolton, P.; Papanikolaou, K.; Bailey, A.; Goodman, R.; Rutter, M. Variable expression of the autism broader phenotype: Findings from extended pedigrees. *J. Child Psychol. Psychiatry* **2000**, *41*, 491–502. [CrossRef] [PubMed]
43. Hill, E.; Berthoz, S.; Frith, U. Brief report: Cognitive processing of own emotions in individuals with autistic spectrum disorder and in their relatives. *J. Autism Dev. Disord.* **2004**, *34*, 229–235. [CrossRef] [PubMed]

44. Ozonoff, S.; Rogers, S.J.; Farnham, J.M.; Pennington, B.F. Can standard measures identify subclinical markers of autism? *J. Autism Dev. Disord.* **1993**, *23*, 429–441. [CrossRef] [PubMed]
45. Szatmari, P.; Jones, M.B.; Tuff, L.; Bartolucci, G.; Fisman, S.; Mahoney, W. Lack of cognitive impairment in first-degree relatives of children with pervasive developmental disorders. *J. Am. Acad. Child Adolesc. Psychiatry* **1993**, *32*, 1264–1273. [CrossRef] [PubMed]
46. Fombonne, E.; Bolton, P.; Prior, J.; Jordan, H.; Rutter, M. A family study of autism: Cognitive patterns and levels in parents and siblings. *J. Child Psychol. Psychiatry* **1997**, *38*, 667–683. [CrossRef] [PubMed]
47. Folstein, S.E.; Santangelo, S.L.; Gilman, S.E.; Piven, J.; Landa, R.; Lainhart, J.; Hein, J.; Wzorek, M. Predictors of cognitive test patterns in autism families. *J. Child Psychol. Psychiatry* **1999**, *40*, 1117–1128. [CrossRef] [PubMed]
48. Hughes, C.; Plumet, M.H.; Leboyer, M. Towards a cognitive phenotype for autism: Increased prevalence of executive dysfunction and superior spatial span amongst siblings of children with autism. *J. Child Psychol. Psychiatry* **1999**, *40*, 705–718. [CrossRef] [PubMed]
49. Briskman, J.; Happé, F.; Frith, U. Exploring the cognitive phenotype of autism: Weak "central coherence" in parents and siblings of children with autism: II. Real-life skills and preferences. *J. Child Psychol. Psychiatry* **2001**, *42*, 309–316. [CrossRef] [PubMed]
50. Happé, F.; Briskman, J.; Frith, U. Exploring the cognitive phenotype of autism: Weak "central coherence" in parents and siblings of children with autism: I. Experimental tests. *J. Child Psychol. Psychiatry* **2001**, *42*, 299–307. [CrossRef] [PubMed]
51. Pilowsky, T.; Yirmiya, N.; Shalev, R.S.; Gross-Tsur, V. Language abilities of siblings of children with autism. *J. Child Psychol. Psychiatry* **2003**, *44*, 914–925. [CrossRef] [PubMed]
52. Dorris, L.; Espie, C.A.E.; Knott, F.; Salt, J. Mind-reading difficulties in the siblings of people with Asperger's syndrome: Evidence for a genetic influence in the abnormal development of a specific cognitive domain. *J. Child Psychol. Psychiatry* **2004**, *45*, 412–418. [CrossRef] [PubMed]
53. Shaked, M.; Gamliel, I.; Yirmiya, N. Theory of mind abilities in young siblings of children with autism. *Autism* **2006**, *10*, 173–187. [CrossRef] [PubMed]
54. Christ, S.E.; Holt, D.D.; White, D.A.; Green, L. Inhibitory control in children with autism spectrum disorder. *J. Autism Dev. Disord.* **2007**, *37*, 1155–1165. [CrossRef] [PubMed]
55. Dalton, K.M.; Nacewicz, B.M.; Alexander, A.L.; Davidson, R.J. Gaze-fixation, brain activation, and amygdala volume in unaffected siblings of individuals with autism. *Biol. Psychiatry* **2007**, *61*, 512–520. [CrossRef] [PubMed]
56. Gamliel, I.; Yirmiya, N.; Sigman, M. The development of young siblings of children with autism from 4 to 54 months. *J. Autism Dev. Disord.* **2007**, *37*, 171–183. [CrossRef] [PubMed]
57. Gamliel, I.; Yirmiya, N.; Jaffe, D.H.; Manor, O.; Sigman, M. Developmental trajectories in siblings of children with autism: Cognition and language from 4 months to 7 years. *J. Autism Dev. Disord.* **2009**, *39*, 1131–1144. [CrossRef] [PubMed]
58. Kawakubo, Y.; Kuwabara, H.; Watanabe, K.-I.; Minowa, M.; Someya, T.; Minowa, I.; Kono, T.; Nishida, H.; Sugiyama, T.; Kato, N.; *et al.* Impaired prefrontal hemodynamic maturation in autism and unaffected siblings. *PLoS ONE* **2009**, *4*, e6881. [CrossRef] [PubMed]
59. Koh, H.C.; Milne, E.; Dobkins, K. Contrast sensitivity for motion detection and direction discrimination in adolescents with autism spectrum disorders and their siblings. *Neuropsychologia* **2010**, *48*, 4046–4056. [CrossRef] [PubMed]
60. Ben-Yizhak, N.; Yirmiya, N.; Seidman, I.; Alon, R.; Lord, C.; Sigman, M. Pragmatic language and school related linguistic abilities in siblings of children with autism. *J. Autism Dev. Disord.* **2011**, *41*, 750–760. [CrossRef] [PubMed]
61. Levy, Y.; Bar-Yuda, C. Language performance in siblings of nonverbal children with autism. *Autism* **2011**, *15*, 341–354. [CrossRef] [PubMed]
62. Sumiyoshi, C.; Kawakubo, Y.; Suga, M.; Sumiyoshi, T.; Kasai, K. Impaired ability to organize information in individuals with autism spectrum disorders and their siblings. *Neurosci. Res.* **2011**, *69*, 252–257. [CrossRef] [PubMed]
63. Fiorentini, C.; Gray, L.; Rhodes, G.; Jeffery, L.; Pellicano, E. Reduced face identity aftereffects in relatives of children with autism. *Neuropsychologia* **2012**, *50*, 2926–2932. [CrossRef] [PubMed]

64. Warren, Z.E.; Foss-Feig, J.H.; Malesa, E.E.; Lee, E.B.; Taylor, J.L.; Newsom, C.R.; Crittendon, J.; Stone, W.L. Neurocognitive and behavioral outcomes of younger siblings of children with autism spectrum disorder at age five. *J. Autism Dev. Disord.* **2012**, *42*, 409–418. [CrossRef] [PubMed]
65. Gerdts, J.A.; Bernier, R.; Dawson, G.; Estes, A. The broader autism phenotype in simplex and multiplex families. *J. Autism Dev. Disord.* **2013**, *43*, 1597–1605. [CrossRef] [PubMed]
66. Malesa, E.; Foss-Feig, J.; Yoder, P.; Warren, Z.; Walden, T.; Stone, W.L. Predicting language and social outcomes at age 5 for later-born siblings of children with autism spectrum disorders. *Autism* **2013**, *17*, 558–570. [CrossRef] [PubMed]
67. Yoder, P.; Stone, W.L.; Walden, T.; Malesa, E. Predicting social impairment and ASD diagnosis in younger siblings of children with autism spectrum disorder. *J. Autism Dev. Disord.* **2009**, *39*, 1381–1391. [CrossRef] [PubMed]
68. Oerlemans, A.M.; Droste, K.; van Steijn, D.J.; de Sonneville, L.M.J.; Buitelaar, J.K.; Rommelse, N.N.J. Co-segregation of social cognition, executive function and local processing style in children with ASD, their siblings and normal controls. *J. Autism Dev. Disord.* **2013**, *43*, 2764–2778. [CrossRef] [PubMed]
69. Pickles, A.; St Clair, M.C.; Conti-Ramsden, G. Communication and social deficits in relatives of individuals with SLI and relatives of individuals with ASD. *J. Autism Dev. Disord.* **2013**, *43*, 156–167. [CrossRef] [PubMed]
70. Robel, L.; Rousselot-Pailley, B.; Fortin, C.; Levy-Rueff, M.; Golse, B.; Falissard, B. Subthreshold traits of the broad autistic spectrum are distributed across different subgroups in parents, but not siblings, of probands with autism. *Eur. Child Adolesc. Psychiatry* **2013**, *23*, 225–233. [CrossRef] [PubMed]
71. Gizzonio, V.; Avanzini, P.; Fabbri-Destro, M.; Campi, C.; Rizzolatti, G. Cognitive abilities in siblings of children with autism spectrum disorders. *Exp. Brain Res.* **2014**, *232*, 2381–2390. [CrossRef] [PubMed]
72. Oerlemans, A.M.; van der Meer, J.M.J.; van Steijn, D.J.; de Ruiter, S.W.; de Bruijn, Y.G.E.; de Sonneville, L.M.J.; Buitelaar, J.K.; Rommelse, N.N.J. Recognition of facial emotion and affective prosody in children with ASD (+ADHD) and their unaffected siblings. *Eur. Child Adolesc. Psychiatry* **2014**, *23*, 257–271. [CrossRef] [PubMed]
73. Lowenthal, R.; Paula, C.S.; Schwartzman, J.S.; Brunoni, D.; Mercadante, M.T. Prevalence of pervasive developmental disorder in Down's syndrome. *J. Autism Dev. Disord.* **2007**, *37*, 1394–1395. [CrossRef] [PubMed]
74. Biao, J. Prevalence of autism spectrum disorder among children aged 8 years—Autism and developmental disabilities monitoring network, 11 Sites, United States, 2010. *Surveill. Summ.* **2014**, *63*, 1–21.
75. Leyfer, O.T.; Tager-Flusberg, H.; Dowd, M.; Tomblin, J.B.; Folstein, S.E. Overlap between autism and specific language impairment: Comparison of Autism Diagnostic Interview and Autism Diagnostic Observation Schedule scores. *Autism Res.* **2008**, *1*, 284–296. [CrossRef] [PubMed]
76. Tsermentseli, S.; O'Brien, J.M.; Spencer, J.V. Comparison of form and motion coherence processing in autistic spectrum disorders and dyslexia. *J. Autism Dev. Disord.* **2008**, *38*, 1201–1210. [CrossRef] [PubMed]
77. Lord, C.; Rutter, M.; DiLavore, P.; Risi, S. *Autism Diagnostic Observation Schedule (ADOS) Manual*; Western Psychological Services: Los Angeles, CA, USA, 2001.
78. Rutter, M.; le Couteur, A.; Lord, C. *ADI-R: Autism Diagnostic Interview–Revised*; Western Psychological Services: Los Angeles, CA, USA, 2003.
79. Rutter, M.; Bailey, A.; Lord, C. *Social Communication Questionnaire*; Western Psychological Services: Los Angeles, CA, USA, 2003.
80. Schopler, E.; Reichler, R.J.; Renner, B.R. *The Childhood Autism Rating Scale*; Western Psychological Services: Los Angeles, CA, USA, 1988.
81. Bernier, R.; Gerdts, J.; Munson, J.; Dawson, G.; Estes, A. Evidence for broader autism phenotype characteristics in parents from multiple-incidence autism families. *Autism Res.* **2012**, *5*, 13–20. [CrossRef] [PubMed]
82. Sebat, J.; Lakshmi, B.; Malhotra, D.; Troge, J.; Lese-Martin, C.; Walsh, T.; Yamrom, B.; Yoon, S.; Krasnitz, A.; Kendall, J.; *et al.* Strong association of de novo copy number mutations with autism. *Science* **2007**, *316*, 445–449. [CrossRef] [PubMed]
83. Pinto, D.; Pagnamenta, A.T.; Klei, L.; Anney, R.; Merico, D.; Regan, R.; Conroy, J.; Magalhaes, T.R.; Correia, C.; Abrahams, B.S.; *et al.* Functional impact of global rare copy number variation in autism spectrum disorders. *Nature* **2010**, *466*, 368–372. [CrossRef] [PubMed]

84. Spiker, D.; Lotspeich, L.; Kraemer, H.C.; Hallmayer, J.; McMahon, W.; Petersen, P.B.; Nicholas, P.; Pingree, C.; Wiese-Slater, S.; Chiotti, C. Genetics of autism: Characteristics of affected and unaffected children from 37 multiplex families. *Am. J. Med. Genet.* **1994**, *54*, 27–35. [CrossRef] [PubMed]
85. Matson, J.L.; Shoemaker, M. Intellectual disability and its relationship to autism spectrum disorders. *Res. Dev. Disabil.* **2009**, *30*, 1107–1114. [CrossRef] [PubMed]
86. Newschaffer, C.J.; Falb, M.D.; Gurney, J.G. National autism prevalence trends from United States special education data. *Pediatrics* **2005**, *115*, e277–e282. [CrossRef] [PubMed]
87. Bölte, S.; Dziobek, I.; Poustka, F. Brief report: The level and nature of autistic intelligence revisited. *J. Autism Dev. Disord.* **2009**, *39*, 678–682. [CrossRef] [PubMed]
88. Messinger, D.; Young, G.S.; Ozonoff, S.; Dobkins, K.; Carter, A.; Zwaigenbaum, L.; Landa, R.J.; Charman, T.; Stone, W.L.; Constantino, J.N.; *et al.* Beyond autism: A baby siblings research consortium study of high-risk children at three years of age. *J. Am. Acad. Child Adolesc. Psychiatry* **2013**, *52*, 300–308. [CrossRef] [PubMed]
89. Yirmiya, N.; Gamliel, I.; Shaked, M.; Sigman, M. Cognitive and verbal abilities of 24- to 36-month-old siblings of children with autism. *J. Autism Dev. Disord.* **2007**, *37*, 218–229. [CrossRef] [PubMed]
90. Yirmiya, N.; Gamliel, I.; Pilowsky, T.; Feldman, R.; Baron-Cohen, S.; Sigman, M. The development of siblings of children with autism at 4 and 14 months: Social engagement, communication, and cognition. *J. Child Psychol. Psychiatry* **2006**, *47*, 511–523. [CrossRef] [PubMed]
91. Cassel, T.D.; Messinger, D.S.; Ibanez, L.V.; Haltigan, J.D.; Acosta, S.I.; Buchman, A.C. Early social and emotional communication in the infant siblings of children with autism spectrum disorders: An examination of the broad phenotype. *J. Autism Dev. Disord.* **2007**, *37*, 122–132. [CrossRef] [PubMed]
92. Iverson, J.M.; Wozniak, R.H. Variation in vocal-motor development in infant siblings of children with autism. *J. Autism Dev. Disord.* **2007**, *37*, 158–170. [CrossRef] [PubMed]
93. Merin, N.; Young, G.S.; Ozonoff, S.; Rogers, S.J. Visual fixation patterns during reciprocal social interaction distinguish a subgroup of 6-month-old infants at-risk for autism from comparison infants. *J. Autism Dev. Disord.* **2007**, *37*, 108–121. [CrossRef] [PubMed]
94. Toth, K.; Dawson, G.; Meltzoff, A.N.; Greenson, J.; Fein, D. Early social, imitation, play, and language abilities of young non-autistic siblings of children with autism. *J. Autism Dev. Disord.* **2007**, *37*, 145–157. [CrossRef] [PubMed]
95. Hutman, T.; Chela, M.K.; Gillespie-Lynch, K.; Sigman, M. Selective visual attention at twelve months: Signs of autism in early social interactions. *J. Autism Dev. Disord.* **2012**, *42*, 487–498. [CrossRef] [PubMed]
96. Mitchell, S.; Brian, J.; Zwaigenbaum, L.; Roberts, W.; Szatmari, P.; Smith, I.; Bryson, S. Early language and communication development of infants later diagnosed with autism spectrum disorder. *J. Dev. Behav. Pediatr.* **2006**, *27*, S69–S78. [CrossRef] [PubMed]
97. Rozga, A.; Hutman, T.; Young, G.S.; Rogers, S.J.; Ozonoff, S.; Dapretto, M.; Sigman, M. Behavioral profiles of affected and unaffected siblings of children with autism: Contribution of measures of mother-infant interaction and nonverbal communication. *J. Autism Dev. Disord.* **2011**, *41*, 287–301. [CrossRef] [PubMed]
98. Sullivan, M.; Finelli, J.; Marvin, A.; Garrett-Mayer, E.; Bauman, M.; Landa, R. Response to joint attention in toddlers at risk for autism spectrum disorder: A prospective study. *J. Autism Dev. Disord.* **2007**, *37*, 37–48. [CrossRef] [PubMed]
99. Bryson, S.E.; Zwaigenbaum, L.; Brian, J.; Roberts, W.; Szatmari, P.; Rombough, V.; McDermott, C. A prospective case series of high-risk infants who developed autism. *J. Autism Dev. Disord.* **2007**, *37*, 12–24. [CrossRef] [PubMed]
100. Georgiades, S.; Szatmari, P.; Zwaigenbaum, L.; Bryson, S.; Brian, J.; Roberts, W.; Smith, I.; Vaillancourt, T.; Roncadin, C.; Garon, N. A prospective study of autistic-like traits in unaffected siblings of probands with autism spectrum disorder. *JAMA Psychiatry* **2013**, *70*, 42–48. [CrossRef] [PubMed]
101. Macari, S.L.; Campbell, D.; Gengoux, G.W.; Saulnier, C.A.; Klin, A.J.; Chawarska, K. Predicting developmental status from 12 to 24 months in infants at risk for autism spectrum disorder: A preliminary report. *J. Autism Dev. Disord.* **2012**, *42*, 2636–2647. [CrossRef] [PubMed]
102. Zwaigenbaum, L.; Bryson, S.; Rogers, T.; Roberts, W.; Brian, J.; Szatmari, P. Behavioral manifestations of autism in the first year of life. *Int. J. Dev. Neurosci.* **2005**, *23*, 143–152. [CrossRef] [PubMed]
103. Stone, W.L.; McMahon, C.R.; Yoder, P.J.; Walden, T.A. EArly social-communicative and cognitive development of younger siblings of children with autism spectrum disorders. *Arch. Pediatr. Adolesc. Med.* **2007**, *161*, 384–390. [CrossRef] [PubMed]

104. Hudry, K.; Chandler, S.; Bedford, R.; Pasco, G.; Gliga, T.; Elsabbagh, M.; Johnson, M.H.; Charman, T. Early language profiles in infants at high-risk for autism spectrum disorders. *J. Autism Dev. Disord.* **2014**, *44*, 154–167. [CrossRef] [PubMed]
105. Goldberg, W.A.; Jarvis, K.L.; Osann, K.; Laulhere, T.M.; Straub, C.; Thomas, E.; Filipek, P.; Spence, M.A. Brief report: Early social communication behaviors in the younger siblings of children with autism. *J. Autism Dev. Disord.* **2005**, *35*, 657–664. [CrossRef] [PubMed]
106. Gangi, D.N.; Ibañez, L.V.; Messinger, D.S. Joint attention initiation with and without positive affect: Risk group differences and associations with ASD symptoms. *J. Autism Dev. Disord.* **2014**, *44*, 1414–1424. [CrossRef] [PubMed]
107. Nichols, C.M.; Ibañez, L.V.; Foss-Feig, J.H.; Stone, W.L. Social smiling and its components in high-risk infant siblings without later ASD symptomatology. *J. Autism Dev. Disord.* **2014**, *44*, 894–902. [CrossRef] [PubMed]
108. Loh, A.; Soman, T.; Brian, J.; Bryson, S.E.; Roberts, W.; Szatmari, P.; Smith, I.M.; Zwaigenbaum, L. Stereotyped motor behaviors associated with autism in high-risk infants: A pilot videotape analysis of a sibling sample. *J. Autism Dev. Disord.* **2007**, *37*, 25–36. [CrossRef] [PubMed]
109. Holmboe, K.; Elsabbagh, M.; Volein, A.; Tucker, L.A.; Baron-Cohen, S.; Bolton, P.; Charman, T.; Johnson, M.H. Frontal cortex functioning in the infant broader autism phenotype. *Infant Behav. Dev.* **2010**, *33*, 482–491. [CrossRef] [PubMed]
110. Damiano, C.R.; Nahmias, A.; Hogan-Brown, A.L.; Stone, W.L. What do repetitive and stereotyped movements mean for infant siblings of children with autism spectrum disorders? *J. Autism Dev. Disord.* **2013**, *43*, 1326–1335. [CrossRef] [PubMed]
111. Bedford, R.; Elsabbagh, M.; Gliga, T.; Pickles, A.; Senju, A.; Charman, T.; Johnson, M.H.; BASIS Team. Precursors to social and communication difficulties in infants at-risk for autism: Gaze following and attentional engagement. *J. Autism Dev. Disord.* **2012**, *42*, 2208–2218. [CrossRef] [PubMed]
112. Esposito, G.; del Carmen Rostagno, M.; Venuti, P.; Haltigan, J.D.; Messinger, D.S. Brief report: Atypical expression of distress during the separation phase of the strange situation procedure in infant siblings at high risk for ASD. *J. Autism Dev. Disord.* **2014**, *44*, 975–980. [CrossRef] [PubMed]
113. Haltigan, J.D.; Ekas, N.V.; Seifer, R.; Messinger, D.S. Attachment security in infants at-risk for autism spectrum disorders. *J. Autism Dev. Disord.* **2011**, *41*, 962–967. [CrossRef] [PubMed]
114. Wan, M.W.; Green, J.; Elsabbagh, M.; Johnson, M.; Charman, T.; Plummer, F.; BASIS Team. Quality of interaction between at-risk infants and caregiver at 12–15 months is associated with 3-year autism outcome. *J. Child Psychol. Psychiatry* **2013**, *54*, 763–771. [CrossRef] [PubMed]
115. Dundas, E.; Gastgeb, H.; Strauss, M.S. Left visual field biases when infants process faces: A comparison of infants at high- and low-risk for autism spectrum disorder. *J. Autism Dev. Disord.* **2012**, *42*, 2659–2668. [CrossRef] [PubMed]
116. Garon, N.; Bryson, S.E.; Zwaigenbaum, L.; Smith, I.M.; Brian, J.; Roberts, W.; Szatmari, P. Temperament and its relationship to autistic symptoms in a high-risk infant sib cohort. *J. Abnorm. Child Psychol.* **2009**, *37*, 59–78. [CrossRef] [PubMed]
117. Christensen, L.; Hutman, T.; Rozga, A.; Young, G.S.; Ozonoff, S.; Rogers, S.J.; Baker, B.; Sigman, M. Play and developmental outcomes in infant siblings of children with autism. *J. Autism Dev. Disord.* **2010**, *40*, 946–957. [CrossRef] [PubMed]
118. Paul, R.; Fuerst, Y.; Ramsay, G.; Chawarska, K.; Klin, A. Out of the mouths of babes: Vocal production in infant siblings of children with ASD. *J. Child Psychol. Psychiatry* **2011**, *52*, 588–598. [CrossRef] [PubMed]
119. Cornew, L.; Dobkins, K.R.; Akshoomoff, N.; McCleery, J.P.; Carver, L.J. Atypical social referencing in infant siblings of children with autism spectrum disorders. *J. Autism Dev. Disord.* **2012**, *42*, 2611–2621. [CrossRef] [PubMed]
120. Curtin, S.; Vouloumanos, A. Speech preference is associated with autistic-like behavior in 18-months-olds at risk for Autism Spectrum Disorder. *J. Autism Dev. Disord.* **2013**, *43*, 2114–2120. [CrossRef] [PubMed]
121. Del Rosario, M.; Gillespie-Lynch, K.; Johnson, S.; Sigman, M.; Hutman, T. Parent-reported temperament trajectories among infant siblings of children with autism. *J. Autism Dev. Disord.* **2014**, *44*, 381–393. [CrossRef] [PubMed]
122. Gliga, T.; Senju, A.; Pettinato, M.; Charman, T.; Johnson, M.H. Spontaneous belief attribution in younger siblings of children on the autism spectrum. *Dev. Psychol.* **2014**, *50*, 903–913. [CrossRef] [PubMed]

123. Patten, E.; Belardi, K.; Baranek, G.T.; Watson, L.R.; Labban, J.D.; Oller, D.K. Vocal patterns in infants with autism spectrum disorder: Canonical babbling status and vocalization frequency. *J. Autism Dev. Disord.* **2014**, *44*, 2413–2428. [CrossRef] [PubMed]
124. Schwichtenberg, A.J.; Young, G.S.; Sigman, M.; Hutman, T.; Ozonoff, S. Can family affectedness inform infant sibling outcomes of autism spectrum disorders? *J. Child Psychol. Psychiatry* **2010**, *51*, 1021–1030. [CrossRef] [PubMed]

5

Clinical Genetic Aspects of Autism Spectrum Disorders

G. Bradley Schaefer

University of Arkansas for Medical Sciences, Arkansas Children's Hospital, 1 Children's Way, Slot 512-22, Little Rock, AR 72202, USA; schaefergb@uams.edu

Academic Editor: Merlin G. Butler

Abstract: Early presumptions opined that autism spectrum disorder (ASD) was related to the rearing of these children by emotionally-distant mothers. Advances in the 1960s and 1970s clearly demonstrated the biologic basis of autism with a high heritability. Recent advances have demonstrated that specific etiologic factors in autism spectrum disorders can be identified in 30%–40% of cases. Based on early reports newer, emerging genomic technologies are likely to increase this diagnostic yield to over 50%. To date these investigations have focused on etiologic factors that are largely mono-factorial. The currently undiagnosed causes of ASDs will likely be found to have causes that are more complex. Epigenetic, multiple interacting loci, and four dimensional causes (with timing as a variable) are likely to be associated with the currently unidentifiable cases. Today, the "Why" is more important than ever. Understanding the causes of ASDs help inform families of important issues such as recurrence risk, prognosis, natural history, and predicting associated co-morbid medical conditions. In the current era of emerging efforts in "personalized medicine", identifying an etiology will be critical in identifying endo-phenotypic groups and individual variations that will allow for tailored treatment for persons with ASD.

Keywords: multifactorial inheritance; genetic testing; diagnostic yield; copy number variants; gene sequencing; genomics

---

1. Introduction

1.1. Autism as a Neuro-Genetic Disorder

Not long after autism was identified in the 1940s as a distinct developmental disorder, the question of causation was discussed. Most of the early theories as to the etiology of autism were framed in the context of the prevailing psychiatric models of the time. Thus many theorized that autism was an acquired condition associated with children raised by cold, emotionally-distant mothers. Given our current understanding of the etiology of autism spectrum disorders (which will be a large focus of this review) it is hard to imagine how these theories gained popular acceptance. One has to also appreciate the extreme guilt that this must have evoked on the parents, and this compounded by the stress of having a special needs child.

From the 1940s to the present, the understanding of the etiology of autism has mirrored the eras of scientific advancement in the field of developmental biology and genetics. Population studies in the 1960s and 1970s provided clear proof of the biologic and genetic basis of autism. Progress in genetic testing in the 1980s and 1990s began to identify specific genetic markers in some patients with autism. The progression from linkage studies to cytogenetic, molecular cytogenetic, molecular and now genomic testing have all been very congruent in identifying genomic "hot spots" associated with autism.

Current understanding recognizes autism as having a strong genetic basis with a complex inheritance pattern. Strong genetic factors are involved. As with all human medical conditions, there is environmental modulation. There is clear etiologic and genetic heterogeneity. Literally hundreds of "autism genes" have been identified. Thus, from an etiologic standpoint, it would be better stated "the autisms" rather than "autism". This understanding will be critical as the science of autism therapies moves forward. Using targeted therapies for specific identified causes of autism holds the promise of improved outcomes and reduced adverse events. For the purposes of this review I will discuss autism spectrum disorders (ASDs) unless otherwise stated. In general, from a clinical genetic standpoint, the evaluation is not different for persons on different parts of the spectrum. The focus of this review is to highlight the genetic factors in autism especially in the light of clinical applications.

1.1.1. Indisputable Evidence of the Genetic Basis of Autism Spectrum Disorders (ASDs)

As noted above, population studies have provided strong evidence of the genetic basis of ASDs [1]. In fact, when compared to other neurodevelopmental disabilities (NDD), autism is one of most—if not the most—heritable NDDs known.

From 2006 to 2008 we reviewed a large portion of the existing published information on the population genetic characteristics of autism spectrum disorders [2,3]. This information provided a very strong indication of the genetic basis of ASDs. Classic parameters of population genetics that supported this included data on twin concordance, heritability, relative risk ratio and sibling risk ratio.

In this review, I will provide a brief summary of this collected body of information. Twin concordance studies showed an estimated 70% concordance among monozygotic twins (reported ranges 36%–95%). In contrast, concordance among dizygotic twins was around 3% (range 0%–31%) or 30% if a broader phenotypic definition was used. Heritability estimates were noted to be 0.8 to 0.9. The estimated relative (sibling) risk ratio is reported to be about 150 for monozygotic twins and 8–10 for dizygotic twins and full siblings [4]. In the realm of the discipline of population genetics this is overwhelming support of a genetic basis to ASDs. These data have been replicated and validated in more recent and larger studies [4–6]. With a broader design and larger sample size, these more recent studies have also added another population parameter not previously noted. A 2–3-fold increased recurrence risk of ASD has been documented in half-siblings (both maternal and paternal) of probands with an ASD [4–7]. The increased occurrence in even less closely related individuals lends very strong support for the genetic basis of autism.

1.1.2. Why Then Is the Genetic Basis of ASDs Still Debated?

Even with such a strong body of evidence as to the genetic basis of ASDs, not everyone is convinced. Significant opposition to this notion exists. There exist multiple factions of people who do not recognize the validity of the commonly accepted medical literature. Common objections voiced include the concern over some link between ASDs and childhood immunizations. Some question how could a "genetic disorder" be increasing in frequency? This is cited in light of the continued increase in the reported incidence of ASD. Over the past 20 years the reported occurrence of ASD has almost quadrupled [8]. Current estimates put the prevalence of ASD at about 1/68 children [9]. The logical question is "How could a condition could be increasing at such a rapid rate and yet have a primary genetic origin?" As one of my partners expressed to me "It is interesting that the incidence of conditions like diabetes and asthma are similarly increasing and yet no one is questioning the genetic basis of these conditions [10].

1.2. Multifactorial Inheritance

Strictly speaking, all human medical conditions could be classified as having a "multi-factorial etiology". This implies that these conditions have both genetic and environmental factors which contribute to the overall phenotype. All conditions have genetic and environmental contributions—depending on the condition, the relative proportion of each varies considerably. *Mendelian inheritance* is the term applied to those conditions in which a single gene mutation has a major phenotypic effect with significantly less environmental influences on the phenotype and in which the inheritance follows a monogenic pattern. For more complex traits, the relative contribution of environmental and genetic factors is more balanced. Conditions are designated as having *multifactorial inheritance* if several characteristics are noted:

1. Clear genetic variability exists yet no uni-factorial mode of inheritance can be identified
2. Family studies indicate an increased risk for near relatives to be affected
3. Complicated pathophysiology or morphogenetic processes are involved
4. Biologic influences of environmental factors

Genetic susceptibility refers to a condition that is predominantly determined by environmental factors with expression and phenotypic variability affected by genetic changes that alter the susceptibility to the environmental factor [11].

Considering the above definitions, ASDs clearly fall into the category of multi-factorial inheritance. The recurrence risk pattern of multi-factorial traits typically demonstrates:

1. An increased recurrence risk in close relatives as compared to the general population frequency
2. A non-linear decrease in frequency with increasing distance of relationship—typically no increased recurrence rates are seen beyond 3rd degree relatives
3. The recurrence risk increases with the number of affected individuals
4. There is an increased risk with increased severity of the condition
5. There is an increased risk if person(s) affected are of the "rarer" gender. (In ASD a distinct gender bias of a 3- to 4-fold rate of affected males has been noted)

Recurrence risk data that had accumulated up until about 2008 matched well with this model. The overall recurrence risk for a sibling of a single proband with ASD was reported as 3%–10%. Further refinement of these risks noted that the estimated recurrence risk for a sibling of an affected person with an ASD was established as 4% if the affected individual was male and 7% if female. If there were more than one affected sibling with an ASD, the recurrence risk for future sibs increased to a remarkable 30%–50%. These numbers have been verified in multiple studies [12].

As already stated, multifactorial inheritance implies both genetic and environmental factors are at work. The established heritability rates of around 0.8 or more implies that the majority of the ASD phenotype is determined by genetic factors. Still, environmental influences need to be acknowledged. The issue of environmental contributors to autism is one of the most highly debated topics in all of the body of medical literature. A discussion of this is beyond the focus of this review.

2. Discussion

A thorough discussion of the genetic aspects of ASDs crosses the gamut of genetic principles to be considered in human diseases and disorders. In this section we will discuss each of these parameters individually. We will also review changes in the reported data in light of changes in reported information before and after about 2008. Table 1 provides a summary of the information below.

2.1. Epidemiology/Population Genetics

Epidemiologic data is extremely helpful in population genetics. Knowing the specifics about occurrence, incidence, prevalence and biases of a condition is important in defining genetic factors and the magnitude of their influence on the trait. The reported overall incidence of ASDs has steadily increased over the past 3 decades. The curve has risen sharply since the year 2000. At that point, the reported incidence of ASDs was 1/150 school-aged children. In 2014 it had risen to 1/68 (a 120% increase). Boys are estimated to be affected 4–5 times as often as girls; with the reported incidence now being 1/42 in boys and 1/189 in girls. With this notable increase in reported cases, recent studies have re-evaluated the population genetics of ASDs. Some have reinforced what has already been known. Others have challenged long-standing assumptions. We will look at each of these individually.

2.1.1. Recurrence Risk

Recent studies [6,13,14] have suggested that the recurrence for siblings in the situation of a single affected proband may be higher than the previously noted 3%–10%. These more recent studies reported risks of 10%–19%. While there has not been a formal weighted analysis yet of these changing numbers, these studies provide sufficient support of using an increased recurrence risk of 10%–20%. In the event of more than one affected sibling with an ASD recent studies have confirmed the estimated 30%–50% recurrence risk for subsequent sibs [14–16]. The newer studies have also reported relative risk ratios (RRR) for full siblings as 6.9–10.3 and significant concordance calculations with RRR estimates of 150 for monozygotic twins as compared to 8.2 for dizygotic twins [4,5].

2.1.2. Heritability

Heritability is defined as the proportion of the observed phenotype that is attributable to genetic factors. Heritability estimates over the past 20 years for ASD have been in the range of 0.7 to 0.9. One recent study [4] has given a much lower estimate of 0.4–0.6. For now these data must be cautiously interpreted in light of most other reports.

2.1.3. Sex Bias (Occurrence Gender)

Historically a reproducible and significant gender bias has been noted in the incidence of most neurodevelopmental disabilities. In general males have been found to have a 4–5-fold increased occurrence of these conditions [17]. This is true for ASDs. This difference is noted more so in those persons with ASD who have milder degrees of cognitive impairment. If individuals with mild cognitive impairment are considered, the gender bias is about 2 times increased in males. In individuals with more severe impairments the bias is 4–7 times increased [18]. The first assumption that would be made in this setting would be that X-linked genes might be associated with this observed increased occurrence in males. Interestingly it has been suggested that only about 10% of the reported male excess can be attributed to X-linked genes. A previously cited study [13] did not identify a gender bias. However, others have confirmed this finding [14,19]. For now it appears safe to assume that there is indeed a 4–5-fold increased incidence of ASDs in males.

2.1.4. Proband Gender Effect (Recurrence)

As previously mentioned, most multi-factorial conditions show a gender bias in their occurrence. Recurrence rates can then also be shown to have a gender specific recurrence rate with the rate being higher if the affected individual is of the less frequent gender. In ASDs the recurrence rate in siblings of an affected male has been stated as 4% as compared to 7% if the affected individual is a female [3]. In more recent studies, this "proband gender effect" on recurrence in siblings has been questioned. Three studies [5,14,19] found no proband gender differences. Two other recent studies [15,20] did observe this phenomenon. From a practical standpoint, if the proband gender effect is indeed real, the small difference that would be present would not be sufficiently large enough to be predicted to be of sufficient magnitude as to affect familial decision making. Thus, while this is an interesting question and worthy of additional investigations, clinical counseling could probably be best given as 10%–20% recurrence risk for either gender.

2.1.5. Reproductive Stoppage and Birth Order

Earlier observations have noted that despite a per pregnancy prediction of a 3%–10% recurrence rate of ASDs, the actual number of observed recurrences was less (2%–3%). This raised the question of reproductive "stoppage" (aka curtailment of reproduction). That is the presumption that once a couple has had a child with an ASD, they are less likely to have other children—regardless. These correlated observations suggested that stoppage might be at work, but without investigative support. Three recent reports [16,21,22] have all objectively confirmed the suspicion of stoppage in families with children with an ASD. Finally, some studies have investigated the association with birth order and ASD. Birth order is an interesting parameter to consider. In actuality birth order effects are predicted to be more of an environmental influence. Two studies have noted no birth order effect in one report [14] *versus* a decrease in ASDs in later siblings. Reported birth order effects, if real, are likely to be related in some degree to the same factors in reproductive curtailment (psycho-social environmental factors).

2.1.6. Parental Age Effects

An association with an advanced paternal age (which is felt to be associated with an increased occurrence of *de novo* mutations) has previously been reported in ASDs [23]. One recent report [14] actually reported the opposite—an association with younger fathers.

Table 1. Summarizes the current parameters of the population aspects of ASDs.

Parameter	Value	Comments
Recurrence risk	10%–20%	Value increased based on newer studies
Relative recurrence ratio		
Monozygotic twins	150	
Dizygotic twins	8	
Full siblings	7–10	
Heritability	0.7–0.9	One recent study estimate of 0.5
Occurrence gender	4–5× higher in males	Few studies have not seen this
Proband gender effect	2× increase if female	Recent studies differ on this effect
Paternal age	Increased	One recent study saw a higher occurrence in younger fathers
Reproductive curtailment (stoppage)	Appears to be real phenomenon	
Birth order	Decreased in later sibs	To be confirmed

2.2. *Genetic Loci and ASDs*

Given the information in the preceding section, a genetic basis for ASDs is unquestionable. As such, the next question is "Can these genetic factors be identified?" In this context a couple of terms should be defined. "*Etiology*" is a specific diagnosis that can be translated into useful clinical information for the family, including providing information about prognosis, recurrence risks, and preferred modes of available therapy [24]. This definition was further refined to include the stipulation that there is "sufficient literature evidence to make a causal relationship of the disorder . . . and if it meets the Schaefer-Bodensteiner definition" [25]. "*Diagnostic yield*" is the proportion of cases in which the etiology can be determined after a complete evaluation. Essentially it is the batting average in finding the etiology of a given condition.

Genetic testing technologies have dramatically improved over the past 3 decades. Each significant advancement in genetic testing technology has produced an increased understanding of the genetic factors that cause ASDs. A rise in the diagnostic yield in defining an etiology for ASD parallels the introduction of these new technologies. A discussion of the causes of ASDs can be framed in the context of the ontogeny of the development of each new modality.

2.2.1. Linkage

Linkage technology was developed and refined, with a further expansion into genome wide association studies. Multiple studies using this technology were reported in cohorts of patients with ASD. A summary of these results is that linkage was identified with most autosomes. A careful review of the cumulative results identified consistent reports of linkage to chromosomal regions 2q, 7q22-31 (with a parent of origin effect), 13q, 15q11-13, 16p and 17q11 (a male specific locus). Better *lod* scores were obtained if a broader phenotypic definition was used. Repeat studies with larger sample sizes did not change these results/conclusions.

Since ASDs shows a clear male predominance, a logical assumption might be that X-linked genes could be playing a major role. However, linkage studies specifically targeting the X chromosome did not identify X-linked genes as accounting for a large portion of the male predominance. Only four minor linkages to the X chromosome were noted. Stated another way, a much smaller proportion of the male preponderance is explained by X-linked genes than initially suspected [26]. This raises an interesting corollary question. If X-linked genes do not explain the male excess in cases, what does? Other possible explanations that have been proposed include (1) Mosaicism/tissue specific expression of X-linked genes; (2) Dysregulation of methylation of brain expressed genes on the X chromosome and (3) Hormonally mediated changes (*i.e.*, differential expression on the "male brain").

2.2.2. Cytogenetics

Microscopically detected chromosome abnormalities have consistently been reported in association with ASD. Refinements of chromosome analysis (prometaphase and later interphase studies) enhance detection rates. Estimated positive findings in ASDs have a reported range of 3%–12% with the best overall estimates being 3%–5% [27–29]. The most commonly seen abnormalities reported are deletions or duplications of the proximal 15q region. Other commonly reported aneuploidies include deletions of 2q37, 7q, 18q, and Xp and duplication of 22q13. An association with whole chromosome aneuploidies such as 47 XXY and 45X/46XY has also been seen.

2.2.3. Fluorescent-*in Situ*-Hybridization (FISH)

Fluorescent-*in situ*-hybridization (FISH) technology became generally available for clinical use in the 1990s. With the introduction of FISH studies, clinical geneticists had another tool beyond just karyotype analysis for identifying mutations in patients. When applied to patients with ASDs the most common single loci FISH findings were found in association with the chromosomal regions 2q, 15q, 17p, 22q11, and 22q13.

2.2.4. Chromosomal Microarray (CMA)

Around the year 2000, molecular cytogenetic techniques were introduced to clinical medicine. Chromosomal microarray (CMA) quickly became a powerful tool for identifying copy number variants (CNVs) in the human genome. When microarray studies are performed in patients with neurodevelopmental disabilities, a significant number of patients will have either small deletions or duplications identified. Currently microarray studies are still one of the highest yield diagnostic tests in these patients. In the process of the study of CNVs in ASDs, a handful of "ASD syndromes" has been identified. These syndromes are recognizable phenotypes that are associated with specific CNVs. These conditions have notable clinical features besides having ASD. Table 2 list a few of the most well-known ASD syndromes associated with small chromosomal deletions or duplications.

Table 2. "Autism Syndromes" Identified by Chromosomal Microarray.

Copy Number Variant	Incidence in Cohorts with ASDs	Eponym	Other Key Features (besides ASD)
1q21.1 del	1%	None	Congenital heart disease (30%)
2q22.3 del dup	<1%	Mowat-Wilson	Hirschprung disease, epilepsy, facial dysmorphisms
16p11.2 del/dup	1%	None	
17p11.2 dup	<1%	Potocki-Lupski	Hypotonia, slow growth, epilepsy
22q11.2 del	<1%	DiGeorge/Shprintzen	Multiple congenital anomalies
22q13.3 del	1%	Phelan-McDermid	Hypotonia, accelerated growth

Over the past 15 years, many studies have been published that have reported on the incidence of CNVs identified by microarrays in patients with ASDs. Cumulatively over 100 different clinically significant changes have been reported in patients with ASDs. Estimates of the prevalence of pathogenic CNVs in ASD range from 8% to 21%. Overall it has been concluded that CMA will identify a known pathogenic CNV in about 10% of all cases of ASD [12]. Prior to the introduction of microarray technology, the overall diagnostic yield for a complete evaluation of a person with ASD was accepted as being around 6%–12%. Thus the introduction of this one test modality greatly enhances the overall diagnostic yield. As will be discussed below, this high yield warrants making CMA a "first-tier" test in the etiologic evaluation of persons with ASD.

2.2.5. Key ASD Loci

One of the fascinating observations that can be made from the data presented in the above section is the consistency of the findings across studies regardless of the testing modality utilized. A review of this information readily identifies several "ASD hot spots". Specifically, certain loci jump out as consistently being identified by linkage, chromosomal studies, FISH and microarray studies. This aggregate information serves as a strong indicator for investigators that key genes that paly a strong role in the occurrence of ASD lie in these regions. Some of the strongest evidence points to strong genetic factors in the pathogenesis of ASD lie in chromosomal regions 2q, 7q, 15q11-13, 16p, 17q, 22q, Xp, and Xq. A more detailed listing of these areas of interest can be found in the ACMG practice guidelines reported in 2013 [12].

2.3. Clinical Genetic Evaluation of ASD

Not surprisingly, the number of requests for consultations by clinical geneticists with the referral indication of ASD has tremendously increased over the past 15 years. Of course this is in part due to the greatly increased reported incidence. In addition, there is an increased awareness among both the lay and medical communities of the recent rapid advances in genetics and genomics. As such, a large number of children with the diagnosis of ASD are being seen for an etiologic evaluation. However, many question the rationale for such evaluations. The question raised is simply "You can't cure the condition, so what good is it in figuring out what caused it?" This is an age old question that geneticists have answered almost since the inception of the discipline. It is critically important to note that an etiologic answer can be helpful to patients and their families in many different ways [30]. Examples of these would include:

(1) Genetic counseling—including providing recurrence risk information
(2) Counseling regarding the natural history of the condition
(3) Anticipation of a later associated co-morbid condition
(4) Prevention of secondary disorders
(5) Availability of prenatal diagnosis
(6) Access to public support systems
(7) Access to syndrome-specific support groups
(8) The reassurance of knowing "Why" in reliving the stress of the unknown
(9) The possibility of a specific treatment strategy—should one be available or developed in the future

2.3.1. Role of Dysmorphology/Clinical Genetics

When a patient is referred for a clinical genetic evaluation for ASD, many families want to know "Why" (discussed above) and "What will happen?" as clinical genetics is not a discipline familiar to many people [31]. A major skill set of a trained clinical geneticist is that of a "dysmorphology assessment". The geneticist has the ability to identify differences in morphology of patients and often to assemble the list of noted findings into a recognizable pattern [32]. The identification of such patterns can then aid in directing the rest of the diagnostic workup.

When a cohort of persons with ASD is evaluated, two sub-groups are easily identified [33]. An estimated 10%–20% of persons with ASD fit into the category of "complex" or syndromic' ASD. These are patients who, besides having ASD, are noted to have recognizable abnormalities of morphogenesis manifest as dysmorphic features, microcephaly, or cerebral dysgenesis [34]. As a whole, this group has a more guarded outcome with a higher degree of cognitive impairment and epilepsy and a greater occurrence of co-morbid medical problems. The second group (those with just ASD) has been referred to by several terms including "simple", "essential", "idiopathic" or "non-syndromic". As a whole this group has a higher heritability, more affected family members, and a higher male: female ratio than the complex group [33].

The initial part of the etiologic evaluation of ASD then is to determine whether or not the patient fits into the syndromic or non-syndromic category. If it is the former the next step is to see if a specific syndromic etiology can be identified. Sometimes this can be accomplished simply as part of the initial history and physical examination. Table 3 lists some of the most important syndromes associated with ASD that should be considered. A related question in this regards is when to do an etiologic evaluation for ASD in a patient who already has a known syndromic diagnosis. For some syndromes the known association with ASD is so strong that one can safely assume that the condition is indeed the cause of the ASD. In these cases no further evaluation is indicated. For other dysmorphic syndromes the reported association is not as convincing and a full evaluation should be considered. For a listing of these two groups the reader is referred to a recent review [12].

Table 3. Important Dysmorphic Syndromes to Consider in the Etiologic Evaluation of ASD.

22q11.2 Deletions (Including DiGeorge and Shprintzen Syndromes)
CHARGE syndrome
Fragile X syndrome
Opitz FG syndrome
Prader Willi/Angelman syndrome
PTEN associated disorders
Rett syndrome
Smith-Magenis syndrome
Sotos syndrome

In the discipline of dysmorphology, there is a well-known relationship between certain types of pigmentary abnormalities and neurodevelopmental disorders [35]. This association is felt to be due to the embryonic neuro-ectodermal cells that both populate the glial elements of the brain and give rise to the melanocytes in the skin. As such part of the dysmorphologic evaluation includes a careful cutaneous examination aided by the use of a Woods lamp to identify even subtle changes in skin pigmentation. In some cases abnormal pigmentation in association with ASD is indicative of a neuro-cutaneous syndrome. The strongest link here is tuberous sclerosis as a clearly identified cause of ASD [36]. Similar to the assumptions with certain dysmorphic syndromes, the co-existent diagnosis of ASD in a person with tuberous sclerosis does not warrant further investigation. Other patients may have pigmentary abnormalities noted in non-random patterns suggestive of somatic mosaicism [37]. In patients with ASD with these types of skin changes, a skin biopsy for cultured fibroblasts may be needed to identify the etiology (Figure 1).

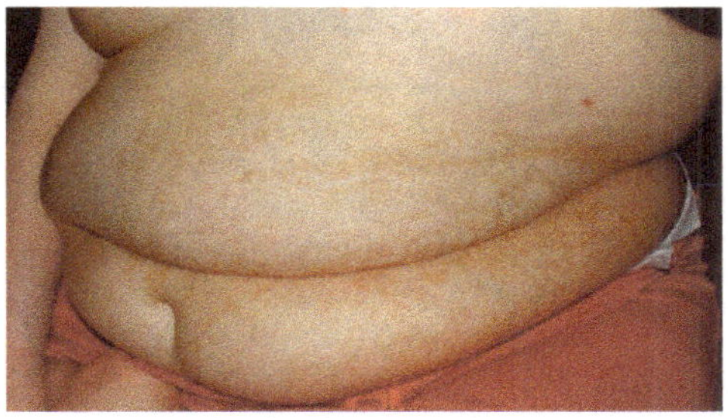

Figure 1. Pigmentary Changes in a Patient with Somatic Mosaicism. Note the linear pattern of the pigmentary changes.

Another important concept to consider is that of "expanded phenotypes". An expanded phenotype refers to the full range of phenotypes seen with mutations (variants) at a specific locus (gene). What is typically seen in the progress of clinical genetics is that mutations in a gene are initially reported in association with a known clinical disorder. Soon after this relationship is defined, the same or similar mutations at the same locus are identified with different phenotypes. Over time a broad range of phenotypes associated with changes in the same gene is defined. For example, mutations in the gene MeCP2 were initially described as the cause of Rett syndrome. As the range of the expanded phenotype was defined, mutations in MeCP2 have also been seen in patients with non-syndromic cognitive impairment and cerebral palsy [38]. Salient to these discussions, 4% of females with idiopathic ASD will have pathogenic mutations in MeCP2 [12]. This highlights a couple of very important concepts. First, it must be recognized that expanded phenotypes exist and need to be appreciated in a diagnostic workup. It is not readily intuitive that MeCP2 testing should be part of an ASD evaluation. The second point is critically important: genotype does not change phenotype. If the patient with ASD is found to have a MeCP2 mutation, the diagnosis does not change to Rett syndrome, simply the cause of the ASD has been identified.

As noted in an earlier section ASD exhibits a familial pattern of multifactorial inheritance. Thus multiple members of the same kindred may be found to have ASD. Even within families, a large degree of variable expression is typically seen. Family members with ASD may differ in their degree of social and cognitive impairment. They may also differ in co-morbid medical conditions. Along the lines of the discussions of expanded phenotypes the same causative mutation may produce different phenotypes. Thus as one investigates the kindred of a person with ASD, other neurodevelopmental and neurobehavioral phenotypes need to be considered. It is not uncommon for a family with a person with ASD to also have persons affected with other conditions. The incidence of other conditions such as depression, schizophrenia, anxiety and even Attention Deficit Hyperactivity Disorder (ADHD) are higher in relatives of persons with ASD [39]. Recent discoveries of other etiologies of ASD have identified some of these links. For example, a copy number variant—deletion 17q12—has been reported with both ASD and schizophrenia in the same family [40].

An interesting question has been raised in regard to the craniofacial appearance of patients with non-syndromic ASD. Specifically, is there an "ASD face"? In a non-published series of studies, myself and one other clinical geneticist reviewed the photographs of 33 children with ASD [41]. We then cataloged any dysmorphic features noted. These findings were tabulated for recurrent features. Those features are listed in Table 4. These photographs plus another 31 photographs of age and gender matched normal children without ASD were presented to three other clinical geneticists in a blinded fashion. They were asked to identify any of the features in the established list in the 64 photographs. Five of the nine features (shortened columella, thick scalp hair, lateral extension of the eyebrows, thickened ala nasae, and prominent nasal root) occurred more often (p value range 0.006–0.02) in the group of children with ASDs. While this is a very interesting observation, it is not clear what, if any, clinical significance it might have.

Table 4. Common Facial Features Noted in Non-syndromic ASD [41].

Thick scalp hair
Lateral extension of the eyebrows
Sloped forehead with prominent brow
Infraorbital hypoplasia
Prominent pre-maxilla
Short columella
Prominent (broad) nasal root
Thickened ala nasae
Prominent philtral ridges
Small ears

Bolded features were noted to occur statistically more often in children with ASD in a blinded study.

2.3.2. Guidelines for the Clinical Genetic Evaluation of ASD

With ever changing advancements in genetic testing technology comes the question of which test to use when. To answer this question the American College of Medical Genetics' Professional Practice and Guidelines Committee developed a framework to aid the geneticists in these evaluations. The initial guidelines were published in 2008 [42] and subsequently revised [12] to reflect further changes in testing technologies and emerging findings in the literature. This report proposes a "tiered" approach to the diagnostic evaluation. The earlier tiers use testing modalities that have a higher diagnostic yield and are less invasive/easier to accomplish than others. In brief, the most recent report notes an expected diagnostic yield of 30%–40%. That is to say that a specific mono-factorial etiology can be identified in patients with ASD in 30%–40% of the cases. For details of these evaluations the reader is referred to the reference provided [12]. While these numbers may seem low to many, they represent a significant increase from the 6%–12% yield reported prior to the year 2000. As such it is recommended that every person with the diagnosis of ASD be offered a clinical genetic consultation. That is not to say that every person with ASD will receive such a work up. Many details factor into the ultimate decision of whether to proceed with testing or not. It is crucial that these families receive detailed pre-evaluation informed consent. They need to understand what the tiered process entails, what the projected costs may be (especially in light of 3rd party payer policies), any potential risks of the testing and, of course, the diagnostic yield. Once the family understands what is involved that can decide whether such an evaluation is appropriate for them.

At the time of this writing, the 2013 guidelines are only a couple of years old. However, the ever advancing science of genetic testing is soon going to necessitate another revision of these recommendations. The advent of relatively inexpensive and rapid genomic testing methods has already been applied to cohorts of patients with ASD [43–46]. Currently a handful of publications have found that whole exome sequencing (WES) and whole genome sequencing (WGS) are expected to significantly increase the diagnostic yield when applied to patients with ASD. A summary of se current reports suggests that WES/WGS may identify an additional 10%–15% of causes of ASD. It is important to note that current sequencing techniques are not very good at detecting the larger copy number variants. Thus these techniques do not obviate the use of chromosomal microarray (CMA). Microarray testing itself is a high yield test identifying an etiology of ASD in about 10% of cases. Together WES and CMA alone may identify the cause of ASD in 20% of cases [45]. Finally, it is also important to note that the diagnostic yields are different for the 2 ASD sub-groups. Not surprisingly, the yield is higher (about double) in the complex/syndromic group.

2.3.3. What about Unknowns?

The recent advances in genetics and genomics have been extremely exciting and gratifying for clinical geneticists. Cases that have defied answers for literally decades are now being understood. As noted above, the increase in diagnostic yield for ASD from around 10% to almost 40% is indeed exciting. However, that still means that 60% of cases will have no answer despite a thorough evaluation. So the questions remain; "What about the unknown cases?" "What could possibly be the cause of the other cases?" We have already alluded to the fact that the application of WES/WGS testing to the diagnostic algorithm will undoubtedly increase the diagnostic yield. It is a little too early yet to definitively say by how much. However, consideration of the several early reports suggests that the application of these modalities in testing may increase the yield to 50%, maybe 60%. At that point it appears that the straight-forward, mono-factorial etiologies will mostly have been identified. The remainder of cases is likely due to more complicated mechanisms. Many such mechanisms have been suggested. Some of these would include:

(1) Mutations in non-coding DNA
(2) Epigenetic disorders including those fitting a MEGDI model—mixed genetics/epigenetics
(3) Multiple contributing loci
(4) Complex gene x gene interactions
(5) Snippets

It is highly likely that further insights into the etiology of ASD will come from investigations into these (and other) mechanisms.

2.4. Metabolic and Mitochondrial Disorders

Among the many genetic causes of ASD, metabolic and mitochondrial disorders deserve a separate discussion. These conditions have been the subject of vigorous debate among genetic and metabolic specialists over the past many years. The importance in sorting out the answers in these conditions lies in the commonly stated point that these conditions are "low yield, but high impact" [12]. Specifically, these conditions have the greatest potential for treatment among the myriad of causes of ASD. They may also present special situations of genetic susceptibility to environmental factors as well as project for a more progressive/deteriorative course.

Many metabolic (*i.e.*, inborn errors of metabolism) and mitochondrial conditions have been reported in association with ASD [47–49]. While some have been reported with the non-syndromic phenotype, many exhibit a variety of other features that stand as clues to the possible cause. Signs and symptoms that suggest such a possible etiology include poor linear growth, laboratory changes (anemia, acid-base abnormalities, lactic acidosis), cyclical vomiting, rashes, tone abnormalities, gastrointestinal problems, refractory epilepsy, changes in sensorium, neuro-regression outside of the typical speech loss of 18–24 months and microcephaly. An especially important situation to consider is developmental regression associated with fever or illness. This type of regression especially with recurrent episodes and multiple organ dysfunctions are clues to a possible mitochondrial disorder. These patients have been noted to have loss of speech after a febrile illness or immunizations with a subsequent encephalopathy. (It is particularly important to note that despite this association, immunizations do not cause ASD. There simply are no reputable studies which show any such plausible link.) In the evaluation of the etiology of a person with ASD, the presence of any of these clues should prompt an extended evaluation to include metabolic and mitochondrial causes.

3. Conclusions

A large body of solid and consistent studies identifies a clear genetic etiology of ASD. Like most complex phenotypes, ASD has a "multi-factorial etiology". This means that both genetic and environmental factors contribute to the overall phenotype. Heritability estimates suggest that genetic factors by far play the largest role. Clinical genetic evaluations currently can identify the cause of ASD in 30%–40% of cases. Early evidence suggests that the addition of genomic techniques to the standardly recommended testing protocol is likely to increase this yield to over 50%. Such evaluations should be offered to families after clear and careful informed consent. Knowledge of the cause of ASD can be very empowering for families. Simply knowing "Why" can be very reassuring and directive for many families. In addition, this provides genetic information for familial risks, prognosis, and awareness of possible associated conditions.

Most importantly, the identification of a genetic etiology of ASD is the first step in establishing "personalized medicine" for these patients. What is currently quite clear is that ASD is not a single condition. It is a collective of conditions with a common, strictly defined neuro-behavioral phenotype.

In reality it is "the ASDs" with literally hundreds of genetic causes identified. The delineation of specific subtypes (endo-phenotypes) of ASD will facilitate the investigation of differential responses to therapies. This coupled with a growing understanding of ASD as a disorder of the synapses should allow for the development of targeted therapies based upon a specific genetic diagnosis. While it is impossible to dogmatically state when this might happen, it is anticipated that this type of focused intervention is just on the horizon.

References

1. Folstein, S.E.; Piven, J. Etiology of autism: Genetic influences. *Pediatrics* **1991**, *87*, 767–773. [PubMed]
2. Schaefer, G.B.; Lutz, R.E. Diagnostic yield in the clinical genetic evaluation of autism spectrum disorders. *Genet. Med.* **2006**, *8*, 549–556. [PubMed]
3. Schaefer, G.B.; Mendelsohn, N.J. Genetics evaluation for the etiologic diagnosis of autism spectrum disorders. *Genet. Med.* **2008**, *10*, 4–12. [CrossRef] [PubMed]
4. Sandin, S.; Lichtenstein, P.; Kuja-Halkola, R.; Larsson, H.; Hultman, C.M.; Reichenberg, A. The familial risk of autism. *JAMA* **2014**, *311*, 1770–1777. [CrossRef] [PubMed]
5. Gronborg, T.K.; Schendel, D.E.; Parner, E.T. Recurrence of autism spectrum disorders in full- and half-siblings and trends over time: A population-based cohort study. *JAMA Pediatr.* **2013**, *167*, 947–953. [CrossRef] [PubMed]
6. Risch, N.; Hoffmann, T.J.; Anderson, M.; Croen, L.A.; Grether, J.K.; Windham, G.C. Familial recurrence of autism spectrum disorder: Evaluating genetic and environmental contributions. *Am. J. Psychiatry* **2014**, *171*, 1206–1213. [CrossRef] [PubMed]
7. Constantino, J.N.; Todorov, A.; Hilton, C.; Law, P.; Zhang, Y.; Molloy, E.; Fitzgerald, R.; Geschwind, D. Autism recurrence in half siblings: Strong support for genetic mechanisms of transmission in ASD. *Mol. Psychiatry* **2013**, *18*, 137–138. [CrossRef] [PubMed]
8. Jensen, C.M.; Steinhausen, H.C.; Lauritsen, M.B. Time trends over 16 years in incidence-rates of autism spectrum disorders across the lifespan based on nationwide Danish register data. *J. Autism Dev. Disord.* **2014**, *44*, 1808–1818. [CrossRef] [PubMed]
9. McCarthy, M. Autism diagnoses in the US rise by 30%, CDC reports. *BMJ* **2014**. [CrossRef] [PubMed]
10. Kahler, S.G. Increasing incidence of autism and genetics. Personal Communication, 2014.
11. Schaefer, G.B.; Thompson, J.N. *Medical Genetics: An Integrated Approach*; McGraw Hill Education: New York, NY, USA, 2014.
12. Schaefer, G.B.; Mendelsohn, N.J.; Professional Practice Guideline Committee. Clinical genetics evaluation in identifying the etiology of autism spectrum disorders: 2013 Guideline revisions. *Genet. Med.* **2013**, *15*, 399–407. [CrossRef] [PubMed]
13. Constantino, J.N.; Zhang, Y.; Frazier, T.; Abbacchi, A.M.; Law, P. Sibling recurrence and the genetic epidemiology of autism. *Am. J. Psychiatry* **2010**, *167*, 1349–1356. [CrossRef] [PubMed]
14. Ozonoff, S.; Young, G.S.; Carter, A.; Messinger, D.; Yirmiya, N.; Zwaigenbaum, L.; Bryson, S.; Carver, L.J.; Constantino, J.N.; Dobkins, K.; *et al.* Recurrence risk for autism spectrum disorders: A baby siblings research consortium study. *Pediatrics* **2011**, *128*, e488–e495. [CrossRef] [PubMed]
15. Werling, D.M.; Geschwind, D.H. Recurrence rates provide evidence for sex-differential, familial genetic liability for autism spectrum disorders in multiplex families and twins. *Mol. Autism* **2015**, *6*, 27. [CrossRef] [PubMed]
16. Wood, C.L.; Warnell, F.; Johnson, M.; Hames, A.; Pearce, M.S.; McConachie, H.; Parr, J.R. Evidence for ASD recurrence rates and reproductive stoppage from large UK ASD research family databases. *Autism Res.* **2015**, *8*, 73–81. [CrossRef] [PubMed]
17. Jacquemont, S.; Coe, B.P.; Hersch, M.; Duyzend, M.H.; Krumm, N.; Bergmann, S.; Beckmann, J.S.; Rosenfeld, J.A.; Eichler, E.E. A higher mutational burden in females supports a "female protective model" in neurodevelopmental disorders. *Am. J. Hum. Genet.* **2014**, *94*, 415–425. [CrossRef] [PubMed]
18. Ritvo, E.R.; Jorde, L.B.; Mason-Brothers, A.; Freeman, B.J.; Pingree, C.; Jones, M.B.; McMahon, W.M.; Petersen, P.B.; Jenson, W.R.; Mo, A. The UCLA-University of Utah epidemiologic survey of autism: Recurrence risk estimates and genetic counseling. *Am. J. Psychiatry* **1989**, *146*, 1032–1036. [PubMed]

19. Messinger, D.S.; Young, G.S.; Webb, S.J.; Ozonoff, S.; Bryson, S.E.; Carter, A.; Carver, L.; Charman, T.; Chawarska, K.; Curtin, S.; *et al.* Early sex differences are not autism-specific: A Baby Siblings Research Consortium (BSRC) study. *Mol. Autism* **2015**, *6*, 32. [CrossRef] [PubMed]
20. Frazier, T.W.; Youngstrom, E.A.; Hardan, A.Y.; Georgiades, S.; Constantino, J.N.; Eng, C. Quantitative autism symptom patterns recapitulate differential mechanisms of genetic transmission in single and multiple incidence families. *Mol. Autism* **2015**, *6*, 58. [CrossRef] [PubMed]
21. Grønborg, T.K.; Hansen, S.N.; Nielsen, S.V.; Skytthe, A.; Parner, E.T. Stoppage in Autism Spectrum Disorders. *J. Autism Dev. Disord.* **2015**, *45*, 3509–3519. [CrossRef] [PubMed]
22. Hoffmann, T.J.; Windham, G.C.; Anderson, M.; Croen, L.A.; Grether, J.K.; Risch, N. Evidence of reproductive stoppage in families with autism spectrum disorder: A large, population-based cohort study. *JAMA Psychiatry* **2014**, *71*, 943–951. [CrossRef] [PubMed]
23. Durkin, M.S.; Maenner, M.J.; Newschaffer, C.J.; Lee, L.C.; Cunniff, C.M.; Daniels, J.L.; Kirby, R.S.; Leavitt, L.; Miller, L.; Zahorodny, W.; *et al.* Advanced parental age and the risk of autism spectrum disorder. *Am. J. Epidemiol.* **2008**, *168*, 1268–1276. [CrossRef] [PubMed]
24. Schaefer, G.B.; Bodensteiner, J.B. Evaluation of the child with idiopathic mental retardation. *Pediatr. Clin. N. Am.* **1992**, *39*, 929–943.
25. Moeschler, J.B.; Shevell, M.; Committee on Genetics. Comprehensive evaluation of the child with intellectual disability or global developmental delays. *Pediatrics* **2014**, *134*, e903–e918. [CrossRef] [PubMed]
26. Hallmayer, J.; Hebert, J.M.; Spiker, D.; Lotspeich, L.; McMahon, W.M.; Peterse, P.B.; Nicholas, P.; Pingree, C.; Lin, A.A.; Cavalli-Sforza, L.L.; *et al.* Autism and the X chromosome: Multipoint sib-pair analysis. *Arch. Gen. Psychiatry* **1996**, *53*, 985–989. [CrossRef] [PubMed]
27. Reddy, K.S. Cytogenetic abnormalities and fragile-X syndrome in Autism Spectrum Disorder. *BMC Med. Genet.* **2005**, *6*, 3. [CrossRef] [PubMed]
28. Shevell, M.I.; Majnemer, A.; Rosenbaum, P.; Abrahamowicz, M. Etiologic yield of autistic spectrum disorders: A prospective study. *J. Child Neurol.* **2001**, *16*, 509–512. [CrossRef] [PubMed]
29. Weidmer-Mikhail, E.; Sheldon, S.; Ghaziuddin, M. Chromosomes in autism and related pervasive developmental disorders: A cytogenetic study. *J. Intellect. Disabil. Res.* **1998**, *42*, 8–12. [CrossRef] [PubMed]
30. Johnson, C.P.; Myers, S.M. Identification and evaluation of children with autism spectrum disorders. *Pediatrics* **2007**, *120*, 1183–1215. [CrossRef] [PubMed]
31. Carter, M.T.; Scherer, S.W. Autism spectrum disorder in the genetics clinic: A review. *Clin. Genet.* **2013**, *83*, 399–407. [CrossRef] [PubMed]
32. Jones, K.L.; Jones, M.C.; del Campo, M. *Smith's Recognizable Patterns of Human Malformations*, 7th ed.; Elsevier, Saunders: Philadelphia, PA, USA, 2013.
33. Miles, J.H.; Hillman, R.E. Value of a clinical morphology examination in autism. *Am. J. Med. Genet.* **2000**, *91*, 245–253. [CrossRef]
34. Wong, V.C.; Fung, C.K.; Wong, P.T. Use of dysmorphology for subgroup classification on autism spectrum disorder in Chinese children. *J. Autism Dev. Disord.* **2014**, *44*, 9–18. [CrossRef] [PubMed]
35. Thomas, I.T.; Frias, J.L.; Cantu, E.S.; Lafer, C.Z.; Flannery, D.B.; Graham, J.G., Jr. Association of pigmentary anomalies with chromosomal and genetic mosaicism and chimerism. *Am. J. Hum. Genet.* **1989**, *45*, 193–205. [PubMed]
36. Guo, X.; Tu, W.J.; Shi, X.D. Tuberous sclerosis complex in autism. *Iran J. Pediatr.* **2012**, *22*, 408–411. [PubMed]
37. Biesecker, L.G.; Spinner, N.B. A genomic view of mosaicism and human disease. *Nat. Rev. Genet.* **2013**, *14*, 307–320. [CrossRef] [PubMed]
38. Hoffbuhr, K.; Devaney, J.M.; LaFleur, B.; Sirianni, N.; Scacheri, C.; Giron, J.; Schuett, J.; Innis, J.; Marino, M.; Philippart, M.; *et al.* MeCP2 mutations in children with and without the phenotype of Rett syndrome. *Neurology* **2001**, *56*, 1486–1495. [CrossRef] [PubMed]
39. Eriksson, M.A.; Westerlund, J.; Anderlid, B.M.; Gillber, C.; Fernell, E. First-degree relatives of young children with autism spectrum disorders: Some gender aspects. *Res. Dev. Disabil.* **2012**, *33*, 1642–1648. [CrossRef] [PubMed]
40. Moreno-De-Luca, D.; SGENE Consortium. Deletion 17q12 is a recurrent copy number variant that confers high risk of autism and schizophrenia. *Am. J. Hum. Genet.* **2010**, *87*, 618–630. [CrossRef] [PubMed]
41. Schaefer, G.B. Personal Communication of unpublished data, 2015.

42. Schaefer, G.B.; Mendelsohn, N.J. Clinical genetics evaluation in identifying the etiology of autism spectrum disorders. *Genet. Med.* **2008**, *10*, 301–305. [CrossRef] [PubMed]
43. Butler, M.G.; Dasouki, M.J.; Zhou, X.P.; Talebizadeh, Z.; Brown, M.; Takahashi, T.N.; Miles, J.H.; Wang, C.H.; Stratton, R.; Pilarski, R.; *et al.* Subset of individuals with autism spectrum disorders and extreme macrocephaly associated with germline PTEN tumour suppressor gene mutations. *J. Med. Genet.* **2005**, *42*, 318–321. [CrossRef] [PubMed]
44. Jiang, Y.H.; Yuen, R.K.; Jin, X.; Wang, M.; Chen, N.; Wu, X.; Ju, J.; Mei, J.; Shi, Y.; He, M.; *et al.* Detection of clinically relevant genetic variants in autism spectrum disorder by whole-genome sequencing. *Am. J. Hum. Genet.* **2013**, *93*, 249–263. [CrossRef] [PubMed]
45. Tammimies, K.; Marshall, C.R.; Walker, S.; Kaur, G.; Thiruvahindrapuram, B.; Lionel, A.C.; Yuen, R.K.; Uddin, M.; Roberts, W.; Weksberg, R.; *et al.* Molecular diagnostic yield of chromosomal microarray analysis and whole-exome sequencing in children with Autism Spectrum Disorder. *JAMA* **2015**, *314*, 895–903. [CrossRef] [PubMed]
46. Yuen, R.K.; Thiruvahindrapuram, B.; Merico, D.; Walker, S.; Tammimies, K.; Hoang, N.; Chrysler, C.; Nalpathamkalam, T.; Pellecchia, G.; Liu, Y.; *et al.* Whole-genome sequencing of quartet families with autism spectrum disorder. *Nat. Med.* **2015**, *21*, 185–191. [CrossRef] [PubMed]
47. Haas, R.H. Autism and mitochondrial disease. *Dev. Disabil. Res. Rev.* **2010**, *16*, 144–153. [CrossRef] [PubMed]
48. Page, T. Metabolic approaches to the treatment of autism spectrum disorders. *J. Autism Dev. Disord.* **2000**, *30*, 463–469. [CrossRef] [PubMed]
49. Zecavati, N.; Spence, S.J. Neurometabolic disorders and dysfunction in autism spectrum disorders. *Curr. Neurol. Neurosci. Rep.* **2009**, *9*, 129–136. [CrossRef] [PubMed]

6

Participatory Art Activities Increase Salivary Oxytocin Secretion of ASD Children

Sanae Tanaka [1,†], Aiko Komagome [2,†], Aya Iguchi-Sherry [3,†], Akiko Nagasaka [4], Teruko Yuhi [5], Haruhiro Higashida [5], Maki Rooksby [6,7], Mitsuru Kikuchi [8], Oko Arai [2], Kana Minami [5,9], Takahiro Tsuji [5,10] and Chiharu Tsuji [5,*]

1 Division of Integrated Art and Sciences and Local Community Support, Research Center for Child Mental Development, Kanazawa University, Kanazawa 920-8640, Japan; tanakast@staff.kanazawa-u.ac.jp

2 The COI Site, Tokyo University of the Arts Tokyo 110-8714, Japan; komagome.aiko@ms.geidai.ac.jp (A.K.); tanaka.oko@ms.geidai.ac.jp (O.A.)

3 Artlink Central, Scotland FK8 1EA, UK; ayaiguchi@icloud.com

4 Department of Childhood Care and Education, Faculty of Social Work, Kinjo University, Hakusan 924-8511, Japan; ngsk-a4@kinjo.ac.jp

5 Department of Basic Research on Social Recognition, Research Center for Child Mental Development, Kanazawa University, Kanazawa 920-8640, Japan; y-teruko@med.kanazawa-u.ac.jp (T.Y.); haruhiro@med.kanazawa-u.ac.jp (H.H.); minami-k@staff.kanazawa-u.ac.jp (K.M.); tsuji-t@u-fukui.ac.jp (T.T.)

6 Adverse Childhood Experiences (ACE) Lab, Institute of Health and Wellbeing, University of Glasgow, Glasgow G12 8RZ, UK; Maki.Rooksby@glasgow.ac.uk

7 Social Brain in Action Lab, Institute of Neuroscience and Psychology, University of Glasgow, Glasgow G12 8QB, UK

8 Department of Psychiatry and Neurobiology, Graduate School of Medical Science, Kanazawa University, Kanazawa 920-8640, Japan; mitsuruk@med.kanazawa-u.ac.jp

9 Department of Health Development Nursing, Institute of Medical, Pharmaceutical and Health Sciences, Kanazawa University, Kanazawa 920-0942, Japan

10 Department of Ophthalmology, Faculty of Medical Sciences, University of Fukui, Fukui 910-1193, Japan

* Correspondence: ctsuji@med.kanazawa-u.ac.jp or higashida.c@gmail.com

† These authors contributed equally to this work.

Abstract: Autism spectrum disorder (ASD) occurs in 1 in 160 children worldwide. Individuals with ASD tend to be unique in the way that they comprehend themselves and others, as well as in the way that they interact and socialize, which can lead to challenges with social adaptation. There is currently no medication to improve the social deficit of children with ASD, and consequently, behavioral and complementary/alternative intervention plays an important role. In the present pilot study, we focused on the neuroendocrinological response to participatory art activities, which are known to have a positive effect on emotion, self-expression, sociability, and physical wellbeing. We collected saliva from 12 children with ASD and eight typically developed (TD) children before and after a visual art-based participatory art workshop to measure the levels of oxytocin, a neuropeptide involved in a wide range of social behaviors. We demonstrated that the rate of increase in salivary oxytocin following art activities in ASD children was significantly higher than that in TD children. In contrast, the change rate of salivary cortisol after participatory art activities was similar between the two groups. These results suggest that the beneficial effects of participatory art activities may be partially mediated by oxytocin release, and may have therapeutic potential for disorders involving social dysfunction.

Keywords: autism spectrum disorder; oxytocin; cortisol; group activity; stress; art

1. Introduction

Autism spectrum disorder (ASD) is estimated to occur in 1 in 160 children worldwide [1]; ASD tends to begin in childhood and tends to persist for life. Deficits in social skills are the defining symptoms of ASD [2], which greatly impede the ability of individuals to function in community settings throughout their lives. Effective social interaction is essential for building friendships and avoiding unnecessary aversive interactions with peers during the early years, while communication with coworkers and customers is necessary for successful work performance in adults. Thus, social deficits are likely to lead ASD individuals to socially withdraw or isolate. Despite these serious consequences of social deficits in ASD, there is currently no medication to attenuate the impairment of social behaviors.

Moreover, in many cases, depression and anxiety accompany social deficits and other core symptoms of ASD such as repetitive behaviors and a narrow range of interests [2,3]. Therefore, numerous studies have focused on the hypothalamic–pituitary–adrenal (HPA) axis with regard to level of cortisol (CORT), which is frequently used as a stress biomarker [4]. The HPA axis is a highly regulated system that enables stress adaptation and diurnal rhythm, and CORT is secreted when the HPA axis is activated [5,6]. Previous studies have shown that in children with ASD, diurnal rhythm of CORT differs from that in typically developed (TD) children; in addition, children with ASD exhibit hyperresponsive CORT secretions in the social evaluative context or social situations [7]. Dysfunction of the HPA axis has been shown to negatively affect mental health in TD children and children with ASD [3,8]. Thus, management of stress in children with ASD may help decrease the risk of a concurrent mental disorder.

Recently, the therapeutic use of oxytocin (OT), which has a diverse role in mammalian social behaviors, has gained increasing attention. OT is a nonapeptide produced by the hypothalamic neurons in the brain. It is released to the bloodstream to reach peripheral organs or within the hypothalamic and other limbic regions of the brain [9]. The involvement of OT in social recognition, selective social bonding, attachment, anxiety, and stress coping has been demonstrated in a considerable amount of animal studies [9,10]. Indeed, mice that have a deficiency in OT release, such as OT null mice or CD38 knockout mice, are unable to recognize previously encountered conspecifics [11,12]. Furthermore, OT has been shown to be important for mate-bonding in monogamous prairie voles [13], as well as in parent-infant bonding in prairie voles, sheep, and primates [14,15]. The OT system is activated in stressful, challenging, and threatening conditions, and functions to facilitate stress coping [9]. OT has also been implicated in human emotions and social behaviors [14]; for instance, physical interaction between parents and infants increase endogenous OT in both the mother and father, and the increase in OT correlates with the level of affectionate behavior of the mother [15].

Exogenously administrated OT has been shown to modulate social behaviors, stress, and anxiety both in healthy individuals and in patients with neuropsychiatric disorders [16]. Moreover, intranasal administration of OT affects social perception, in that it improves discrimination of facial expressions [17,18] and increases the gaze to the eye region [19]. In addition, OT application has been previously shown to enhance feelings of trust [20] and generosity [21]. Thus, the peripheral application of OT has been considered a potentially effective therapeutic treatment for autism and schizophrenia; however, recent clinical trials have shown conflicting results [22]. Although this is in part due to the underpowered design of the trials, the use of exogenous OT as a therapeutic agent is questionable given it has low blood brain barrier permeability and metabolic stability in plasma [23]. Therefore, nonpharmacological interventions that increase endogenous OT are needed to ameliorate the social deficit of patients with ASD, especially those that can effectively stimulate the release of OT in the brain.

The World Health Organization (WHO) recently summarized how art-based interventions can help improve health and well-being, as well as contribute to the prevention of, and recovery from mental and physical illness [24]. Participatory art, in which participants engage in creative activities during social interaction, is known for its beneficial effects on physical health and emotional well-being [25,26]. In fact, the experience of participating in the creative process itself improves mental health conditions, thereby building resilience, boosting social and communicative skills, and improving self-confidence [26–28]. More broadly, such activities are included in social prescribing, an emerging intervention modality that has garnered interest and attention in the academic and clinical communities [29]. With participatory art, as well as social prescribing, the approach to treating various health ailments is holistic and practical, whereby activities such as art, exercising, and gardening are supervised by trained specialists, many of whom are nonclinicians [30]. Because ASD is a neurodevelopmental disorder for which no specific intervention has been established, such activities may provide valuable coping mechanisms across the life span for those affected and their families.

In the present study, we conducted the preliminary study to investigate whether the salivary OT level changes following participation in visual art-based activities in ASD and typically developed (TD) children. Because ASD individuals often struggle to adapt to changes or a new environment, we also measured the salivary CORT level, which is often used as a psychological stress biomarker. To the best of our knowledge, this is the first study to assess the neuroendocrinological changes in individuals who have taken part in participatory art activities.

2. Materials and Methods

2.1. Participants

For this study, 10 TD children (aged 8–9 years) and 13 children (8–13 years) with ASD were recruited. All the children were volunteers; however, all children did not participate in all five sessions of visual art-based participatory workshops, and the data from children who participated less than twice were not used for analysis. Four boys and 4 girls, aged 8–9 years, who were TD and 11 boys and 1 girl, aged 8–13 years, who had ASD were analyzed (Table 1). ASD was diagnosed by children's psychiatrists or pediatricians, who used criteria from the American Psychiatric Association's Diagnostic and Statistical Manual of Mental Disorders, Fourth Edition, Text Revision (DSM-IV-TR) or Fifth Edition (DSM-V) or from the International Statistical Classification of Diseases and Related Health Problems, 10th edition (ICD-10). The evaluations included IQ testing, behavioral observation, and questionnaires; depending on the child, the Childhood Autism Rating Scale (CARS), Autism Diagnostic Observation Schedule (ADOS), Diagnostic Interview for Social and Communication Disorders (DISCO), or Pervasive Developmental Disorders Autism Society Japan Rating Scale (PARS) was used.

Table 1. Age, mean scores of Early Symptomatic Syndromes Eliciting Neurodevelopmental Clinical Examinations-Questionnaire (ESSENCE-Q) and education for each group of children.

	TD	ASD
Numbers	8 (male: 4, female: 4)	12 (male: 11, female: 1)
Age	96–119 months mean: 107, SD: 6.9	113–162 months mean: 135, SD: 16.7
ESSENCE-Q	Yes: 0.4, Maybe/A Little: 0.1/0.3	Yes: 2.83, Maybe/A Little: 1.58/2.83
Education	regular class	regular or special needs classes or special education support classes

The participants' parents were asked to respond to the Early Symptomatic Syndromes Eliciting Neurodevelopmental Clinical Examinations-Questionnaire (ESSENCE-Q) in order to screen the current status of TD children and children with ASD. The ESSENCE-Q is a brief screening questionnaire established specifically for the purpose of shortening the identification process of a wide variety of neurodevelopmental problems [31].

Among the children with ASD, 10 were enrolled in either regular or special needs classes at local schools in Japan. The other 2 children in this group were students at special support education schools.

2.2. Ethics Statement

The study was approved as a noninvasive medical study by Kanazawa University Graduate School of Medicine in 2018 (approval number #2790-2). The study was performed according to the Declaration of Helsinki and the Ethical Guidelines for Clinical Studies of the Ministry of Health, Labor and Welfare of Japan. After the children and their parents had been given a complete explanation of the study, they provided written informed consent. The participants were informed that they could choose not to supply their saliva on each occasion, even after agreeing to participate in the study.

2.3. Visual Art-Based Participatory Art Workshop

During the visual art-based participatory art workshops, participants created their own original stories and made characters and props with different kind of materials. Then participants used the Smoovie application on an iPad (Apple, Inc., Cupertino, CA, USA) to make their own movies with short stop-motion animation. The subjects of their stories varied from their everyday life to the objects that surrounded them; the theme of the project was fully participant led. The aim of this workshop was to let the participants express themselves as freely as possible and not to make them feel as if they were working on a school task or a job. We provided arts and crafts materials that stimulated different senses—paper (colored, textured, plain; different weights of paper), fabric (patterned, textured), tape (washi tape, colored tape), soft clay (colored, neutral), soft construction material (bubble wrap, wrapping material, cardboard), glue (hot glue gun, glue stick), paint, colored pens, and decorative material (sequins, gems, buttons).

The facilitators and supporters of the art workshop set up a comfortable venue, prepared the tools, explained how to use them, and provided a variety of materials. The art workshops conducted in this study were facilitated by a visual artist and supported by the art faculty, students from the University of the Arts, and a staff member who is licensed in special education. During the activity, the organizers interacted with the participants as and when appropriate and encouraged them throughout the creative processes of generating ideas and producing animations.

2.4. Assessment

The visual art-based participatory art workshops were held five times between 22 July–10 August in 2018 and 2019. The workshops in 2018 were held from 14:30–16:30, while those in 2019 were held from 14:00–15:30. Sessions for TD children and ASD children were organized separately. The saliva samples were collected within 10 min of arrival, and just after the participatory art was finished. The percentage of salivary OT or CORT for each session was determined as (concentration after session/concentration before session) × 100. The total number of sessions analyzed before and after the art workshop and the percentage after the workshops for TD and ASD group were 33 and 42, respectively. The personal average percentage after the workshops was calculated as a mean percentage of all the sessions that each child participated (8 subjects for TD group and 12 subjects for ASD group).

2.5. Saliva Collection and Analysis

The saliva samples (0.3–1.0 mL) were collected in a sterile 50 mL polypropylene tube (Greiner Bio-one Co. Ltd., Tokyo, Japan), and were immediately placed in ice for storage at −20 °C. Three to 5 days later, the samples were thawed and centrifuged twice at 4 °C at 1500× g for 10 min. The samples were divided into 1.5-mL microtubes, each containing 100 μL, and kept again at −80 °C until required for the assay. The salivary OT level was measured using a 96-plate commercial OT-ELISA kit (Enzo Life Sciences, Farmingdale, NY, USA), as described previously [32–34]. The measurements were performed in duplicate. Samples (100 μL) without fractionation were treated according to the manufacturer's instructions. The optical density of the samples and standards was measured at wavelengths of 405 nm by a microplate reader (Bio-Rad, Richmond, CA, USA). The salivary CORT level was measured using a cortisol enzyme immunoassay kit (Salimetrics, State College, PA, USA) as previously described [35].

Samples (25 μL) were treated according to the manufacturer's instructions. The optical density of the samples and standards were measured at wavelengths of 450 nm by a microplate reader (Bio-Rad, Richmond, CA, USA). Measurements were performed in duplicate. Sample concentrations were calculated according to the relevant standard curve. The intraassay and interassay coefficients were <12.4% and <12.1%, respectively.

2.6. *Statistical Analysis*

Statistical analysis was performed using Prism 8 software (GraphPad Software Inc., San Diego, CA, USA). Wilcoxon rank-sum tests were used to compare the levels of salivary OT or CORT of TD children with children with ASD before and after each visual art-based workshop session. The Mann–Whitney *U* test was used to compare the average percentage of OT or CORT of TD children with children with ASD after each session. Two-tailed student's *t* test was used to assess the personal average percentage of salivary OT or CORT after each session in which a child participated. All data were calculated as means ± standard errors of the means. In all analyses, $p < 0.05$ was considered statistically significant.

3. Results

The salivary OT level after each session of visual art-based participatory art workshop showed a significant decrease in the TD group (before, 161.5 ± 19.4 pg/mL, after 136.6 ± 16.0 pg/mL; $p = 0.015$) (Figure 1a), whereas there was no significant difference in the ASD group (before 167.9 ± 17.9 pg/mL, after 175.5 ± 16.4 pg/mL; $p = 0.880$) (Figure 1a). However, the average percentage of salivary OT after each session of the ASD group was significantly higher than that of the TD group (TD, 90.8% ± 6.9%; ASD, 127.9% ± 11.8%; $p = 0.024$) (Figure 1b). Also, the personal average percentage of salivary OT after each participated session of the ASD group was significantly higher than that of the TD group (TD, 88.4% ± 4.8%; ASD, 134.5% ± 15.6%; $p = 0.03$) (Figure 1c).

The concentrations of salivary cortisol were not significantly different before and after the participatory art workshop in either the TD or ASD group (Figure 2a). No significant difference was observed between the TD and ASD groups with regards to the average percentage after each session, and/or in the average percentage of personal salivary CORT after each session (Figure 2b,c).

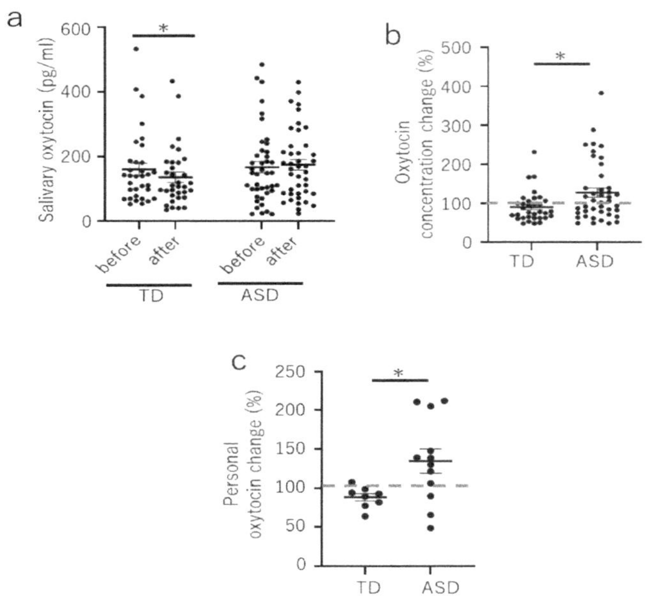

Figure 1. The salivary oxytocin levels before and after participatory art workshops. (**a**). Salivary oxytocin level before and after each session in the typically developed (TD) children and those with autism spectrum disorder (ASD). Note that not all children attended all five sessions of the art workshop (total number of sessions analyzed: 33 for the TD children and 42 for the children with ASD). (**b**). Percentage of salivary oxytocin in the TD children and those with ASD after each session. Note that not all children attended all five sessions of the art workshop (total number of sessions analyzed—33 for the TD children and 42 for the children with ASD). (**c**). Personal average percentage of salivary oxytocin level after each session in the TD and ASD groups (number of children assessed: TD, $n = 8$; ASD, $n = 12$). Data are mean ± sem. * $p < 0.05$.

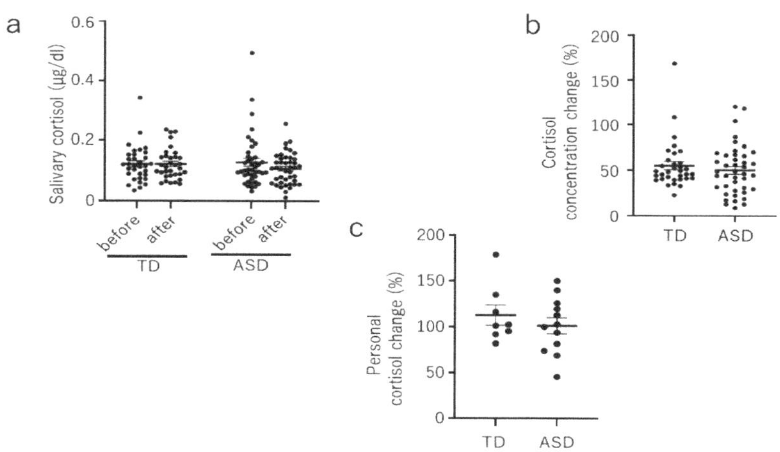

Figure 2. The salivary cortisol level before and after participatory art workshop. (**a**). Salivary cortisol level before and after each session in the TD and ASD groups. Note that not all children attended all five sessions of the art workshop (total number of sessions analyzed—33 for the TD children and 42 for the children with ASD). (**b**). Percentage of salivary cortisol after each session in the TD and ASD groups. Note that not all children attended all five sessions of the art workshop (total number of sessions analyzed—33 for the TD children and 42 for the children with ASD). (**c**). Personal average percentage of salivary cortisol level after each session in the TD and ASD groups (number of children assessed: TD, $n = 8$; ASD, $n = 12$). Data are mean ± sem.

4. Discussion

The current trial was a pioneering study to assess salivary OT and CORT concentrations in ASD and TD children in response to a positive social activity, participatory arts. Although we could not detect a statistical difference in OT levels after each session in the ASD group, the average percentage of salivary OT after each session, and the personal average percentage of salivary OT after each session were increased in ASD children. However, no significant difference in the cortisol level was detected before and after participatory art activities in either the ASD or TD group. Since the cortisol level did not change significantly during the participatory art activities, we suggest that OT is released as a result of positive social activities, rather than a response to stress.

Because all the children participated voluntarily in the visual art-based participatory art workshop, the TD children were expected not to feel anxious or stressed about their participation, and we initially assumed that their OT levels would increase after participatory art activities. However, the OT level decreased instead. As the CORT level in TD children did not change significantly, the decrease in the OT level may not be a result of the stress response. Because both groups of children enjoyed the art activities, the results suggest that the TD children may have felt driven to complete their artwork, which corresponded with a decrease in the OT level afterwards. A decrease in OT levels has been suggested to reflect a reduction in social qualities of attention or, more broadly, in social interaction [36]. In our case, the decrease in the TD group may correspond to a shift in attention upon completion of their work. The children with ASD, on the other hand, required the experience to form a part of their routine over the course of the workshop attendance and may have gained more pleasure out of the process of creativity. It has been reported that attention systems are disrupted and atypical in children with ASD [37]. It is possible that our participants with ASD required more sessions than the TD children in order to understand the structure of the workshops and to focus on their creative activities. Alternatively, there might have been an increase in the OT level in TD children during the activities, but the time course may have differed from that observed in the children with ASD. Larger sample sizes and further follow up will allow a better understanding of the process.

Our preliminary study had several limitations. First, the study was designed to examine the immediate OT response of participatory art activity. Although the percentage change of OT level was increased in ASD children, we failed to show a statistical difference in the salivary OT level before and after each of the workshop due to the modest sample size and the large variance in the OT concentration. Therefore, it is necessary to conduct a further trial with a larger sample size of ASD children to obtain reliable data. Second, we did not include any psychological, emotional, or behavioral measurement that may be relevant to the OT response. As shown in Figure 1c, there is a diverse variability in the personal percentage change in ASD children compared to the TD children; as a result, we need to conduct a further study to elucidate the correlation between the traits of children and the OT responsiveness to participatory art activities. Third, it is worth pointing out that our study did not include a control condition in order to disentangle the potential effect of participatory art from other more generic activities involving crafting or animation making. Such a control could have simply involved being in the premise for the workshop sessions, as in a wait-list group. However, each workshop typically required the entire duration of the children's visit in terms of staff cover and their families who need to fit in taking and collecting their children. Staffs and participants were all volunteers and we faced several practical difficulties which prevented from adding this important aspect to our design this time. We will be mindful for exploring options for adding the control in our future work.

The WHO recently summarized how art interventions can help improve health and well-being, and can help to prevent both mental and physical illness [24]. They also stated that while art is conceptually difficult to define, it is important to verify the effectiveness of art. Indeed, although a wide variety of studies use diverse methodologies, these are often based on psychological tests or subjective feedback. Our study aimed to capture the fluctuations in the neuroendocrine response to participatory art activities. In the future study, we will investigate the association of the neuroendocrine response and the traits of children in order to elucidate for whom and in what aspect participatory art activities can be effective. We will also evaluate the effectiveness of participatory arts activities in the long term. Further, experience in multi-sensory processing has been showing some promising results in children with autism spectrum disorders [38]. Given that crafting and creative activities are familiar and popular in typical as well as atypical development, it would be an important agenda to study the therapeutic role of multi-sensory experiences involved in activities such as participatory art. Ultimately, we would like to utilize our research findings related to the use of neuroendocrine responses in combination with psychological, emotional, or behavioral measurement to establish a method to verify the effectiveness of participatory art activities.

In the current study, ELISA was used to measure the saliva OT concentrations; however, with this technique, there remains the issue of antibody specificity. The antibody may not only detect the free form of the target analyte, but different forms, such as precursors and metabolites, or a form within other protein complexes. These phenomena may partially explain the differences in values observed between different ELISA kits, as well as between ELISA and HPLC-MS or radio immunoassay. Indeed, our detected OT concentration range is one digit higher than that reported by other studies [15,39,40]. However, since we have detected the relative change in salivary OT in the context of physical interaction and/or in social interaction [32,34,41], although the values may not be reflecting the absolute physiological value of free OT, the relative change in monitored values are likely to be comparable.

In conclusion, the current experiment was designed to assess salivary OT and CORT concentrations in ASD and TD children in response to participation in visual art-based activities, since art is known to improve mental and physical health and overall quality of life. We demonstrated increased OT release after participatory art activities that was unrelated to the stress response. Thus, our case study is the first to show the biological link between the social experience of participatory art and its positive psychosocial effects.

Author Contributions: S.T., A.K., A.I.-S. have contributed equally to this work. S.T. and C.T. recruited the participants; S.T., A.K., A.I.-S., M.R. and C.T. conceived and designed the experiments; S.T., A.K., A.I.-S., M.R., A.N., K.M., M.K., and O.A. performed and organized art workshop; T.Y. performed saliva assay; T.T., C.T., H.H. analyzed the data and data interpretation; H.H. contributed to provide analytical tools; C.T. prepared the initial draft and M.R. and C.T. revised the manuscript. All authors have read and agreed to the published version of the manuscript.

References

1. Elsabbagh, M.; Divan, G.; Koh, Y.J.; Kim, Y.S.; Kauchali, S.; Marcin, C.; Montiel-Nava, C.; Patel, V.; Paula, C.S.; Wang, C.; et al. Global prevalence of autism and other pervasive developmental disorders. *Autism Res.* **2012**, *5*, 160–179. [CrossRef]
2. Geschwind, D.H. Advances in autism. *Annu. Rev. Med.* **2009**, *60*, 367–380. [CrossRef]
3. Simonoff, E.; Pickles, A.; Charman, T.; Chandler, S.; Loucas, T.; Baird, G. Psychiatric disorders in children with autism spectrum disorders: Prevalence, comorbidity, and associated factors in a population-derived sample. *J. Am. Acad. Child. Adolesc. Psychiatry* **2008**, *47*, 921–929. [CrossRef]
4. Hellhammer, D.H.; Wust, S.; Kudielka, B.M. Salivary cortisol as a biomarker in stress research. *Psychoneuroendocrinology* **2009**, *34*, 163–171. [CrossRef]
5. Chrousos, G.P. Stress and disorders of the stress system. *Nat. Rev. Endocrinol.* **2009**, *5*, 374–381. [CrossRef]
6. de Kloet, E.R.; Joels, M.; Holsboer, F. Stress and the brain: From adaptation to disease. *Nat. Rev. Neurosci.* **2005**, *6*, 463–475. [CrossRef]
7. Taylor, J.L.; Corbett, B.A. A review of rhythm and responsiveness of cortisol in individuals with autism spectrum disorders. *Psychoneuroendocrinology* **2014**, *49*, 207–228. [CrossRef]
8. Shirtcliff, E.A.; Essex, M.J. Concurrent and Longitudinal Associations of Basal and Diurnal Cortisol with Mental Health Symptoms in Early Adolescence. *Dev. Psychobiol.* **2008**, *50*, 690–703. [CrossRef]
9. Jurek, B.; Neumann, I.D. The Oxytocin Receptor: From Intracellular Signaling to Behavior. *Physiol. Rev.* **2018**, *98*, 1805–1908. [CrossRef]
10. Modi, M.E.; Young, L.J. The oxytocin system in drug discovery for autism: Animal models and novel therapeutic strategies. *Horm. Behav.* **2012**, *61*, 340–350. [CrossRef]

11. Ferguson, J.N.; Young, L.J.; Hearn, E.F.; Matzuk, M.M.; Insel, T.R.; Winslow, J.T. Social amnesia in mice lacking the oxytocin gene. *Nat. Genet.* **2000**, *25*, 284–288. [CrossRef]
12. Jin, D.; Liu, H.X.; Hirai, H.; Torashima, T.; Nagai, T.; Lopatina, O.; Shnayder, N.A.; Yamada, K.; Noda, M.; Seike, T.; et al. CD38 is critical for social behaviour by regulating oxytocin secretion. *Nature* **2007**, *446*, 41–45. [CrossRef]
13. Tabbaa, M.; Paedae, B.; Liu, Y.; Wang, Z. Neuropeptide Regulation of Social Attachment: The Prairie Vole Model. *Compr. Physiol.* **2016**, *7*, 81–104. [CrossRef]
14. Feldman, R. Oxytocin and social affiliation in humans. *Horm. Behav.* **2012**, *61*, 380–391. [CrossRef]
15. Feldman, R.; Gordon, I.; Schneiderman, I.; Weisman, O.; Zagoory-Sharon, O. Natural variations in maternal and paternal care are associated with systematic changes in oxytocin following parent-infant contact. *Psychoneuroendocrinology* **2010**, *35*, 1133–1141. [CrossRef]
16. Andari, E.; Hurlemann, R.; Young, L.J. A Precision Medicine Approach to Oxytocin Trials. *Curr. Top. Behav. Neurosci.* **2018**, *35*, 559–590. [CrossRef]
17. Domes, G.; Heinrichs, M.; Michel, A.; Berger, C.; Herpertz, S.C. Oxytocin improves "mind-reading" in humans. *Biol. Psychiatry* **2007**, *61*, 731–733. [CrossRef]
18. Savaskan, E.; Ehrhardt, R.; Schulz, A.; Walter, M.; Schachinger, H. Post-learning intranasal oxytocin modulates human memory for facial identity. *Psychoneuroendocrinology* **2008**, *33*, 368–374. [CrossRef]
19. Yamasue, H.; Domes, G. Oxytocin and Autism Spectrum Disorders. *Curr. Top. Behav. Neurosci.* **2018**, *35*, 449–465. [CrossRef]
20. Kosfeld, M.; Heinrichs, M.; Zak, P.J.; Fischbacher, U.; Fehr, E. Oxytocin increases trust in humans. *Nature* **2005**, *435*, 673–676. [CrossRef]
21. Zak, P.J.; Stanton, A.A.; Ahmadi, S. Oxytocin increases generosity in humans. *PLoS ONE* **2007**, *2*, e1128. [CrossRef]
22. Young, L.J.; Barrett, C.E. Neuroscience. Can oxytocin treat autism? *Science* **2015**, *347*, 825–826. [CrossRef]
23. Gulliver, D.; Werry, E.; Reekie, T.A.; Katte, T.A.; Jorgensen, W.; Kassiou, M. Targeting the Oxytocin System: New Pharmacotherapeutic Approaches. *Trends Pharmacol. Sci.* **2019**, *40*, 22–37. [CrossRef]
24. Fancourt, D.; Finn, S. *What is the Evidence on the Role of the Arts in Improving Health and Well-Being? A Scoping Review*; (Health Evidence Network (HEN) Synthesis Report 67); WHO Regional Office for Europe: Copenhagen, Denmark, 2019.
25. Hacking, S.; Secker, J.; Kent, L.; Shenton, J.; Spandler, H. Mental health and arts participation: The state of the art in England. *J. R Soc. Promot. Health* **2006**, *126*, 121–127. [CrossRef]
26. Bone, T.A. Art and Mental Health Recovery: Evaluating the Impact of a Community-Based Participatory Arts Program through Artist Voices. *Community Ment Health J.* **2018**, *54*, 1180–1188. [CrossRef]
27. Hacking, S.; Secker, J.; Spandler, H.; Kent, L.; Shenton, J. Evaluating the impact of participatory art projects for people with mental health needs. *Health Soc. Care Community* **2008**, *16*, 638–648. [CrossRef]
28. Stickley, T.; Wright, N.; Slade, M. The art of recovery: Outcomes from participatory arts activities for people using mental health services. *J. Ment. Health* **2018**, *27*, 367–373. [CrossRef]
29. Bickerdike, L.; Booth, A.; Wilson, P.M.; Farley, K.; Wright, K. Social prescribing: Less rhetoric and more reality. A systematic review of the evidence. *BMJ Open* **2017**, *7*, e013384. [CrossRef]
30. Toma, M.; Morris, J.; Kelly, C.; Jinal-Snape, D. *The Impact of Art Attendance and Participation on Health and Wellbeing: Systematic Literature Review (Work Package 1)*; Glasgow Centre for Population Health: Glasgow, UK, 2014.
31. Hatakenaka, Y.; Fernell, E.; Sakaguchi, M.; Ninomiya, H.; Fukunaga, I.; Gillberg, C. ESSENCE-Q-a first clinical validation study of a new screening questionnaire for young children with suspected neurodevelopmental problems in south Japan. *Neuropsychiatr. Dis. Treat.* **2016**, *12*, 1739–1746. [CrossRef]
32. Tsuji, S.; Yuhi, T.; Furuhara, K.; Ohta, S.; Shimizu, Y.; Higashida, H. Salivary oxytocin concentrations in seven boys with autism spectrum disorder received massage from their mothers: A pilot study. *Front. Psychiatry* **2015**, *6*, 58. [CrossRef]
33. MacLean, E.L.; Gesquiere, L.R.; Gee, N.; Levy, K.; Martin, W.L.; Carter, C.S. Validation of salivary oxytocin and vasopressin as biomarkers in domestic dogs. *J. Neurosci. Methods* **2018**, *293*, 67–76. [CrossRef]
34. Yuhi, T.; Ise, K.; Iwashina, K.; Terao, N.; Yoshioka, S.; Shomura, K.; Maehara, T.; Yazaki, A.; Koichi, K.; Furuhara, K.; et al. Sex Differences in Salivary Oxytocin and Cortisol Concentration Changes during Cooking in a Small Group. *Behav. Sci.* **2018**, *8*, 101. [CrossRef]

35. Kumazaki, H.; Warren, Z.; Corbett, B.A.; Yoshikawa, Y.; Matsumoto, Y.; Higashida, H.; Yuhi, T.; Ikeda, T.; Ishiguro, H.; Kikuchi, M. Android Robot-Mediated Mock Job Interview Sessions for Young Adults with Autism Spectrum Disorder: A Pilot Study. *Front. Psychiatry* **2017**, *8*. [CrossRef]
36. Nishizato, M.; Fujisawa, T.X.; Kosaka, H.; Tomoda, A. Developmental changes in social attention and oxytocin levels in infants and children. *Sci. Rep. UK* **2017**, *7*. [CrossRef]
37. Guillon, Q.; Hadjikhani, N.; Baduel, S.; Roge, B. Visual social attention in autism spectrum disorder: Insights from eye tracking studies. *Neurosci. Biobehav. Rev.* **2014**, *42*, 279–297. [CrossRef]
38. Case-Smith, J.; Weaver, L.L.; Fristad, M.A. A systematic review of sensory processing interventions for children with autism spectrum disorders. *Autism* **2015**, *19*, 133–148. [CrossRef]
39. Schladt, T.M.; Nordmann, G.C.; Emilius, R.; Kudielka, B.M.; de Jong, T.R.; Neumann, I.D. Choir versus Solo Singing: Effects on Mood, and Salivary Oxytocin and Cortisol Concentrations. *Front. Hum. Neurosci.* **2017**, *11*, 430. [CrossRef]
40. Jong, T.R.; Menon, R.; Bludau, A.; Grund, T.; Biermeier, V.; Klampfl, S.M.; Jurek, B.; Bosch, O.J.; Hellhammer, J.; Neumann, I.D. Salivary oxytocin concentrations in response to running, sexual self-stimulation, breastfeeding and the TSST: The Regensburg Oxytocin Challenge (ROC) study. *Psychoneuroendocrinology* **2015**, *62*, 381–388. [CrossRef]
41. Yuhi, T.; Kyuta, H.; Mori, H.A.; Murakami, C.; Furuhara, K.; Okuno, M.; Takahashi, M.; Fuji, D.; Higashida, H. Salivary Oxytocin Concentration Changes during a Group Drumming Intervention for Maltreated School Children. *Brain Sci.* **2017**, *7*, 152. [CrossRef]

7

Clock Genes and Altered Sleep–Wake Rhythms: Their Role in the Development of Psychiatric Disorders

Annaëlle Charrier [1,*], Bertrand Olliac [2,3], Pierre Roubertoux [4] and Sylvie Tordjman [1,5]

1 Pôle Hospitalo-Universitaire de Psychiatrie de l'Enfant et de l'Adolescent (PHUPEA), Université de Rennes 1, Centre Hospitalier Guillaume-Régnier, 154 Rue de Châtillon, Rennes 35000, France; s.tordjman@yahoo.fr
2 Pôle Universitaire de Psychiatrie de l'Enfant et de l'Adolescent, Centre Hospitalier Esquirol, Limoges 87025, France; Bertrand.Olliac@chu-limoges.fr
3 INSERM, U1094, Tropical Neuroepidemiology, Limoges 87000, France
4 Aix Marseille Université, INSERM, GMGF UMR_S 910, Marseille 13385, France; pierre.roubertoux@univ-amu.fr
5 Laboratoire Psychologie de la Perception (LPP), Université Paris Descartes, CNRS UMR 8158, Paris 75270, France
* Correspondence: a.charrier@ch-guillaumeregnier.fr

Academic Editor: Merlin G. Butler

Abstract: In mammals, the circadian clocks network (central and peripheral oscillators) controls circadian rhythms and orchestrates the expression of a range of downstream genes, allowing the organism to anticipate and adapt to environmental changes. Beyond their role in circadian rhythms, several studies have highlighted that circadian clock genes may have a more widespread physiological effect on cognition, mood, and reward-related behaviors. Furthermore, single nucleotide polymorphisms in core circadian clock genes have been associated with psychiatric disorders (such as autism spectrum disorder, schizophrenia, anxiety disorders, major depressive disorder, bipolar disorder, and attention deficit hyperactivity disorder). However, the underlying mechanisms of these associations remain to be ascertained and the cause–effect relationships are not clearly established. The objective of this article is to clarify the role of clock genes and altered sleep–wake rhythms in the development of psychiatric disorders (sleep problems are often observed at early onset of psychiatric disorders). First, the molecular mechanisms of circadian rhythms are described. Then, the relationships between disrupted circadian rhythms, including sleep–wake rhythms, and psychiatric disorders are discussed. Further research may open interesting perspectives with promising avenues for early detection and therapeutic intervention in psychiatric disorders.

Keywords: clock genes; circadian rhythm; circadian clocks network; synchronization of oscillators; sleep-wake rhythm; psychiatric disorders; schizophrenia; autism spectrum disorder; mood disorders; attention deficit hyperactivity disorder

1. Introduction: Circadian Rhythms and Their Molecular Mechanisms

The function of the body is subject to different biological rhythms, the circadian one being keyed to a cycle of a 24-h day corresponding approximately to the 24-h light/dark cycle of the Earth's rotation. In fact, the range of the internal clock period for healthy adults is 24 h and 11 $\pm$ 16 min but it is set back to a 24-h cycle each day by exposure to morning light and to external clocks [1]. This rhythm regulates most of our biological and behavioral functions. Its dysregulation leads to sleep disorders and major physiological disturbances. In psychiatric disorders, sleep problems (especially reduced total sleep with insomnia, longer sleep latency, nocturnal and early morning awakenings) are highly prevalent symptoms. Insomnia is the most frequent sleep problem reported in psychiatric disorders [2]. In autism, a prevalence of insomnia from 50% to 80% has been reported [3–6] compared to 9–50% in age-matched typically developing children [7–11]. However, the interpretation of these results has to take into consideration the high prevalence of insomnia (30%) in typically developing individuals [12–14]. It is noteworthy that sleep disorders are not specific to autism spectrum disorder (ASD) given that they are observed in ASD individuals with intellectual disability (ID), ID individuals without ASD, and individuals with brain injury as well as ID, suggesting a possible overlap between ASD and ID. Concerning schizophrenia, a genome-wide association study (GWAS) shows genetic correlations between sleep disorders and schizophrenia and between the late evening chronotype and risk of schizophrenia [15]. No rigorous study of prevalence of sleep disorders was conducted in bipolar spectrum disorder and depression-related disorders but altered patterns of clock genes were reported in these disorders [16,17]. Conversely, high rates of sleep problems and mental disorders have been reported in shift workers, including insomnia, fatigue, anxiety and depression [18–24]. It is noteworthy that altered patterns of clock genes were also reported in shift workers [25–27].

The objective of this article is an attempt to clarify the relationships between psychiatric disorders, altered expression of clock genes and endogenous circadian rhythm disturbances (especially altered sleep–wake rhythms). Is the disruption of circadian rhythms, and therefore of sleep–wake rhythms, a prerequisite for the genesis of psychiatric disorders? What roles do the clock genes play in the disruption of endogenous circadian rhythms? After describing the molecular mechanisms of circadian rhythms, their relationships with psychiatric disorders are discussed, focusing in particular on bipolar disorder, anxiety, depression, attention deficit disorder, schizophrenia and autism spectrum disorder (a rich literature review on this topic was available for these psychiatric disorders, which was not the case for other disorders such as addictions or dementia).

1.1. *Daily and Circadian Rhythms*

There are different categories of physiological rhythms with different time scales, such as ultradian, tidal, circadian, lunar, and seasonal rhythms. A daily rhythm is a regular and predictable phenomenon which is defined as a series of significant physiological changes over 24 h. The biological rhythm consists of two components: the first is exogenous and modulated by environmental factors such as light–dark alternations, sleep–wake, hot–cold, and seasonal change [28–31]; the second is endogenous and linked to genetic factors (studies in identical twins showed that they had identical biological rhythms [32]). Homologous genes involved in the animal's activity–rest cycle have been described in humans. It has been observed that the individual tendency to get up and go to bed more or less early was associated with a polymorphism of the *circadian locomotor output cycles kaput* (*Clock*) gene. Socio-ecological exogenous factors modulate rhythms and are called synchronizers. Endogenous factors, genetic by nature, underpin the internal biological clock which is responsible for an internal time synchronization coordinating the circadian variations of biochemical, physiological and behavioral parameters.

Circadian rhythms are the best known biological rhythms at the molecular level. The alternation of activity and rest over a period of 24 h (or rest-activity cycle) was observed in drosophila, fish and mammals including rodents (rats, mice, hamsters) and humans. In mammals, this circadian rhythm is generated by a master central clock, mainly reset by ambient light, and is located in the suprachiasmatic nuclei (SCN) of the hypothalamus [33,34]. Circadian regulation of all biological functions is processed through direct or indirect signals (cyclic hormone production) between the suprachiasmatic nuclei and different body structures (brain regions, organs). The body has peripheral clocks located in each organ (heart, lung, liver, muscles, kidneys, retina, etc.) that optimize the function of each organ according to the environmental context allowing therefore adaptation of the organism to environmental changes. Thus, the circadian clocks network has an adaptive function [35]. Both central and peripheral clocks are detectable though both cyclic gene expression and rhythmic physiological processes. These peripheral clocks work independently but must be re-synchronized continuously through the brain's master clock acting as a real conductor. Furthermore, the neurohormone melatonin is involved in the synchronization (i.e., adjustment of the timing of existing oscillations) of peripheral oscillators; the nocturnal synthesis and release of melatonin by the pineal gland are controlled by the SCN master clock and inhibited by light exposure [36].

1.2. Clock Genes

The first gene known as being responsible for the circadian rhythm was found in drosophila; it is the *period* (*Per*) gene [37]. Subsequent research has highlighted another gene involved in the circadian rhythm: the *timeless* (*Tim*) gene [38–41].

Chemical mutagenesis performed in mammals such as mice allowed identification of the first clock genes: the *Clock* gene [42] (or *Npas2* in neuronal tissue), whose mutation was responsible for a lengthened rest–activity cycle. Other clock genes were then identified in the circadian regulation of the mouse: the *brain and muscle ARNT-like protein 1* (*Bmal1*) gene as a *Clock* partner, *Per1* and *Per2* genes, and *cryptochrome-1* (*Cry1*) and *Cry2* genes (genes encoding proteins involved in blue light reception in non-mammalian species).

The role of melatonin on the circadian oscillatory rhythms, and in particular as a neuroendocrine synchronizer of molecular oscillatory systems has been documented [36,43–46]. Studies in animal models showed that melatonin is involved in the regulation of circadian expression of several clock genes, such as *Per1*, *Per2*, *Bmal1*, *reverse erythroblastosis virus* (*REV-ERBα*), *Clock* and *Cry1*, in both central and peripheral melatonin target tissues. For example, in rat and mouse models, it has been shown that melatonin induces rhythmic expression of *Per1*, *Bmal1*, *Clock* and *Cry1* in the pituitary (*pars tuberalis*) [47,48]. It is noteworthy that *Per1* expression is undetectable in melatonin-deficient mice [49,50] and pinealectomy abolishes rhythmic expression of *Per1* in the *Pars tuberalis* (PT) and desynchronizes *Per1* and *Per2* expression in the SCN [51,52]. Moreover, melatonin synchronizes circadian oscillations in the cardiovascular system by influencing circadian rhythmic expression of both *Per1* and *Bmal1* in the rat heart [53]. In the pituitary of sheep, melatonin stimulates *Cry1* expression and suppresses other clock genes expression [54]. These effects are probably mediated by melatonin (MT) receptors, such as the MT1 receptors. Indeed, in the *pars tuberalis* of MT1 knockout mice, expression of *Per1*, *Bmal1*, *Clock* and *Cry1* was dramatically reduced but not changed in MT2 knockout mice [54]. Furthermore, in the hypothalamic SCN of rats, melatonin treatment induces phase advance of the nuclear receptor *REV-ERBα* expression [55]. In adipose tissue, melatonin synchronizes metabolic and hormonal function [56] by regulating *Per2*, *Clock* and *REV-ERBα* [57] (*REV-ERBα* is required for the daily balance of carbohydrate and lipid metabolism [58]). Finally, melatonin regulates oscillation of *Clock* genes in healthy and cancerous human breast epithelial cells [59] and induces a shift in the 24-h oscillatory expression of *Per2* and *Bmal1* in cultured fetal adrenal gland [60]. Taken together, these studies underline the major role of melatonin in the regulation of clock genes expression allowing the synchronization of central and peripheral oscillators.

In humans, homologues of *Clock*, *Bmal1*, *Per* and *Cry* were identified. The *Clock* gene, the only cloned circadian rhythm gene, is located on chromosome 4 [61]. There are other clock genes involved in circadian regulation, such as *retinoic acid receptor-related orphan receptor* (*ROR*)*-A* and *ROR-B*, *REV-ERB*, and *casein kinase-1* (*Ck1*)ε and *Ck1δ*, which control transcription of *Bmal1* gene. Additionally, the *albumin-D-site-binding protein* (*Dbp*) is also a circadian clock-controlled gene, involved in the circadian transcriptional regulation of several metabolic enzymes and some transcription factors. Some studies [25–27] report altered expression of certain clock genes in cases of shift workers (*Per1* and *Per2*), and free-running/constant conditions (*Per1*). However, most of the clock genes are affected in case of sleep-deprivation studies [62,63], highlighting the interaction between clock genes and sleep reported by Franken et al. [64,65]. Indeed, clock genes contribute to the homeostatic aspect of sleep regulation and mutations in some clock genes modify the markers of sleep homeostasis and an increase in homeostatic sleep drive alters clock genes expression in the forebrain [64]. It is noteworthy that the expression of clock genes is ubiquitous in humans (central nervous system, spleen, thymus, intestine, heart, lung, etc.), but also in animals (clock genes are found in most cell types among vertebrates).

1.3. Molecular Working of the Cellular Circadian Clock

The discoveries of the different clock genes led to the proposal of a molecular clock model based on a feedback loop running over 24 h [66]. The molecular mechanisms underlying the circadian rhythms are rather similar regardless of the species. They include enhancer elements, repressor elements and control loops involving phosphorylation-dephosphorylation, methylation, acetylation reactions and the specific protein dimerization [67,68]. In mammals, this molecular circadian system is present in the hypothalamic central clock, the suprachiasmatic nuclei, and in secondary clocks within the brain and peripheral organs. Light perceived by the retina leads to changes in transcription of certain genes of the circadian rhythm in the master clock and shows the ability of the body to adjust to a change in the cycle of the photoperiodic environment. This master clock synchronizes multiple peripheral circadian oscillators via mechanisms that remain to be better ascertained.

The molecular loop of the circadian clock seems to imply in a general way two types of mechanisms: transcriptional (transcriptional regulation of genes at the DNA level, i.e., their copy in the form of RNA messenger) and post-transcriptional (regulating steps downstream of the transcription) (see Figure 1 [69]).

Transcriptional mechanisms: these mechanisms can be summarized by autoregulatory feedback loops. The first is a primary negative feedback loop: they rely on a pair of positive elements and a pair of negative elements. In mammals, the positive elements are two proteins, CLOCK and BMAL1 transcription factors which heterodimerize each other. The two negative elements are also two proteins, PERIOD (PER) and CRYPTOCHROME (CRY). In a neuron of the suprachiasmatic nucleus, there is little PER and CRY in the morning. The CLOCK–BMAL1 complex activates maximally the transcription of *Per* and *Cry* genes. However, the PER and CRY proteins do not accumulate immediately due to their instability, which allows the cycle not to be interrupted prematurely. Following interactions with other proteins they are gradually stabilized during the day, then they heterodimerize and finally migrate into the nucleus [70], where they inhibit the transcriptional activity of the CLOCK–BMAL1 heterodimer and thus their own transcription [71,72]. The *Per* and *Cry* genes being less and less active, the PER and CRY proteins are less and less produced. Their amount reaches a maximum at the beginning of night, and then decreases. At the same time, the CLOCK–BMAL1 heterodimer gradually regains its activity during the night. Thus, the molecular mechanism of the clock consists principally in a feedback loop comprising a positive component (with the CLOCK–BMAL1 heterodimer) and a negative component (with the PER–CRY heterodimer). A complete cycle of this loop lasts about 24 h. CLOCK and BMAL1 heterodimers are also involved in a daily transcription of many clock-controlled genes (CCGs) in different peripheral tissues [73–75]. In addition to the primary feedback loop, another regulatory feedback loop is formed by the orphan nuclear receptors REV-ERBα and RORα. In the nucleus, REV-ERBα competes with RORα for binding to the ROR-responsive element (RORE) in the *Bmal1* promoter. Whereas RORα activates transcription of *Bmal1*, REV-ERBα represses it. Consequently, the cyclic expression of *Bmal1* is achieved by both positive and negative regulation of RORs and REV-ERBs, respectively. This secondary feedback loop is called the "stabilizing loop".

Post-transcriptional mechanisms: the proper functioning of the circadian loop requires that PER and CRY proteins disappear in due course, once they have served their purpose. As long as they inhibit the activity of positive elements (CLOCK and BMAL1), a new cycle cannot start. Several post-transcriptional processes thus affect the ability of PER and CRY to act on CLOCK and BMAL1. The most studied aspect is the modification of these proteins by phosphorylation and dephosphorylation. Several kinase proteins include PER and/or CRY among their targets, and each one of the two proteins can be phosphorylated on many distinct sites. They accelerate or slow down their transfer to the proteasome. Proteins to be degraded are "marked" by ubiquitin. Post-transcriptional regulations of the clock proteins of the main molecular loop make it possible to ensure intracellular traffic, functionality and degradation of clock proteins which are crucial for the functioning of the molecular loop over 24 h [76].

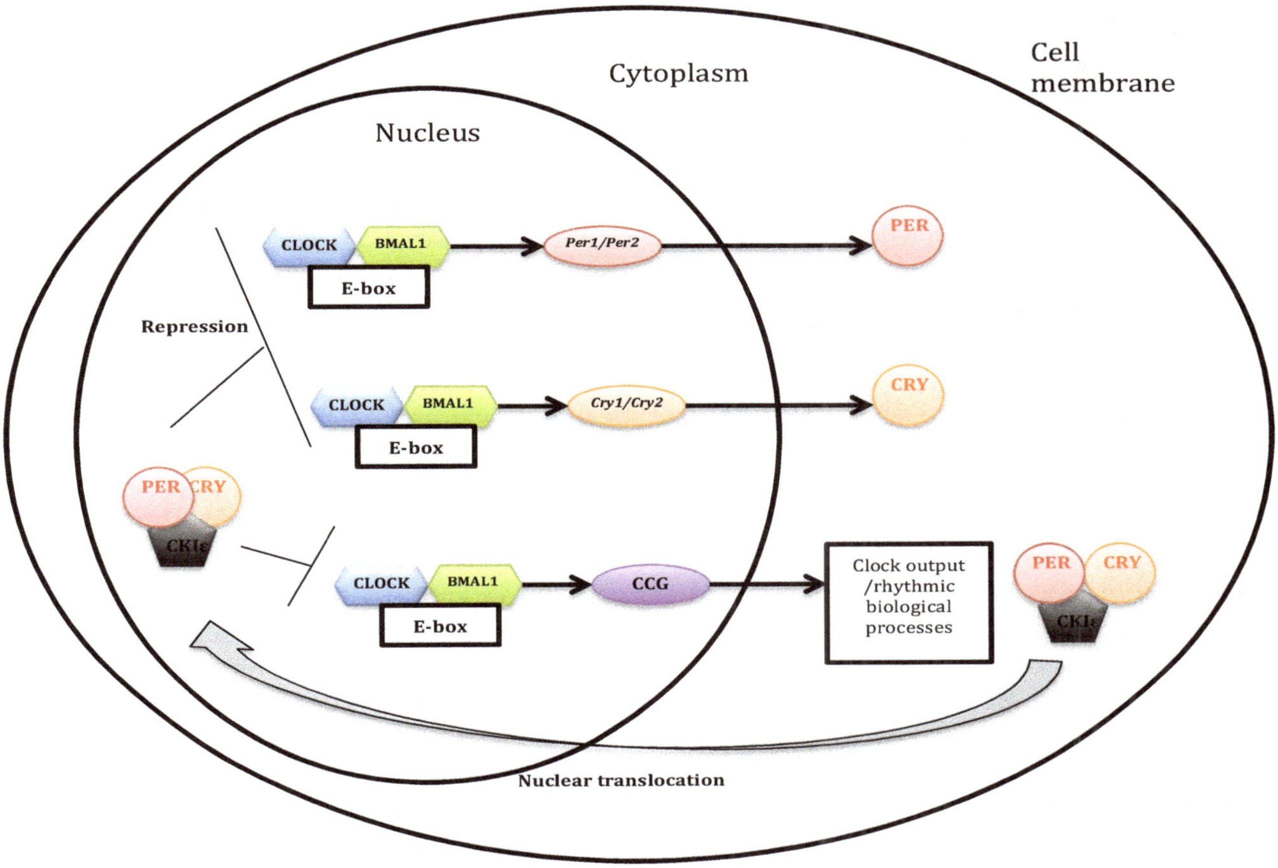

Figure 1. Model of the mammalian cell-autonomous oscillator (based on Lowrey and Takahashi, 2011) [69]. The transcriptional activators *circadian locomotor output cycles kaput* (CLOCK) and *brain and muscle ARNT-like protein 1* (BMAL1) stimulate the expression of *cryptochrome-1* (*Cry*) and *period* (*Per*) genes. The protein products of these genes are associated in the cytoplasm to form dimers that go into the core. There, they serve two functions: first, the repression of their own transcription, via the inhibition of CLOCK–BMAL1; and second, the activation of *Bmal1* gene, by a mechanism that remains to be discovered. These proteins are thus two regulating loops, one negative and the other positive. CLOCK and BMAL1 activate also the so-called clock-controlled genes (CCG) whose products transmit the rhythm information to the rest of the body via the output channels of the clock. Some proteins modulate the progression of control loops. Thus, casein kinase Iε (CKIε) can phosphorylate PER proteins, which destabilizes them and prevents their translocation into the nucleus.

2. Relationships between Circadian Rhythms and Psychiatric Disorders

Several hypotheses can be raised regarding the relationships between the development of psychiatric disorders and problems of circadian rhythms, including altered sleep–wake rhythms:

(1) First, sleep problems may lead to cognitive impairments due to the effects of sleep deprivation and fatigue on learning and attention capacities, long-term memory, language development and emotions [77–82];

(2) Recent studies in cognitive and developmental psychology have highlighted the importance of rhythmicity and synchrony of motor, emotional, and inter-personal rhythms in early development of social communication; the synchronization of rhythms allows tuning and adaptation to the external environment [83]. Impaired circadian rhythms with an absence of synchronization of

the circadian clocks network might alter the functioning of motor, emotional and interpersonal rhythms, leading to social communication impairments and vulnerability to psychiatric disorders with social communication deficit such as ASD or schizophrenia (for a review of literature on the importance of rhythmicity and synchrony of motor, emotional, and inter-personal rhythms in early development of social communication, see [83,84]). In addition, circadian rhythms involve sequences of continuities/discontinuities that might be important for typical fetal and child development in order to provide a secure environment (through stable and predictable regularities) but also variations allowing the individual to adapt to changes. Impaired circadian rhythms with no, little or irregular variability might lead to anxiety and difficulties in adapting to changes associated with restricted and repetitive interests observed in some psychiatric disorders described in this article such as ASD, schizophrenia and anxiety disorder;

(3) Clock genes control critical periods of brain development [85] and therefore, abnormal expression of clock genes might participate to neurodevelopmental disorders such as psychiatric disorders. It is noteworthy that only a few days of circadian rhythm impairments may impact the maturation and specialization of some brain structures at specific developmental periods; these abnormalities can alter the temporal organization of brain maturation and development [86];

(4) Circadian rhythm impairments may alter transcriptional and splicing regulation of Parvalbumin (PV) neurons, knowing that PV knockout mice (PV−/−) or heterozygous (PV+/−) mice showed autism behavioral phenotype [87]. More generally, circadian rhythm impairments may affect gene expression involved in synapse formation and brain maturation;

(5) Also, clock-controlled genes (CCGs) may have pleiotropic effects outside the molecular clock and have therefore more widespread impact on cognition, mood, and reward-related behaviors [88];

(6) Finally, circadian rhythm impairments (provoked or not by sleep problems) may also alter the adaptation of the individual to his/her environment and therefore his/her state of homeostasis. In this perspective, psychiatric disorders might reflect a loss of synchronization between the external environment's rhythms and the individual's internal rhythms, leading to major problems of adaptation for the individual and the appearance of psychiatric disorders. Single-nucleotide polymorphisms (SNPs) in core circadian clock genes have been associated with autism spectrum disorder [89], attention deficit hyperactivity disorder [90,91], anxiety disorder [92], major depressive disorder [93–95], bipolar disorder [95–97] and schizophrenia [98–101]. However, the causal relationship for these associations remains to be better ascertained. Circadian clock genes may affect specific aspects of psychiatric disorders through circadian control or through distinct regulation of downstream effectors.

The suprachiasmatic nuclei (SCN) coordinate the rhythms of other brain regions and peripheral organs like a pacemaker [102]. The sleep–wake cycle is the most documented example of the activity of the SCN, but endocrine, metabolic and immunological activities are also conducted by the SCN. For example, the glucocorticoids are regulated by the circadian cycle and affect the circadian rhythms of the amygdala [103,104]. Also, they regulate directly the clock genes [105,106].

We will explore the current state of research on this subject through five psychiatric disorders: bipolar disorder, anxiety and depression, attention deficit disorder, schizophrenia, and autism spectrum disorders.

2.1. Bipolar Spectrum Disorder

The mechanisms underlying the association between alterations in circadian rhythms and mood disorders are still unclear. However, current scientific studies provide food for thought. According to Jackson et al. [107], sleep disorder is the most common prodrome of mania and one of the six most common prodromes of depression in bipolar disorder (bipolar type I disorder is defined as an isolated manic episode, and bipolar type II disorder is defined as manic and depressive episodes) [108]. Between mood episodes, the sleep–wake cycle remains disrupted in patients with bipolar disorder who have some difficulty falling asleep and frequent night awakenings [109]. These patients have a significantly more eventide sleep pattern than control subjects, in other words, they go to bed later and have more difficulty getting up early compared to healthy controls [110].

McClung [111] studied the involvement of the *Clock* gene in manic episodes in mice. She compared *Clock* mutant mice to mice with a normal *Clock* gene. Mice in which the gene had been modified had mania-like behavior. Those mice were hyperactive, less anxious and less depressed. They slept less and showed greater brain activity in response to sugar water, cocaine and a mild electrical stimulation of the brain. When researchers added lithium in their water, these mice did not show their manic behavior anymore and started to act like the mice with a normal *Clock* gene. A lithium salt treatment could affect circadian rhythms by modulating the expression of clock genes [112–115]. Indeed, lithium salts might inhibit the expression of *glycogen synthase kinase 3β (GSK-3β)* gene [116], a gene involved in the brain's biological clock [117]. Kaladchibachi demonstrated that both genetic and pharmacological reduction of *GSK-3* activity in mice have a specific effect on the circadian transcriptional oscillation consisting of *mPer2* period lengthening, indicating a delay in phase [116]. Moreover, it has been shown that *GSK-3β* is rhythmically expressed in the SCN and liver of mice, and that it undergoes a daily cycle in phosphorylation in vivo. Lithium chloride treatment inhibits the *GSK-3β* expression and results in a phase delay of *Clock* gene expression in fibroblasts [118]. Bipolar spectrum disorder has been associated with variations in the *Clock* gene. A single-nucleotide polymorphism (SNP) in the 3-flanking region of the *Clock* gene (3111 T to C) is associated with a higher recurrence rate of bipolar episodes [16]. This SNP was also associated in bipolar disorder and/or antidepressant treatment with sleep problems (insomnia and decreased need for sleep) [17,119]. Some studies reported other clock genes associated with bipolar disorder (such as *Bmal1* and *Per3)* [96]. Furthermore, a SNP in *Bmal1* and a SNP in *Tim* have also been identified as having a link with bipolar disorder [99]. One South Indian study showed that the occurrence of the five repeat alleles of *Per3* may be a risk factor for bipolar disorder onset in this ethnic group [120]. The coding region of *Per3* gene contains a variable number tandem-repeat (VNTR) polymorphisms which has been associated with diurnal preference, sleep structure and sleep homeostasis in healthy individuals. In a homogeneous sample of patients with bipolar type I disorder (occurrence of one or more manic episodes or mixed episodes), they observed that *Per3* VNTR influenced age of onset: earlier onset in homozygote carriers of *Per35* variant, later onset in homozygotes for *Per34*, and intermediate onset in heterozygotes. Sjöholm et al. [121] studied four single-nucleotide polymorphisms (SNPs) of *Cry2* gene in a cohort of bipolar patients, some with fast cycles. They observed that *Cry2* is associated with rapid cycling in bipolar disorder patients. Rapid cycling in bipolar disorder is defined according to the 5th version of Diagnostic and Statistical Manual of Mental Disorders (DSM-5) as four or more mood episodes in any combination or order within any year in the course of the illness. The A allele of rs10838524 (*Cry2* SNP) was significantly overrepresented among bipolar disorder cases with rapid cycling compared to controls. There was a significant trend in the association between the A allele of rs10838524 and rapid cycling ($p = 0.0076$) and this allele increased the risk for rapid cycling both in a homozygote and a heterozygote form (that is dominant model) compared to controls. Two closely related clock genes, retinoid-related orphan receptors α (*RORA*) and β (*RORB*) are involved in a number of pathways including neurogenesis, stress response, and modulation of circadian rhythms. A study reports that four intronic *RORB* SNPs showed positive associations with the pediatric bipolar phenotype and suggests that clock genes in general and *RORB* in particular may be important candidates for further investigation in the search for the molecular basis of bipolar disorder [122]. Further studies are necessary to better assess the role of *RORB* in bipolar spectrum disorder and explore if this gene is particularly relevant for this disorder compared to other clock genes.

Several genetic studies suggest that certain polymorphisms of clock genes are more common in bipolar disorder than in the general population [123,124]. The clock genes might therefore be viewed as genetic vulnerability factors to bipolar disorder [125]. These results need to be examined further.

The litterature review on clock genes and bipolar spectrum disorder is presented in Table 1.

Table 1. Clock genes and bipolar spectrum disorder. RORα: retinoid-related orphan receptors α; RORβ: retinoid-related orphan receptors β.

Studies	Measure	Individuals with Psychiatric Disorder and/or Organisms Models (*n*)	Controls (*n*)	Results
Kaladchibachi et al. [116]	Cyclical expression of clock genes (*Per2*)	Mouse embryonic fibroblasts (MEFs)	-	Genetic depletion of glycogen synthase kinase 3 (GSK3) activity results in a significant delay in the cycling period of *Per2*.
McGrath et al. [122]	Genotyping and analysis of 312 single-nucleotide polymorphisms (SNPs) in *RORA* and 43 SNPs in *RORB*	Bipolar disorder (BD) children (*n* = 305)	Healthy parents (*n* = 306) Healthy individuals (*n* = 140)	Four intronic *RORB* SNPs showed positive associations with the pediatric bipolar phenotype.
Lavebratt et al. [94]	Assessment of *Cry2* gene expression before and after one night of sleep deprivation	BD individuals (*n* = 13)	Healthy individuals (*n* = 8)	*Cry2* mRNA levels are reduced and unresponsive to sleep deprivation in depressed patients with bipolar disorder.
Sjöholm et al. [121]	Analysis of four *Cry2* single-nucleotide polymorphisms	BD individuals in Sweden (*n* = 577); BD type I (*n* = 497); BD type II (*n* = 60); BD with rapid cycling (*n* = 155)	Healthy individuals (*n* = 1044)	Association between the circadian gene *Cry2* and rapid cycling in bipolar disorder.
Karthikeyan et al. [120]	Genotyping and analysis of *Per3* in blood samples	Bipolar type I disorder individuals in South India (*n* = 311)	Healthy individuals (*n* = 346)	The occurrence of the five repeat allele of *Per3* may be a risk factor for bipolar type I disorder onset in this ethnic group.

2.2. *Anxiety and Depression-Related Disorders*

2.2.1. Anxiety Disorder

A team of French researchers has evaluated a range of behaviors associated with psychiatric illnesses in mice in which two genes of the circadian clock, *Cry1* and *Cry2*, were investigated [126]. Their work highlighted the causal relationship between the disruption of encoding genes for cryptochrome proteins 1 and 2 (*Cry1* and *Cry2*) and behaviors associated with anxiety. Mice deficient for CRY 1 and 2 proteins show behavioral alterations characterized among other things by an abnormally high level of anxiety. These results indicate clearly that in addition to their critical roles in regulating the molecular clock; these proteins are directly involved in the control of emotional states.

2.2.2. Major Depressive Disorder (MDD)

Sleep problems, in particular insomnia or hyperinsomnia, are parts of depression criteria and have been hypothesized to be under genetic control. Major depressive disorder, as well as seasonal affective disorder (winter depression and summer depression) and bipolar type I disorder provide excellent models for studying the molecular mechanisms of mood disorder. An important study published in 2013 first demonstrated dysfunctioning clock genes in brains from depressed humans compared to healthy controls [127]. Involvement of the clock genes in depression is also evident from several genetic studies. It has been reported that polymorphisms of clock genes appear in depressed patients [93,128–132].

Several SNPs in the *Clock* gene (T3111C, 3117 G to T, 3125 A to G) has been reported [127,128,133] to be associated with major depression and sleep disturbances (but some studies did not found any association between T3111C and sleep problems; [134,135]). More precisely, the two rare SNPs (3117 G to T and 3125 A to G) were associated with alternating phases of good sleep and insomnia over the course of a few days [133].

A Swedish team, Lavebratt et al. [94] reported in healthy controls a marked diurnal variation in *Cry2* mRNA levels; total sleep deprivation induced a 2.0-fold increase in *Cry2* mRNA levels. In patients with depressive state of bipolar disorder, sleep deprivation induced significantly decreased *Cry2* mRNA expression compared with healthy controls. In addition, *Cry2* mRNA levels were found to be lowered in blood mononuclear cells from depressed patients with bipolar disorder after total sleep deprivation in comparison to healthy controls, and *Cry2* gene variation was associated with winter depression in both Swedish and Finnish patients [94]. Deletion of *Cry2* gene lengthened the circadian period by approximately 48 min. This study [94] suggests that a *Cry2* locus is associated with vulnerability for depression, and that mechanisms of action involve dysregulation of *Cry2* expression. Associations between the gene *Cry2* and winter depression, but also dysthymia and bipolar type I disorder as seen previously, support the view that the *Cry2* gene has a role in mood disorders.

Shi et al. [132] found genetic polymorphisms in circadian genes, especially *Clock* and *Per3*, in major depressive disorder individuals. Authors propose that the impact of the *Clock* and *Per3* SNPs on transcription and/or expression may not be on the core circadian oscillator in humans, but on global output transcriptional pathways, that are mediated sex-dependently by the circadian system.

The litterature review on clock genes and depression related disorders is presented in Table 2.

2.2.3. Familial Advanced Sleep Phase Syndrome (FASPS)

A good example of an abnormal circadian system in humans is the familial advanced sleep phase syndrome (FASPS), described in three families by Jones et al. [136]. FASPS is often associated with depression and anxiety. Affected individuals have a lead of a few hours of their sleep patterns and rhythms of temperature and melatonin, and a shorter period than healthy individuals in constant conditions. The joint efforts of several laboratories of the University of Utah in Salt Lake City have recently led to the description of *Per2* mutation in one of those families affected by FASPS. The mutation caused a substitution of serine by glycine in the *Per2* gene at position 662 [137]; this serine that can normally be phosphorylated by casein kinase Iε (CKIε). Inhibiting the action of CKIε accelerates the clock, which is indeed what is observed in FASPS patients. FASPS are also to be caused by a T44A missense mutation in human CK1δ, which causes hypophosphorylation of *Per2* [138,139]. Transgenic mice over-expressing the *hPer2* mutation exhibit shorter free-running periods, mimicking FASPS [140], and their phenotype is sensitive to CK1δ: increased dosage of CK1δ shortens their period further.

Recently, a team has identified a new mutation in the *hCry2* gene associated with FASPS. The mutation leads to replacement of an alanine residue at position 260 with a threonine. In mice, the *Cry2* mutation causes a shortened circadian period and reduced phase-shift to early–night light pulse associated with phase-advanced behavioral rhythms in the light-dark cycle [141].

2.2.4. Seasonal Affective Disorder (SAD) and Delayed Sleep Phase Syndrome (DSPS)

Environmental changes like the seasons can be associated with depressive episodes in the inability of the circadian clock to adjust appropriately. Seasonal affective disorder (SAD) is defined as recurrent depressive disorder characterized by a seasonal pattern with, generally, an appearance in the fall or winter, apart from triggering external factor, and spontaneous disappearance in the spring or summer, even in the absence of treatment. SAD affects about 5% of the general population [142]. Lewy evokes the idea of a "phase delay of the endogenous circadian oscillator in relation to sleep-wake rhythm" [143], the equivalent of a delayed sleep phase syndrome (DSPS), as the cause of SAD. Genetic variants in *Npas2*, *Per2*, and *Bmal1* have been found to combine with the development of SAD [93,144].

Iwase et al. [145] reported that the SNP T3111C in the *Clock* gene was associated with morning or evening preference for activity and its frequency was decreased in DSPS. Futures studies are required to investigate the possible contribution of T3111C to DSPS susceptibility.

Table 2. Clock genes and depression related disorders.

Studies	Measure	Individuals with Psychiatric Disorder (n)	Controls (n)	Results
Takimoto et al. [146]	Daily variation of melatonin and cortisol, and daily expression of clock genes (*Per*, *Bmal1* and *Clock*) in whole blood cells	Individuals with circadian rhythm sleep disorder (n = 1)	Healthy male individuals (n = 12)	The peak phase of *Per1*, *Per2*, and *Per3* appeared in the early morning, whereas that of *Bmal1* and *Clock* appeared in the midnight hours in healthy male individuals.
Partonen et al. [93]	Analysis of sequence variations (single-nucleotide polymorphisms) in three core clock genes: *Per2*, *Bmal*, and *Npas2*	Depressed individuals (n = 189)	Healthy individuals (n = 189)	Variations in the three circadian clock genes *Per2*, *Bmal*, and *Npas2* are associated with winter depression.
Utge et al. [147]	Analysis of 113 single-nucleotide polymorphisms of 18 genes of the circadian system	Depressed individuals (n = 384)	Healthy individuals (n = 1270)	Significant association between *Tim* variants and depression with fatigue in females, and association to depression with early morning awakening in males.
Lavebratt et al. [94]	Genotyping of single nucleotide polymorphism of the *Cry2* gene	Depressed individuals with bipolar disorder (n = 204)	Healthy individuals (n = 2017)	The *Cry2* gene was significantly associated with winter depression in both samples.
Kovanen et al. [130]	Genotyping of 48 single-nucleotide polymorphisms in *Cry1* and *Cry2* gene	Individuals with dysthymia (n = 136)	Healthy individuals (n = 3871)	Four *Cry2* genetic variants (rs10838524, rs7121611, rs7945565, rs1401419) are significantly associated with dysthymia.
Hua et al. [131]	Genotyping of single nucleotide polymorphisms (SNPs) of *Cry1* rs2287161, *Cry2* rs10838524 and *Tef* *(thyrotroph embryonic factor)* rs738499	Chinese individuals with major depressive disorder (MDD) (n = 105)	Chinese healthy individuals (n = 485)	The polymorphisms of *Cry1* rs2287161and *Tef* rs738499 are associated to major depressive disorder.
Shi et al. [132]	Genotyping of 32 genetic variants from eight clock genes	Major depressive disorder individuals (n = 592)	Healthy individuals (n = 776)	Genetic polymorphisms in circadian genes, especially *Clock* and *Per3*, influence risk of developing depression in a sex- and stress-dependent manner.

2.3. Attention Deficit Hyperactivity Disorder (ADHD)

Many sleep disorders are associated with attention deficit hyperactivity disorder (ADHD), both in adults and children. In particular, the following sleep problems occurring at sleep–wake transition were observed: bed-time refusal, delayed sleep-onset, and early awakenings [148]. Differences in sleep problems were found as a function of ADHD subtype: children with ADHD inattentive type (ADHD-I) had the fewest sleep problems and did not differ from controls, children with ADHD combined type (ADHD-C) had more sleep problems than controls and children with ADHD-I. Daytime sleepiness was greatest in ADHD-I and was associated with sleeping more (not less) than normal [149].

Several studies reported genetic associations between polymorphism (rs1801260) at the 3′-untranslated region (3′-UTR) of the *Clock* gene and psychiatric disorders [17,90] (see Table 3). Concerning the association between the rs1801260 polymorphism and ADHD, Kissling et al. [90] found at least one T-mutation being the risk allele in Caucasians of western European origin and German background.

Xu et al. [91] conducted a study which investigated a previously reported discovery of an association between a single nucleotide polymorphism in the 3′-UTR region of the *Clock* gene (rs1801260) in two independent samples of ADHD probands from UK and Taiwan (aged 5 to 15).

They found a significant over-transmission of the T allele of rs1801260 SNP, which is associated as a risk allele for delayed sleep phase syndrome [145] in ADHD cases in the Taiwanese population. No association was observed between this polymorphism and ADHD in the UK sample. However, they did find evidence for increased transmission of the T allele of rs1801260 in the Taiwanese samples. Their findings support the hypothesis that genetic variation in the 3′-UTR region of *Clock* gene might be a risk factor for the development of ADHD, particularly in the Taiwanese sample studied. Therefore, more functional polymorphisms of this region should be investigated in other independent studies using larger samples.

Table 3. Clock genes and attention deficit hyperactivity disorder (ADHD).

Studies	Measure	Individuals with Psychiatric Disorder (n)	Controls (n)	Results
Kissling et al. [90]	Analysis of polymorphism (rs1801260) at the 3′-untranslated region of the *Clock* gene	ADHD individuals (n = 143)	Healthy individuals (n = 143)	Significant association ($p < 0.001$) between genotype and ADHD-scores of the adult ADHD assessments, and the rs1801260 polymorphism with at least one T-mutation is the risk allele.
Xu et al. [91]	Analysis of polymorphism (rs1801260) at the 3′-untranslated region of the *Clock* gene in ADHD using within-family transmission disequilibrium test	Two clinical ADHD samples: United Kingdom (UK) sample: (n = 180); Taiwan sample: (n = 212)	Both parents or mother alone or father alone UK sample: (n = 296); Taiwan sample: (n = 326)	Increased transmission of the T allele of the rs1801260 polymorphism in Tawainese samples.

2.4. Schizophrenia

Schizophrenia is often associated with sleep alterations [88,150], observed also in untreated patients [151]. Patients with schizophrenia have a desynchronization between the sleep–wake rhythms and melatonin profiles [88,152,153], the rhythms of body temperature [154], and serum levels of tryptophan and prolactin [155]. These anomalies suggest strongly disturbed circadian rhythms in these patients [156]. Studies of polymorphisms of clock genes or alterations in the regulation of these genes in schizophrenia are rare. The litterature review on clock genes and schizophrenia is presented in Table 4.

The expression of *Per1* mRNA in the temporal lobe in individuals with schizophrenia decreases significantly compared with age-matched healthy controls [98]. Another study suggested that *Per3* but not *Per2* abnormalities were associated with schizophrenia [99]. In a sample of 145 Japanese individuals with schizophrenia compared with healthy controls, it was reported that the T3111C polymorphism of the *Clock* gene presented a transmission bias. The T3111C polymorphism of the *Clock* gene might be associated with aberrant dopaminergic transmission in the suprachiasmatic nucleus, which is presumably involved in the pathophysiology of schizophrenia [157]. More recently, two studies focused on white blood cells and fibroblast from smaller samples: Sun et al. [100] reported altered expressions of *Per1*, *Per2*, *Per3* and *Npas2* in white blood cells in individuals with schizophrenia. Indeed, compared with healthy controls, schizophrenia patients presented disruptions in diurnal rhythms of the expression of *Per1*, *Per3*, and *Npas2*, accompanied by a delayed phase in the expression of *Per2* and by a decreasing in *Per3* and *Npas2* expression. Johansson et al. [101] reported a loss of rhythmic expression of *Cry1* and *Per2* in fibroblasts from individuals with schizophrenia compared to cells from healthy controls.

Table 4. Clock genes and schizophrenia. REV-ERBα: reverse erythroblastosis virus; Dbp: albumin-D-site-binding protein.

Studies	Measure	Individuals with Psychiatric Disorder (n)	Controls (n)	Results
Takao et al. [157]	Analysis of 3111C single nucleotide polymorphism of the *Clock* gene	Individuals with schizophrenia (n = 145)	Healthy individuals (n = 128)	Individuals with schizophrenia had a significantly higher frequency of the C allele compared to controls.
Sun et al. [100]	Relative expression of clock gene mRNA: *Per1*, *Per2* and *Per3* in blood samples	Individuals with schizophrenia (n = 13)	Healthy controls (n = 15)	Individuals with schizophrenia presented disruptions in diurnal rhythms of the expression of *Per1*, *Per3*, and *Npas2* compared with healthy controls, accompanied by a delayed phase in the expression of *Per2* and by a decrease in *Per3* and *Npas2* expression.
Johansson et al. [101]	Analysis of *Clock*, *Bmal1*, Per1, *Per2*, *Cry1*, *Cry2*, *REV-ERBα* and *Dbp* in fibroblasts from skin samples	Individuals with chronic schizophrenia under neuroleptic medication (n = 11)	Healthy individuals (n = 11)	Loss of rhythmic expression of *Cry1* and *Per2* in fibroblasts from individuals with schizophrenia compared to cells from healthy controls.

To date, the associations between clock genes and schizophrenia are not clear.

2.5. Autism Spectrum Disorder (ASD)

Surveys of parents show that the prevalence of sleep problems in ASD is 50%–80% compared to 9%–50% in age-matched typically developing children [7–14]. Recent results showing abnormal melatonin secretion in ASD children may change the initial disregard of these disorders and suggest a possible key role of the clock and circadian regulations in ASD. Several independent groups detected abnormal melatonin levels in ASD [158–163]. These studies conducted on independent autism samples and using different methodologies indicate that abnormally low melatonin level is a frequent trait in ASD. More precisely decreased nocturnal as well as diurnal levels have been reported in individuals with ASD; trial studies support therapeutic benefits of melatonin use in ASD [83,84,161]. Nevertheless, both the underlying cause of this anomaly and its relationship with ASD (cause or consequence?) remain still unexplained.

Many studies have advocated a genetic etiology for autism [164] involving in particular synaptic genes related to synaptic cell adhesion molecules NLGN3, NLGN4, and NRXN1 and a postsynaptic scaffolding protein SHANK3. This protein complex is crucial for the maintenance of functional synapses as well as the adequate balance between neuronal excitation and inhibition. Among the factors that could modulate this pathway there are genes controlling circadian rhythms. However, no direct association has been reported between clock genes and NLGN3, NLGN4, NRXN1 and SHANK3 in humans, but epistasis mechanisms cannot be ruled out. SHANK3 expression is modulated by melatonin concentration and the modulation is brain structure-dependent [165]. Concerning relationships between sleep disorders and NLGN3, NLGN4, NRXN1 and SHANK3 could be a pleiotropic effect on sleep of genes associated with brain disorganization. It is noteworthy that possible interplay of synaptic and clock genes may increase the risk of ASD [166]. The involvement of clock genes in ASD was first suggested by Wimpory et al. [167] who stated the hypothesis that anomalies in clock genes operating as timing genes in high frequency oscillator systems may underline timing deficits that could be important in the development of autism spectrum disorder, notably in autistic communication impairment. To test this hypothesis, Nicholas et al. [89] screened single-nucleotide polymorphisms in 11 clock/clock-related genes in 110 individuals with ASD and their parents.

A significant allelic association was detected for *Per1* and *Npas2*. It should be noted that it was a small population and results were not significant after correction for multiple testing. However, the association between *clock* genes and ASD was confirmed by a more recent study [168] reporting also mutations in other circadian clock genes (*Per2, Per3, Clock, Bmal1, Tim, Cry1, Cry2, Dbp* and *Ck1ε*) in ASD patients. Taken together, these findings suggest that the circadian rhythm abnormalities observed in ASD may be linked to abnormalities of the circadian clock genes. Finally, it is noteworthy that clock genes are related to the protein association network described in ASD by Roubertoux and Tordjman [169] either through direct gene × gene interactions or protein × protein interactions.

The litterature review on clock genes and autism spectrum disorder is presented in Table 5.

Table 5. Clock genes and autism spectrum disorder (ASD).

Studies	Measure	Individuals with Psychiatric Disorder (*n*)	Controls (*n*)	Results
Nicholas et al. [89]	Screening of eleven clock/clock-related genes	High-functioning ASD individuals ($n = 110$)	Healthy parents ($n = 220$)	Significant association for two single-nucleotide polymorphisms in *Per1* and in *Npas2*.
Yang et al. [168]	Direct sequencing analysis of the coding regions of 18 canonical clock genes and clock-controlled genes	ASD individuals with sleep disorders ($n = 14$); ASD individuals without sleep disorders ($n = 14$)	Healthy individuals ($n = 23$)	Mutations in circadian-relevant genes (specifically *Per1, Per2, Per3, Clock, Npas2, Bmal1, Tim, Cry1, Cry2, Dbp* and *Ck1ε*) affecting gene function are more frequent in individuals with ASD than in controls.

3. Conclusions

Circadian clocks enable organisms to anticipate temporal organization of biological functions in relation to periodic changes of the environment, and to adapt consequently their behavior. The genes *Clock, Per, Cry* and *Bmal1* are currently the major clock genes identified in humans as being involved in the rhythmicity and timing of biological rhythms at the molecular level. Their alteration involves changes to the 24-h rhythm through poor synchronization between the endogenous circadian rhythms and the sleep-wake cycle, and act especially on sleep disorders. These are often early symptoms of altered sleep–wake rhythms at the onset of psychiatric disorders, especially for mood disorders. Furthermore, impairments in the four major clock genes (*Clock, Per, Cry* and *Bmal1*) were found for bipolar disorder, depression-related disorders, autism spectrum disorder, and impairments in some of these major clock genes were also reported for schizophrenia (*Clock, Per* and *Cry*), anxiety disorder (*Cry*) and attention deficit hyperactivity disorder (*Clock*). In addition, other *clock* genes were associated with these psychiatric disorders, such as *Npas2* (winter depression, autism spectrum disorder and schizophrenia), *RORA* and *RORB* (bipolar disorder) or *Tim, Dbp* and *Ck1ε* (autism spectrum disorder). The associations of identical clock genes with these different psychiatric disorders suggest that they may share similar pathways and etiopathogenic mechanisms. It highlights the interest and need to study these mental disorders through a transnosographic and multidimensional approach focusing on depression, anxiety and stress responses.

The cascading effects resulting from altered clock genes, poorly understood so far, could participate in sleep problems and the emergence of symptoms present in certain psychiatric disorders through, as discussed in the article, impaired regulation of circadian rhythms and emotional states with neurodevelopmental effects (including impaired control of the temporal organization of brain maturation, neurogenesis, synapses formation/functioning and brain specialization at specific developmental periods). Inversely, sleep problems can alter the expression of clock genes and contribute, as seen in this article, to the development of psychiatric disorders through cognitive effects of sleep deprivation and fatigue. More generally, alteration of clock genes (directly or indirectly through sleep problems) might lead to desynchronized and abnormal circadian rhythms (including sleep/wake rhythm but also other circadian rhythms such as neuroendocrine or body temperature rhythms) impairing in turn the synchronization between external and internal rhythms and therefore the adaptation of the individual to his/her internal and external environment with the development of psychiatric disorders. Future studies are required to better ascertain the underlying mechanisms of the relationships between clock genes, sleep disturbances and psychiatric disorders. Further research may open interesting perspectives with promising avenues for early detection and therapeutic intervention in psychiatric disorders.

Author Contributions: Annaëlle Charrier, Bertrand Olliac, Pierre Roubertoux and Sylvie Tordjman wrote the paper.

References

1. Czeisler, C.A.; Duffy, J.F.; Shanahan, T.L.; Brown, E.N.; Mitchell, J.F.; Rimmer, D.W.; Ronda, J.M.; Silva, E.J.; Allan, J.S.; Emens, J.S.; et al. Stability, precision, and near-24-hour period of the human circadian pacemaker. *Science* **1999**, *284*, 2177–2181. [CrossRef] [PubMed]
2. Singh, K.; Zimmerman, A.W. Sleep in Autism Spectrum Disorder and Attention Deficit Hyperactivity Disorder. *Semin. Pediatr. Neurol.* **2015**, *22*, 113–125. [CrossRef] [PubMed]
3. Lai, M.C.; Lombardo, M.V.; Baron-Cohen, S. Autism. *Lancet* **2014**, *383*, 896–910. [CrossRef]
4. Kotagal, S.; Broomall, E. Sleep in children with autism spectrum disorder. *Pediatr. Neurol.* **2012**, *47*, 242–251. [CrossRef] [PubMed]
5. Onore, C.; Careaga, M.; Ashwood, P. The role of immune dysfunction in the pathophysiology of autism. *Brain Behav. Immun.* **2012**, *26*, 383–392. [CrossRef] [PubMed]
6. Kohyama, J. Possible neuronal mechanisms of sleep disturbances in patients with autism spectrum disorders and attention-deficit/hyperactivity disorder. *Med. Hypotheses* **2016**, *97*, 131–133. [CrossRef] [PubMed]
7. Allik, H.; Larsson, J.O.; Smedje, H. Sleep patterns of school-age children with Asperger syndrome or high-functioning autism. *J. Autism Dev. Disord.* **2006**, *36*, 585–595. [CrossRef] [PubMed]
8. Richdale, A.L.; Schreck, K.A. Sleep problems in autism spectrum disorders: Prevalence, nature, and possible biopsychosocial aetiologies. *Sleep Med. Rev.* **2009**, *13*, 403–411. [CrossRef] [PubMed]
9. Polimeni, M.A.; Richdale, A.L.; Francis, A.J. A survey of sleep problems in autism, Asperger's disorder and typically developing children. *J. Intellect. Disabil. Res.* **2005**, *49*, 260–268. [CrossRef] [PubMed]
10. Doo, S.; Wing, Y.K. Sleep problems of children with pervasive developmental disorders: Correlation with parental stress. *Dev. Med. Child. Neurol.* **2006**, *48*, 650–655. [CrossRef] [PubMed]
11. Giannotti, F.; Cortesi, F.; Cerquiglini, A. An investigation of sleep characteristics, electroencephalogram abnormalities and epilepsy in developmentally regressed and non-regressed children with autism. *J. Autism Dev. Disord.* **2008**, *38*, 1888–1897. [CrossRef] [PubMed]
12. Stoleru, S.; Nottelmann, E.D.; Belmont, B.; Ronsaville, D. Sleep problems in children of affectively ill mothers. *J. Child. Psychol. Psychiatry Allied Discip.* **1997**, *38*, 831–841. [CrossRef]
13. Brown, W.D. Insomnia: Prevalence and daytime consequences. In *Sleep: A Comprehensive Handbook*; Lee-Chiong, T., Ed.; John Wiley and Sons: Hoboken, NJ, USA, 2006; pp. 93–98.
14. Ahmed, A.E.; Al-Jahdali, H.; Fatani, A.; Al-Rouqi, K.; Al-Jahdali, F.; Al-Harbi, A.; Baharoon, S.; Ali, Y.Z.; Khan, M.; Rumayyan, A. The effects of age and gender on the prevalence of insomnia in a sample of the Saudi population. *Ethn. Health* **2016**, 1–10. [CrossRef] [PubMed]
15. Lane, J.M.; Vlasac, I.; Anderson, S.G.; Kyle, S.D.; Dixon, W.G.; Bechtold, D.A.; Gill, S.; Little, M.A.; Luik, A.; Loudon, A.; et al. Genome-wide association analysis identifies novel loci for chronotype in 100,420 individuals from the UK Biobank. *Nat. Commun.* **2016**, *7*, 10889. [CrossRef] [PubMed]
16. Benedetti, F.; Dallaspezia, S.; Fulgosi, M.C.; Lorenzi, C.; Serretti, A.; Barbini, B.; Colombo, C.; Smeraldi, E. Actimetric evidence that CLOCK 3111 T/C SNP influences sleep and activity patterns in patients affected by bipolar depression. *Am. J. Med. Genet. B Neuropsychiatr. Genet.* **2007**, *144B*, 631–635. [CrossRef] [PubMed]
17. Serretti, A.; Benedetti, F.; Mandelli, L.; Lorenzi, C.; Pirovano, A.; Colombo, C.; Smeraldi, E. Genetic dissection of psychopathological symptoms insomnia in mood disorders and *CLOCK* gene polymorphism. *Am. J. Med. Genet. B Neuropsychiatr. Genet.* **2003**, *121B*, 35–38. [CrossRef] [PubMed]

18. Scott, A.J.; Monk, T.H.; Brink, L.L. Shiftwork as a Risk Factor for Depression: A Pilot Study. *Int. J. Occup. Environ. Health* **1997**, *3*, S2–S9. [PubMed]
19. Bildt, C.; Michelsen, H. Gender differences in the effects from working conditions on mental health: A 4-year follow-up. *Int. Arch. Occup. Environ. Health* **2002**, *75*, 252–258. [CrossRef] [PubMed]
20. Costa, G. Shift work and occupational medicine: An overview. *Occup. Med.* **2003**, *53*, 83–88. [CrossRef]
21. Muecke, S. Effects of rotating night shifts: Literature review. *J. Adv. Nurs.* **2005**, *50*, 433–439. [CrossRef] [PubMed]
22. Bara, A.C.; Arber, S. Working shifts and mental health–findings from the British Household Panel Survey (1995–2005). *Scand. J. Work Environ. Health* **2009**, *35*, 361–367. [CrossRef] [PubMed]
23. Pallesen, S.; Bjorvatn, B.; Mageroy, N.; Saksvik, I.B.; Waage, S. Measures to counteract the negative effects of night work. *Scand. J. Work Environ. Health* **2010**, *36*, 109–120. [CrossRef] [PubMed]
24. Harma, M.; Kecklund, G. Shift work and health—How to proceed? *Scand. J. Work Environ. Health* **2010**, *36*, 81–84. [CrossRef] [PubMed]
25. James, F.O.; Cermakian, N.; Boivin, D.B. Circadian rhythms of melatonin, cortisol, and *clock* gene expression during simulated night shift work. *SLEEP* **2007**, *30*, 11–1427. [CrossRef]
26. Husse, J.; Hintze, S.C.; Eichele, G.; Lehnert, H.; Oster, H. Circadian Clock Genes *Per1* and *Per2* Regulate the Response of Metabolism-Associated Transcripts to Sleep Disruption. *PLoS ONE* **2012**, *7*, 12–52983. [CrossRef] [PubMed]
27. Taniyama, Y.; yamauchi, T.; takeuchi, S.; Kuroda, Y. *PER1* polymorphism associated with shift work disorder. *Sleep Biol. Rhythm.* **2015**, *13*, 342–347. [CrossRef]
28. Duffy, J.F.; Kronauer, R.E.; Czeisler, C.A. Phase-shifting human circadian rhythms: Influence of sleep timing, social contact and light exposure. *J. Physiol.* **1996**, *495*, 289–297. [CrossRef] [PubMed]
29. Dawson, D.; Lack, L.; Morris, M. Phase resetting of the human circadian pacemaker with use of a single pulse of bright light. *Chronobiol. Int.* **1993**, *10*, 94–102. [CrossRef] [PubMed]
30. Honman, K.; Honman, S.; Nakamura, K.; Sasaki, M.; Endo, T.; Takahashi, T. Differential effects of bright light and social cues on reentrainment of human circadian rhythms. *Am. J. Physiol.* **1995**, *268*, R528–R535.
31. Klerman, E.B.; Rimmer, D.W.; Dijk, D.J.; Kronauer, R.E.; Rizzo, J.F.I.; Czeisler, C.A. Nonphotic entrainment of the human circadian pacemaker. *Am. J. Physiol.* **1998**, *274*, R991. [PubMed]
32. Reinberg, A.; Touitou, Y.; Restoin, A.; Migraine, C.; Levi, F.; Montagner, H. The genetic background of circadian and ultradian rhythm patterns of 17-hydroxycorticosteroids: A cross-twin study. *J. Endocrinol.* **1985**, *105*, 247–253. [CrossRef] [PubMed]
33. Moore, R.Y. Circadian rhythms: Basic neurobiology and clinical applications. *Annu. Rev. Med.* **1997**, *48*, 253–266. [CrossRef] [PubMed]
34. Reppert, S.M.; Weaver, D.R. Coordination of circadian timing in mammals. *Nature* **2002**, *418*, 935–941. [CrossRef] [PubMed]
35. Johnson, C.H. Testing the Adaptive Value of Circadian Systems. *Methods Enzymol.* **2005**, *393*, 818–837. [PubMed]
36. Pevet, P.; Challet, E. Melatonin: Both master clock output and internal time-giver in the circadian clock network. *J. Physiol. Paris* **2011**, *105*, 170–182. [CrossRef] [PubMed]
37. Konopka, R.J.; Benzer, S. Clock mutants of Drosophila melanogaster. *Proc. Natl. Acad. Sci. USA* **1971**, *58*, 2112–2116. [CrossRef]
38. Edery, I.; Rutila, J.E.; Rosbash, M. Phase shifting of the circadian clock by induction of the Drosophila period protein. *Science* **1994**, *263*, 237–240. [CrossRef] [PubMed]
39. Sehgal, A.; Price, J.L.; Man, B.; Young, M.W. Loss of circadian behavioral rhythms and per RNA oscillations in the Drosophila mutant timeless. *Science* **1994**, *263*, 1603–1606. [CrossRef] [PubMed]
40. Gekakis, N.; Saez, L.; Delahaye-Brown, A.M.; Myers, M.P.; Sehgal, A.; Young, M.W.; Weitz, C.J. Isolation of timeless by PER protein interaction: Defection interaction between timeless protein and long-period mutant *per1*. *Science* **1995**, *270*, 811–815. [CrossRef] [PubMed]
41. Myers, M.; Wager-Smith, K.; Rothenfluh-Hilfiker, A.; Young, M. Light-induced degradation of TIMELESS and entrainment of the Drosophila circadian clock. *Science* **1996**, *271*, 1736–1740. [CrossRef] [PubMed]
42. Vitaterna, M.H.; King, D.P.; Chang, A.M.; Kornhauser, J.M.; Lowrey, J.D. Mutagenesis and mapping of a mouse gene, Clock, essential for circadian behavior. *Science* **1994**, *264*, 719–725. [CrossRef] [PubMed]

43. Pevet, P.; Bothorel, B.; Slotten, H.; Saboureau, M. The chronobiotic properties of melatonin. *Cell. Tissue Res.* **2002**, *309*, 183–191. [CrossRef] [PubMed]
44. Slotten, H.A.; Krekling, S.; Sicard, B.; Pévet, P. Daily infusion of melatonin entrains circadian activity rhythms in the diurnal rodent Arvicanthis ansorgei. *Behav. Brain Res.* **2002**, *133*, 11–19. [CrossRef]
45. Slotten, H.A.; Pitrosky, B.; Krekling, S.; Pévet, P. Entrainment of circadian activity rhythms in rats to melatonin administered at T cycles different from 24 hours. *Neurosignals* **2002**, *11*, 73–80. [CrossRef] [PubMed]
46. Johnston, J.D.; Messager, S.; Barrett, P.; Hazlerigg, D.G. Melatonin action in the pituitary: Neuroendocrine synchronizer and developmental modulator? *J. Neuroendocrinol.* **2003**, *15*, 405–408. [CrossRef] [PubMed]
47. Dardente, H.; Menet, J.S.; Poirel, V.J.; Streincher, D.; Gauer, F.; Vivien-Roels, B.; Klosen, P.; Pévet, P.; Masson-Mévet, M. Melatonin induces *Cry*1 expression in the pars tuberalis of the rat. *Mol. Brain Res.* **2003**, *114*, 101–106. [CrossRef]
48. Von Gall, C.; Weaver, D.R.; Moek, J.; Jilg, A.; Stehle, J.H.; Korf, H.W. Melatonin plays a crucial role in the regulation of rhythmic *clock* gene expression in the mouse pars tuberalis. *Ann. N. Y. Acad. Sci.* **2005**, *1040*, 508–511. [CrossRef] [PubMed]
49. Stehle, J.H.; von Gall, C.; Korf, H.W. Organisation of the circadian system in melatonin- proficient C3H and melatonin-deficient C57BL mice: A comparative investigation. *Cell. Tissue Res.* **2002**, *309*, 173–182. [CrossRef] [PubMed]
50. Von Gall, C.; Garabette, M.L.; Kell, C.A.; Frenzel, S.; Dehghani, F.; Schumm-Draeger, P.M.; Weaver, D.R.; Korf, H.W.; Hastings, M.H.; Stehle, J.H. Rhythmic gene expression in pituitary depends on heterologous sensitization by the neurohormone melatonin. *Nat. Neurosci.* **2002**, *5*, 234–238. [CrossRef] [PubMed]
51. Messager, S.; Garabette, M.L.; Hastings, M.H.; Hazlerigg, D.G. Tissue-specific abolition of Per1 expression in the pars tuberalis by pinealectomy in the Syrian hamster. *Neuroreport* **2001**, *12*, 579–582. [CrossRef] [PubMed]
52. Agez, L.; Laurent, V.; Guerrero, H.Y.; Pévet, P.; Masson-Pévet, M.; Gauer, F. Endogenous melatonin provides an effective circadian message to both the suprachiasmatic nuclei and the pars tuberalis of the rat. *J. Pineal Res.* **2009**, *46*, 95–105. [CrossRef] [PubMed]
53. Zeman, M.; Herichova, I. Melatonin and *clock* genes expression in the cardiovascular system. *Front. Biosci.* **2013**, *5*, 743–753. [CrossRef]
54. Johnston, J.D.; Tournier, B.B.; Andersson, H.; Masson-Pevet, M.; Lincoln, G.A.; Hazlerigg, D.G. Multiple effects of melatonin on rhythmic *clock* gene expression in the mammalian pars tuberalis. *Endocrinology* **2006**, *147*, 959–965. [CrossRef] [PubMed]
55. Agez, L.; Laurent, V.; Pevet, P.; Gauer, F. Melatonin affects nuclear orphan receptors mRNA in the rat suprachiasmatic nuclei. *Neuroscience* **2007**, *144*, 522–530. [CrossRef] [PubMed]
56. Alonso-Vale, M.I.; Andreotti, S.; Mukai, P.Y.; Borges-Silva, C.D.; Peres, S.B.; Cipolla-Neto, J.; Lima, F.B. Melatonin and the circadian entrainment of metabolic and hormonal activities in primary isolated adipocytes. *J. Pineal Res.* **2008**, *45*, 422–429. [CrossRef] [PubMed]
57. Kennaway, D.J.; Owens, J.A.; Voultsios, A.; Wight, N. Adipokines and adipocyte function in Clock mutant mice that retain melatonin rhythmicity. *Obesity* **2012**, *20*, 295–305. [CrossRef] [PubMed]
58. Delezie, J.; Dumont, S.; Dardente, H.; Oudart, H.; Gréchez-Cassiau, A.; Klosen, P.; Teboul, M.; Delaunay, F.; Pévet, P.; Challet, E. The nuclear receptor REV-ERBα is required for the daily balance of carbohydrate and lipid metabolism. *FASEB J.* **2012**, *26*, 3321–3335. [CrossRef] [PubMed]
59. Xiang, S.; Mao, L.; Duplessis, T.; Yuan, L.; Dauchy, R.; Dauchy, E.; Blask, D.E.; Frasch, T.; Hill, S.M. Oscillation of clock and clock controlled genes induced by serum shock in human breast epithelial and breast cancer cells: Regulation by melatonin. *Breast Cancer Epub.* **2012**, *6*, 137–150.
60. Torres-Farfan, C.; Mendez, N.; Abarzua-Catalan, L.; Vilches, N.; Valenzuela, G.J.; Seron-Ferre, M. A circadian clock entrained by melatonin is ticking in the rat fetal adrenal. *Endocrinology* **2011**, *152*, 1891–1900. [CrossRef] [PubMed]
61. Steeves, T.D.; King, D.P.; Zhao, Y.; Sangoram, A.M.; Du, F.; Bowcock, A.M.; Moore, R.Y.; Takahashi, J.S. Molecular cloning and characterization of the human *CLOCK* gene: Expression in the suprachiasmatic nuclei. *Genomics* **1999**, *57*, 189–200. [CrossRef] [PubMed]
62. Wisor, J.P.; Pasumarthi, R.; Gerashchenko, D.; Thompson, C.; Pathak, S.; Sancar, A.; Kilduff, T.S. Sleep Deprivation Effects on Circadian *Clock* Gene Expression in the Cerebral Cortex Parallel Electroencephalographic Differences Among Mouse Strains. *J. Neurosci.* **2008**, *28*, 28–7193. [CrossRef] [PubMed]

63. Cedernaes, J.; Osler, M.E.; Voisin, S.; Broman, J.; Vogel, H.; Dickson, S.L.; Zierath, J.R.; Schiöth, H.B.; Benedict, C. Acute sleep loss induces tissue-specific epigenetic and transcriptional alterations to circadian clock genes in men. *J. Clin. Endocrinol. Metab.* **2015**, *100*, 9. [CrossRef] [PubMed]
64. Franken, P.; Thomason, R.; Heller, H.C.; O'Hara, B.F. A non-circadian role for clock-genes in sleep homeostasis: A strain comparison. *BMC Neurosci.* **2007**, *8*, 87. [CrossRef] [PubMed]
65. Franken, P.; Dijk, D.J. Circadian *clock* genes and sleep homeostasis. *Eur. J. Neurosci.* **2009**, *29*, 1820–1829. [CrossRef] [PubMed]
66. Panda, S.; Antoch, M.P.; Miller, B.H.; Su, A.I.; Schook, A.B.; Straume, M.; Schultz, P.G.; Kay, S.A.; Takahashi, J.S.; Hogenesch, J.B. Coordinated transcription of key pathways in the mouse by the circadian clock. *Cell* **2002**, *109*, 307–320. [CrossRef]
67. Hardin, P.E. Activating inhibitors and inhibiting activators: A day in the life of a fly. *Curr. Opin. Neurobiol.* **1998**, *8*, 642–647. [CrossRef]
68. Dunlap, J.C. Molecular bases for circadian clocks. *Cell* **1999**, *96*, 271–290. [CrossRef]
69. Lowrey, P.L.; Takahashi, J.S. Genetics of Circadian Rhythms in Mammalian Model Organisms. *Adv. Genet.* **2011**, *74*, 175–230. [PubMed]
70. Lee, C.; Etchegaray, J.P.; Cagampang, F.R.; Loudon, A.S.; Reppert, S.M. Posttranslational mechanisms regulate the mammalian circadian clock. *Cell* **2001**, *107*, 855–867. [CrossRef]
71. Kume, K.; Zylka, M.J.; Sriram, S.; Shearman, L.P.; Weaver, D.R. mCRY1 and mCRY2 are essential components of the negative limb of the circadian clock feedback loop. *Cell* **1999**, *98*, 193–205. [CrossRef]
72. Shearman, L.P.; Sriram, S.; Weaver, D.R.; Maywood, E.S.; Chaves, I. Interacting molecular loops in the mammalian circadian clock. *Science* **2000**, *288*, 1013–1019. [CrossRef] [PubMed]
73. Marcheva, B.; Ramsey, K.M.; Buhr, E.D.; Kobayashi, Y.; Su, H.; Ko, C.H.; Bass, J. Disruption of the clock components CLOCK and BMAL1 leads to hypoinsulinaemia and diabetes. *Nature* **2010**, *466*, 627–631. [CrossRef] [PubMed]
74. Janich, P.; Pascual, G.; Merlos-Suárez, A. The circadian molecular clock creates epidermal stem cell heterogeneity. *Nature* **2011**, *480*, 209–214. [CrossRef] [PubMed]
75. Paschos, G.K.; Ibrahim, S.; Song, W.; Kunieda, T.; Grant, G.; Reyes, T.M.; Fitzgerald, G.A. Obesity in mice with adipocyte-specific deletion of clock component Arntl. *Nat. Med.* **2012**, *18*, 12–1768. [CrossRef] [PubMed]
76. Takahashi, J.S.; Hong, H.K.; Ko, C.H.; McDearmon, E.L. The genetics of mammalian circadian order and disorder: Implications for physiology and disease. *Nat. Rev. Genet.* **2008**, *9*, 764–775. [CrossRef] [PubMed]
77. Jiang, F.; Van Dyke, R.D.; Zhang, J.; Li, F.; Gozal, D.; Shen, X. Effect of chronic sleep restriction on sleepiness and working memory in adolescents and young adults. *J. Clin. Exp. Neuropsychol.* **2011**, *33*, 892–900. [CrossRef] [PubMed]
78. Wang, G.; Grone, B.; Colas, D.; Appelbaum, L.; Mourrain, P. Synaptic plasticity in sleep: Learning, homeostasis and disease. *Trends Neurosci.* **2011**, *34*, 452–463. [CrossRef] [PubMed]
79. Berger, R.H.; Miller, A.L.; Seifer, R.; Cares, S.R.; Le Bourgeois, M.K. Acute sleep restriction effects on emotion responses in 30- to 36-month-old children. *J. Sleep Res.* **2012**, *21*, 235–246. [CrossRef] [PubMed]
80. Deliens, G.; Gilson, M.; Peigneux, P. Sleep and the processing of emotions. *Exp. Brain Res.* **2014**, *232*, 5–1403. [CrossRef] [PubMed]
81. Coogan, A.N.; Baird, A.L.; Popa-Wagner, A.; Thome, J. Circadian rhythms and attention deficit hyperactivity disorder: The what, the when and the why. *Prog. Neuropsychopharmacol. Biol. Psychiatry.* **2016**, *67*, 74–81. [CrossRef] [PubMed]
82. Seegers, V.; Touchette, E.; Dionne, G.; Petit, D.; Seguin, J.R.; Montplaisir, J.; Vitaro, F.; Falissard, B.; Boivin, M.; Tremblay, R.E. Short persistent sleep duration is associated with poor receptive vocabulary performance in middle childhood. *J. Sleep Res.* **2016**, *25*, 325–332. [CrossRef] [PubMed]
83. Tordjman, S.; Davlantis, K.S.; Georgieff, N.; Geoffray, M.M.; Speranza, M.; Anderson, G.M.; Xavier, J.; Botbol, M.; Oriol, C.; Bellissant, E.; et al. Autism as a disorder of biological and behavioral rhythms: Toward new therapeutic perspectives. *Front. Pediatr.* **2015**, *3*, 1. [CrossRef] [PubMed]
84. Tordjman, S.; Najjar, I.; Bellissant, E.; Anderson, G.M.; Barburoth, M.; Cohen, D.; Jaafari, N.; Schischmanoff, O.; Fagard, O.; Lagdas, I.; et al. Advances in the research of melatonin in autism spectrum disorders: Literature review and new perspectives. *Int. J. Mol. Sci.* **2013**, *14*, 20508–20542. [CrossRef] [PubMed]
85. Kobayashi, Y.; Ye, Z.; Hensch, T.K. Clock genes control cortical critical period timing. *Neuron* **2015**, *86*, 264–275. [CrossRef] [PubMed]

86. Geoffray, M.M.; Nicolas, A.; Speranza, M.; Georgieff, N. Are circadian rhythms new pathways to understand Autism spectrum disorder? *J. Neuropsychol* **2016**, in press.
87. Wöhr, M.; Orduz, D.; Gregory, P.; Moreno, H.; Khan, U.; Vörckel, K.J.; Wolfer, D.P.; Welzl, H.; Gall, D.; Schiffmann, S.N.; et al. Lack of parvalbumin in mice leads to behavioral deficits relevant to all human autism core symptoms and related neural. *Transl. Psychiatry* **2015**, *5*, 525. [CrossRef] [PubMed]
88. Wulff, K.; Dijk, D.J.; Middleton, B.; Foster, R.G.; Joyce, E.M. Sleep and circadian rhythm disruption in schizophrenia. *Br. J. Psychiatry J. Ment. Sci.* **2012**, *200*, 308–316. [CrossRef] [PubMed]
89. Nicholas, B.; Rudrasingham, V.; Nash, S.; Kirov, G.; Owen, M.J.; Wimpory, D.C. Association of *Per1* and *Npas2* with autistic disorder: Support for the clock genes/social timing hypothesis. *Mol. Psychiatry* **2007**, *12*, 581–592. [CrossRef] [PubMed]
90. Kissling, C.; Retz, W.; Wiemann, S.; Coogan, AN.; Clement, RM.; Hunnerkopf, R.; Conner, A.C.; Freitag, C.M.; Rösler, M.; Thome, J. A polymorphism at the 3′-untranslated region of the *CLOCK* gene is associated with adult attention-deficit hyperactivity disorder. *Am. J. Med. Genet. B Neuropsychiatr. Genet.* **2008**, *147*, 333–338. [CrossRef] [PubMed]
91. Xu, X.; Breen, G.; Chen, C.K.; Huang, Y.S.; Wu, Y.Y.; Asherson, P. Association study between a polymorphism at the 3′-untranslated region of *CLOCK* gene and attention deficit hyperactivity disorder. *Behav. Brain Funct.* **2010**, *6*, 48. [CrossRef] [PubMed]
92. Sipila, T.; Kananen, L.; Greco, D.; Donner, J.; Silander, K.; Terwilliger, J.D. An association analysis of circadian genes in anxiety disorders. *Biol. Psychiatry* **2010**, *67*, 1163–1170. [CrossRef] [PubMed]
93. Partonen, T.; Treutlein, J.; Alpman, A.; Frank, J.; Johansson, C.; Depner, M.; Aron, L.; Rietschel, M.; Wellek, S.; Soronen, P. Three circadian clock genes Per2, Arntl, and Npas2 contribute to winter depression. *Ann. Med.* **2007**, *39*, 229–238. [CrossRef] [PubMed]
94. Lavebratt, C.; Sjöholm, L.K.; Soronen, P.; Paunio, T.; Vawter, M.P.; Bunney, W.E.; Adolfsson, R.; Forsell, Y.; Wu, J.C.; Kelsoe, J.R.; et al. CRY2 Is Associated with Depression. *PLoS ONE* **2010**, *5*, e9407. [CrossRef] [PubMed]
95. Soria, V.; Martinez-Amoros, E.; Escaramis, G.; Valero, J.; Perez-Egea, R.; Garcia, C. Differential association of circadian genes with mood disorders: CRY1 and NPAS2 are associated with unipolar major depression and CLOCK and VIP with bipolar disorder. *Neuropsychopharmacology* **2010**, *35*, 1279–1289. [CrossRef] [PubMed]
96. Nievergelt, C.M.; Kripke, D.F.; Barrett, T.B.; Burg, E.; Remick, R.A.; Sadovnick, A.D. Suggestive evidence for association of the circadian genes PERIOD3 and ARNTL with bipolar disorder. *Am. J. Med. Genet. B Neuropsychiatr. Genet.* **2006**, *141B*, 234–241. [CrossRef] [PubMed]
97. Shi, J.; Wittke-Thompson, J.K.; Badner, J.A.; Hattori, E.; Potash, J.B.; Willour, V.L. Clock genes may influence bipolar disorder susceptibility and dysfunctional circadian rhythm. *Am. J. Med. Genet. B Neuropsychiatr. Genet.* **2008**, *147B*, 1047–1055. [CrossRef] [PubMed]
98. Aston, C.; Jiang, L.; Sokolov, B.P. Microarray analysis of postmortem temporal cortex from patients with schizophrenia. *J. Neurosci. Res.* **2004**, *77*, 858–866. [CrossRef] [PubMed]
99. Mansour, H.A.; Wood, J.; Logue, T.; Chowdari, K.V.; Dayal, M.; Kupfer, D.J.; Monk, T.H.; Devlin, B.; Nimgaonkar, V.L. Association study of eight circadian genes with bipolar I disorder, schizoaffective disorder and schizophrenia. *Genes Brain Behav.* **2006**, *5*, 150–157. [CrossRef] [PubMed]
100. Sun, H.Q.; Li, S.X.; Chen, F.B.; Zhang, Y.; Li, P.; Jin, M.; Sun, Y.; Wang, F.; Mi, W.F.; Shi, L.; et al. Diurnal neurobiological alterations after exposure to clozapine in first-episode schizophrenia patients. *Psychoneuroendocrinology* **2016**, *64*, 108–116. [CrossRef] [PubMed]
101. Johansson, A.S.; Owe-Larsson, B.; Hetta, J.; Lundkvist, G.B. Altered circadian clock gene expression in patients with schizophrenia. *Schizophr. Res.* **2016**, *174*, 17–23. [CrossRef] [PubMed]
102. Buhr, E.D.; Takahashi, J.S. Molecular components of the Mammalian circadian clock. *Handb. Exp. Pharmacol.* **2013**, *217*, 3–27.
103. Oster, H.; Damerow, S.; Kiessling, S.; Jakubcakova, V.; Abraham, D.; Tian, J.; Hoffmann, M.W.; Eichele, G. The circadian rhythm of glucocorticoids is regulated by a gating mechanism residing in the adrenal cortical clock. *Cell. Metab.* **2006**, *4*, 163–173. [CrossRef] [PubMed]
104. Son, G.H.; Chung, S.; Choe, H.K.; Kim, H.D.; Baik, S.M.; Lee, H.; Lee, H.W.; Choi, S.; Sun, W.; Kim, H.; et al. Adrenal peripheral clock controls the autonomous circadian rhythm of glucocorticoid by causing rhythmic steroid production. *Proc. Natl. Acad. Sci. USA* **2008**, *105*, 20970–20975. [CrossRef] [PubMed]

105. Yamamoto, T.; Nakahata, Y.; Tanaka, M.; Yoshida, M.; Soma, H.; Shinohara, K.; Yasuda, A.; Mamine, T.; Takumi, T. Acute physical stress elevates mouse PERIOD1 mRNA expression in mouse peripheral tissues via a glucocorticoid-responsive element. *J. Biol. Chem.* **2005**, *280*, 42036–42043. [CrossRef] [PubMed]
106. Dulcis, D.; Jamshidi, P.; Leutgeb, S.; Spitzer, N.C. Neurotransmitter switching in the adult brain regulates behavior. *Science* **2013**, *340*, 449–453. [CrossRef] [PubMed]
107. Jackson, A.; Cavanagh, J.; Scott, J. A systematic review of manic and depressive prodromes. *J. Affect. Disord.* **2003**, *74*, 209–217. [CrossRef]
108. American Psychiatric Association. *Diagnostic and Statistical Manual of Mental Disorders*, 5th ed.; American Psychiatric Association: Washington, DC, USA, 2015.
109. Millar, A.; Espie, C.A.; Scott, J. The sleep of remitted bipolar outpatients: A controlled naturalistic study using actigraphy. *J. Affect. Disord.* **2004**, *80*, 145–153. [CrossRef]
110. Mansour, H.A.; Wood, J.; Chowdari, K.V.; Dayal, M.; Thase, M.E.; Kupfer, D.J.; Monk, T.H.; Devlin, B.; Nimgaonkar, V.L. Circadian phase variation in bipolar I disorder. *Chronobiol. Int.* **2005**, *22*, 571–584. [CrossRef] [PubMed]
111. McClung, C.A. Role for the *Clock* gene in bipolar disorder. *Cold Spring Harb. Symp. Quant. Biol.* **2007**, *72*, 637–644. [CrossRef] [PubMed]
112. Klemfuss, H. Rhythms and the pharmacology of lithium. *Pharmacol. Ther.* **1992**, *56*, 53–78. [CrossRef]
113. Abe, M.; Herzog, E.D.; Block, G.D. Lithium lengthens the circadian period of individual suprachiasmatic nucleus neurons. *Neuroreport* **2000**, *11*, 3261–3264. [CrossRef] [PubMed]
114. Yin, L.; Wang, J.; Klein, P.S.; Lazar, M.A. Nuclear receptor REV-ERBα is a critical lithium-sensitive component of the circadian clock. *Science* **2006**, *311*, 1002–1005. [CrossRef] [PubMed]
115. Li, J.; Lu, W.Q.; Beesley, S.; Loudon, A.S.; Meng, Q.J. Lithium impacts on the amplitude and period of the molecular circadian clockwork. *PLoS ONE* **2012**, *7*, 33292. [CrossRef] [PubMed]
116. Kaladchibachi, S.A.; Doble, B.; Anthopoulos, N.; Woodgett, J.R.; Manoukian, A.S. Glycogen synthase kinase 3, circadian rythms, and bipolar disorder: A molecular link in the therapeutic action of lithium. *J. Circadian Rythm.* **2007**, *5*, 3. [CrossRef] [PubMed]
117. Gould, T.D.; Manji, H.K. Glycogen synthase kinase-3: A putative molecular target for lithium mimetic drugs. *Neuropsychopharmacology* **2005**, *30*, 1223–1237. [CrossRef] [PubMed]
118. Iitaka, C.; Miyazaki, K.; Akaike, T.; Ishida, N. A role for glycogen synthase kinase-3β in the mammalian circadian clock. *J. Biol. Chem.* **2005**, *280*, 29397–29402. [CrossRef] [PubMed]
119. Serretti, A.; Cusin, C.; Benedetti, F.; Mandelli, L.; Pirovano, A.; Zanardi, R.; Colombo, C.; Smeraldi, E. Insomnia improvement during antidepressant treatment and *CLOCK* gene polymorphism. *Am. J. Med. Genet. B Neuropsychiatr. Genet.* **2005**, *137B*, 36–39. [CrossRef] [PubMed]
120. Karthikeyan, K.; Marimuthu, G.; Ramasubramanian, C.; Arunachal, G.; Bahammam, A.; Spence, D.W.; Cardinali, D.P.; Brown, G.M.; Pandi-Perumal, S.R. Association of *Per3* length polymorphism with bipolar disorder and schizophrenia. *Neuropsychiatr. Dis. Treat.* **2014**, *10*, 2325–2330. [PubMed]
121. Sjöholm, L.; Backlund, L.; Cheteh, E.H.; Ek, I.R.; Frisén, L.; Schalling, M.; Ösby, U.; Lavebratt, C.; Nikamo, P. CRY2 is associated with rapid cycling in bipolar disorder patients. *PLoS ONE* **2010**, *5*, e12632. [CrossRef] [PubMed]
122. McGrath, C.L.; Glatt, S.L.; Sklar, P.; Le-Niculescu, H.; Kuczenski, R.; Doyle, A.E.; Biederman, J.; Mick, E.; Faraone, S.V.; Niculescu, A.B.; et al. Evidence for genetic association of RORB with bipolar disorder. *BMC Psychiatry* **2009**, *9*, 70. [CrossRef] [PubMed]
123. Kato, T. Molecular genetics of bipolar disorder and depression. *Psychiatry Clin. Neurosci.* **2007**, *61*, 3–19. [CrossRef] [PubMed]
124. Kato, T.; Kakiuchi, C.; Iwamoto, K. Comprehensive gene expression analysis in bipolar disorder. *Can. J. Psychiatry* **2007**, *52*, 763–771. [PubMed]
125. McClung, C.A. Circadian genes, rhythm and biology of mood disorder. *Pharmacol. Ther.* **2007**, *114*, 222–232. [CrossRef] [PubMed]
126. DeBundel, D.; Gangarossa, G.; Biever, A.; Bonnefont, X.; Valjent, E. Cognitive dysfunction, elevated anxiety, and reduced cocaine response in circadian clock-deficient cryptochrome knockout mice. *Front. Behav. Neurosci.* **2013**, *7*, 152.

127. Li, J.Z.; Bunney, B.G.; Meng, F.; Hagenauer, M.H.; Walsh, D.M.; Vawter, M.P.; Evans, S.J.; Choudary, P.V.; Cartagena, P.; Barchas, J.D.; et al. Circadian patterns of gene expression in the human brain and disruption in major depressive disorder. *Proc. Natl. Acad. Sci. USA* **2013**, *110*, 9950–9955. [CrossRef] [PubMed]
128. Kripke, D.F.; Nievergelt, C.M.; Joo, E.; Shekhtman, T.; Kelsoe, J.R. Circadian polymorphisms associated with affective disorders. *J. Circadian Rhythm.* **2009**, *7*, 2. [CrossRef] [PubMed]
129. Wang, J.; Nuccio, S.R.; Yang, J.Y.; Wu, X.; Bogoni, A.; Willner, A.E. High-speed addition/subtraction/complement/doubling of quaternary numbers using optical nonlinearities and DQPSK signals. *Opt. Lett.* **2012**, *37*, 1139–1141. [CrossRef] [PubMed]
130. Kovanen, L.; Kaunisto, M.; Donner, K.; Saarikoski, S.T.; Partonen, T. *CRY2* genetic variants associate with dysthymia. *PLoS ONE* **2013**, *8*, 71450. [CrossRef] [PubMed]
131. Hua, P.; Liu, W.; Chen, D.; Zhao, Y.; Chen, L.; Zhang, N.; Wang, C.; Guo, S.; Wang, L.; Xiao, H.; et al. *Cry1* and *Tef* gene polymorphisms are associated with major depressive disorder in the Chinese population. *J. Affect. Disord.* **2014**, *157*, 100–103. [CrossRef] [PubMed]
132. Shi, S.Q.; White, M.J.; Borsetti, H.M.; Pendergast, J.S.; Hida, A.; Ciarleglio, C.M.; de Verteuil, P.A.; Cadar, A.G.; Cala, C.; McMahon, D.G.; et al. Molecular analyses of circadian gene variants reveal sex-dependent links between depression and clocks. *Transl. Psychiatry* **2016**, *6*, e748. [CrossRef] [PubMed]
133. Pirovano, A.; Lorenzi, C.; Serretti, A.; Ploia, C.; Landoni, S.; Catalano, M.; Smeraldi, E. Two new rare variants in the circadian "clock" gene may influence sleep pattern. *Genet. Med.* **2005**, *7*, 455–457. [CrossRef] [PubMed]
134. Desan, P.H.; Oren, D.A.; Malison, R.; Price, L.H.; Rosenbaum, J.; Smoller, J.; Charney, D.S.; Gelernter, J. Genetic polymorphism at the *CLOCK* gene locus and major depression. *Am. J. Med. Genet.* **2000**, *96*, 418–421. [CrossRef]
135. Serretti, A.; Gaspar-Barba, E.; Calati, R.; Cruz-Fuentes, C.S.; Gomez-Sanchez, A.; Perez-Molina, A.; de Ronchi, D. 3111T/C clock gene polymorphism is not associated with sleep disturbances in untreated depressed patients. *Chronobiol. Int.* **2010**, *27*, 265–277. [CrossRef] [PubMed]
136. Jones, C.R.; Campbell, S.S.; Zone, S.E.; Cooper, F.; DeSano, A.; Murphy, P.J.; Jones, B.; Czajkowski, L.; Ptácek, L.J. Familial advanced sleep-phase syndrome: A short-period circadian rhythm variant in humans. *Nat. Med.* **1999**, *5*, 1062–1065. [PubMed]
137. Toh, K.L.; Jones, C.R.; He, Y.; Eide, E.J.; Hinz, W.A.; Virshup, D.M.; Ptácek, L.J.; Fu, Y.H. An hPer2 phosphorylation site mutation in familial advanced sleep-phase syndrome. *Science* **2001**, *291*, 1040–1043. [CrossRef] [PubMed]
138. Xu, Y.; Padiath, Q.S.; Shapiro, R.E.; Jones, C.R.; Wu, S.C.; Saigoh, N.; Saigoh, K.; Ptacek, L.J.; Fu, Y.H. Functional consequences of a CKIδ mutation causing familial advanced sleep phase syndrome. *Nature* **2005**, *434*, 640–644. [CrossRef] [PubMed]
139. Meng, Q.-J.; Logunova, L.; Maywood, E.S.; Gallego, M.; Lebiecki, J.; Brown, T.M.; Loudon, A.S.I. Setting clock speed in mammals: The CK1ε *tau* mutation in mice accelerates the circadian pacemaker by selectively destabilizing PERIOD proteins. *Neuron* **2008**, *58*, 78–88. [CrossRef] [PubMed]
140. Xu, Y.; Toh, K.L.; Jones, C.R.; Shin, J.Y.; Fu, Y.H. Modeling of a human circadian mutation yields insights into clock regulation by PER2. *Cell* **2007**, *128*, 59–70. [CrossRef] [PubMed]
141. Hirano, A.; Shi, G.; Jones, C.R.; Lipzen, A.; Pennacchio, L.A.; Xu, Y.; Hallows, W.C.; McMahon, T.; Yamazaki, M.; Ptáček, L.J.; et al. A Cryptochrome 2 mutation yields advanced sleep phase in humans. *Hum. Biol. Med. Neurosci.* **2016**, *10*, 7554. [CrossRef] [PubMed]
142. Wehr, T.A. A circadian signal of change of season in patients with seasonal affective disorder. *Arch. Gen. Psychiatry* **2001**, *58*, 1108–1114. [CrossRef] [PubMed]
143. Lewy, A.J.; Bauer, V.K.; Cutler, N.L.; Sack, R.L.; Ahmed, S.; Thomas, K.H.; Blood, M.L.; Jackson, J.M. Morning versus eveninglight treatment of patients with winter depression. *Arch. Gen. Psychiatry* **1998**, *55*, 890–896. [CrossRef] [PubMed]
144. Johansson, C.; Willeit, M.; Smedh, C.; Ekholm, J.; Paunio, T.; Kieseppa, T.; Lichtermann, D.; Praschak-Rieder, N.; Neumeister, A.; Nilsson, L.G. Circadian clock-related polymorphisms in seasonal affective disorder and their relevance to diurnal preference. *Neuropsychopharmacology* **2003**, *28*, 734–739. [CrossRef] [PubMed]
145. Iwase, T.; Kajimura, N.; Uchiyama, M.; Ebisawa, T.; Yoshimura, K.; Kamei, Y.; Shibui, K.; Kim, K.; Kudo, Y.; Katoh, M.; et al. Mutation screening of the human *Clock* gene in circadian rhythm sleep disorders. *Psychiatry Res.* **2002**, *109*, 121–128. [CrossRef]

146. Takimoto, M.; Hamada, A.; Tomoda, A.; Ohdo, S.; Ohmura, T.; Sakato, H.; Kawatani, J.; Jodoi, T.; Nakagawa, H.; Terazono, H.; et al. Daily expression of clock genes in whole blood cells in healthy subjects and a patient with circadian rhythm sleep disorder. *Am. J. Physiol.* **2005**, *289*, R1273–R1279. [CrossRef] [PubMed]
147. Utge, S.J.; Soronen, P.; Loukola, A.; Kronholm, E.; Ollila, H.M.; Pirkola, S.; Porkka-Heiskanen, T.; Partonen, T.; Paunio, T. Systematic analysis of circadian genes in a population-based sample reveals association of TIMELESS with depression and sleep disturbance. *PLoS ONE* **2010**, *5*, e9259. [CrossRef] [PubMed]
148. Konofal, E.; Lecendreux, M.; Mouren-Siméoni, M.C. Mise au point des études cliniques sur le rapport veille-sommeil dans le trouble déficit de l'attention/hyperactivité de l'enfant. *Ann. Medico-Psychol.* **2002**, *2*, 105–117. [CrossRef]
149. Dickerson Mayes, S.; Calhoun, S.L.; Bixler, E.O.; Vgontzas, A.N.; Mahr, F.; Hillwig-Garcia, J.; Elamir, B.; Edhere-Ekezie, L.; Parvin, M. ADHD Subtypes and Comorbid Anxiety, Depression, and Oppositional-Defiant Disorder: Differences in Sleep Problems. *J. Pediatr. Psychol.* **2009**, *34*, 328–337. [CrossRef] [PubMed]
150. Monti, J.M.; BaHammam, A.S.; Pandi-Perumal, S.R.; Bromundt, V.; Spence, D.W.; Cardinali, D.P.; Brown, G.M. Sleep and circadian rhythm dysregulation in schizophrenia. *Prog. Neuro Psychopharmacol. Biol. Psychiatry* **2013**, *43*, 209–216. [CrossRef] [PubMed]
151. Chouinard, S.; Poulin, J.; Stip, E.; Godbout, R. Sleep in untreated patients with schizophrenia: A meta-analysis. *Schizophr. Bull.* **2004**, *30*, 957–967. [CrossRef] [PubMed]
152. Afonso, P.; Figueira, M.L.; Paiva, T. Sleep-promoting action of the endogenous melatonin in schizophrenia compared to healthy controls. *Int. J. Psychiatry Clin. Pract.* **2011**, *15*, 311–315. [CrossRef] [PubMed]
153. Bromundt, V.; Koster, M.; Georgiev-Kill, A.; Opwis, K.; Wirz-Justice, A.; Stoppe, G.; Cajochen, C. Sleep-wake cycles and cognitive functioning in schizophrenia. *Br. J. Psychiatry J. Ment. Sci.* **2011**, *198*, 269–276. [CrossRef] [PubMed]
154. Morgan, R.; Cheadle, A.J. Circadian body temperature in chronic schizophrenia. *Br. J. Psychiatry J. Ment. Sci.* **1976**, *129*, 350–354. [CrossRef]
155. Rao, M.L.; Gross, G.; Strebel, B.; Halaris, A.; Huber, G.; Braunig, P.; Marler, M. Circadian rhythm of tryptophan, serotonin, melatonin, and pituitary hormones in schizophrenia. *Biol. Psychiatry* **1994**, *35*, 151–163. [CrossRef]
156. Lamont, E.W.; Coutu, D.L.; Cermakian, N.; Boivin, D.B. Circadian rhythms and clock genes in psychotic disorders. *Isr. J. Psychiatry Relat. Sci.* **2010**, *47*, 27–35. [PubMed]
157. Takao, T.; Tachikawa, H.; Kawanishi, Y.; Mizukami, K.; Asada, T. *CLOCK* gene T3111C polymorphism is associated with Japanese schizophrenics: A preliminary study. *Eur. Neuropsychopharmacol.* **2007**, *17*, 273–276. [CrossRef] [PubMed]
158. Rivto, E.R.; Ritvo, R.; Yuwiler, A.; Brothers, A.; Freeman, B.J.; Plotkin, S. Elevated daytime melatonin concentrations in autism: A pilot study. *Eur. Child Adolesc. Psychiatry* **1993**, *2*, 75.
159. Nir, I.; Meir, D.; Zilber, N.; Knobler, H.; Hadjez, J.; Lerner, Y. Brief report: Circadian melatonin, thyroid-stimulating hormone, prolactin, and cortisol levels in serum of young adults with autism. *J. Autism Dev. Disord.* **1995**, *25*, 641. [CrossRef] [PubMed]
160. Kulman, G.; Lissoni, P.; Rovelli, F.; Roselli, M.G.; Brivio, F.; Sequeri, P. Evidence of pineal endocrine hypofunction in autistic children. *Neuroendocrinol. Lett.* **2000**, *21*, 31. [PubMed]
161. Tordjman, S.; Anderson, G.M.; Pichard, N.; Charbuy, H.; Touitou, Y. Nocturnal excretion of 6-sulphatoxymelatonin in children and adolescents with autistic disorder. *Biol. Psychiatry* **2005**, *57*, 134. [CrossRef] [PubMed]
162. Tordjman, S.; Anderson, G.M.; Bellissant, E.; Botbol, M.; Charbuy, H.; Camus, F.; Graignic, R.; Kermarrec, S.; Fougerou, C.; Cohen, D.; et al. Day and nighttime excretion of 6-sulphatoxymelatonin in adolescents and young adults with autistic disorder. *Psychoneuroendocrinology* **2012**, *37*, 1990–1997. [CrossRef] [PubMed]
163. Melke, J.; Goubran-Botros, H.; Chaste, P.; Betancur, C.; Nygren, G.; Anckarsäter, H.; Rastam, M.; Ståhlberg, O.; Gillberg, I.C.; Delorme, R.; et al. Abnormal melatonin synthesis in autism spectrum disorders. *Mol. Psychiatry* **2007**, *13*, 90–98. [CrossRef] [PubMed]
164. Freitag, C.M. The genetics of autistic disorders and its clinical relevance: A review of the literature. *Mol. Psychiatry* **2007**, *12*, 2. [CrossRef] [PubMed]
165. Sarowar, T.; Chhabra, R.; Vilella, A.; Boeckers, T.M.; Zoli, M.; Grabrucker, A.M. Activity and circadian rhythm influence synaptic Shank3 protein levels in mice. *J. Neurochem.* **2016**, *138*, 887–895. [CrossRef] [PubMed]

166. Bourgeron, T. The Possible Interplay of Synaptic and Clock Genes in Autism Spectrum Disorders. *Cold Spring Harb. Symp. Quant. Biol.* **2007**, *72*, 645–654. [CrossRef] [PubMed]
167. Wimpory, D.; Nicholas, B.; Nash, S. Social timing, clock genes and autism: A new hypothesis. *J. Intellect. Disabil. Res.* **2002**, *46*, 352. [CrossRef] [PubMed]
168. Yang, Z.; Matsumoto, A.; Nakayama, K.; Jimbo, E.F.; Kojima, K.; Nagata, K.; Iwamoto, S.; Yamagata, T. Circadian-relevant genes are highly polymorphic in autism spectrum disorder patients. *Brain Dev.* **2016**, *38*, 91–99. [CrossRef] [PubMed]
169. Roubertoux, P.L.; Tordjman, S. The autism spectrum disorders (ASD): From the clinics to the molecular analysis. In *Organism Models of Autism Spectrum Disorders*; Roubertoux, P.L., Ed.; Springer: New York, NY, USA, 2015; pp. 29–66.

8

Tele-Assisted Behavioral Intervention for Families with Children with Autism Spectrum Disorders

Flavia Marino, Paola Chilà, Chiara Failla, Ilaria Crimi, Roberta Minutoli, Alfio Puglisi, Antonino Andrea Arnao, Gennaro Tartarisco, Liliana Ruta, David Vagni † and Giovanni Pioggia *,†

Institute for Biomedical Research and Innovation (IRIB), National Research Council of Italy (CNR), 98164 Messina, Italy; flavia.marino@cnr.it (F.M.); paola.chila@irib.cnr.it (P.C.); chiara.failla@irib.cnr.it (C.F.); ilaria.crimi@irib.cnr.it (I.C.); roberta.minutoli@irib.cnr.it (R.M.); alfio.puglisi@irib.cnr.it (A.P.); antoninoandrea.arnao@cnr.it (A.A.A.); gennaro.tartarisco@cnr.it (G.T.); liliana.ruta@cnr.it (L.R.); david.vagni@cnr.it (D.V.)

* Correspondence: giovanni.pioggia@cnr.it

† These authors contributed equally to the study.

Abstract: Background: Telehealth is useful for both autism spectrum disorder (ASD) diagnosis and treatment, but studies with a direct comparison between teletherapy and traditional in-person therapy are limited. Methods: This randomized control trial—ISRCTN (International Standard Randomised Controlled Trial Number) primary clinical trial registry ID ISRCTN15312724—was aimed at comparing the effect of a tele-assisted and in-person intervention based on a behavioral intervention protocol for families with children affected by ASDs. Forty-two parents with children with autism (30 months to 10 years old) were randomly assigned to 12 sessions of an applied behavioral analysis (ABA) intervention implemented in an individual and group setting, either with or without the inclusion of tele-assistance. Pre- and postintervention assessments were conducted using the Home Situation Questionnaire (HSQ-ASD) and the Parental Stress Index (PSI/SF). Results: Substantial improvements in the perception and management of children's behavior by parents, as well as in the influence of a reduction in parent stress levels on said children's behavior through the use of a tele-assisted intervention, were obtained. Conclusions: This randomized controlled trial demonstrates the evidence-based potential for telehealth to improve treatment of ASDs.

Keywords: telehealth; ASD; ABA; behavioral intervention; RCT

1. Introduction

Social communication deficits and restricted and repetitive interests and behaviors are the core symptom domains of autism spectrum disorders (ASDs) [1,2]. In addition, language, perceptual and sensory processing abnormalities, as well as delays in ASD detection and access to care during the crucial toddler years, remain unique challenges [3,4]. Nevertheless, intensive evidence-based treatments supported by parent-mediated interventions are crucial to obtain improvements in the developmental trajectories and functional outcomes of children with ASDs [5]. Telehealth represents a new technology able to emphasize the strengths of current treatment methods [4,6], mainly because it offers: (i) possible remote diagnostic methods with a consequent reduction in the delay in ASD detection; (ii) a continuous and ubiquitous access to care for families with children with autism; (iii) the chance to directly involve family members in the child's development by actively applying effective parent-mediated interventions.

Telehealth is defined by the Global Health Observatory (GHO) of the WHO as the delivery of healthcare services, where patients and providers are separated by distance [7]. Information and communication technologies are used to interact directly with both clinicians and algorithms. Telehealth is also used for exchanging information to enable the diagnosis and treatment of diseases and injuries, as well as for improving patient access to quality, cost-effective, health services, wherever they may be. It is especially relevant for vulnerable groups [7].

Telehealth is a delivery model demonstrating the potential to deliver early intervention services effectively and efficiently, thereby improving access and reducing the impact of resources shortages in underserved areas. The use of a telehealth delivery model facilitates interdisciplinarity and services coordination, and it also makes possible the consultation with specialists not available within a local community [8].

Despite the undeniable advantages of telehealth and the interest in exploring the feasibility of implementing telehealth-supported behavioral interventions, the number of papers suggesting its effectiveness with children or adults with ASDs are extremely limited in the literature [3,6,9–12]. Recent findings of a scoping review [3] show the potential for telehealth to improve access for the assessment and diagnosis of ASDs, even in the very early diagnostic stages. A recent systematic literature review analyzed 28 studies reporting how telehealth is useful for both diagnosis and treatment in the case of ASDs [9], and the authors concluded that more research is needed before considering telehealth as an efficacious evidence-based treatment model. This seems mainly due to the shortage of direct comparisons between on-site and online teletherapy with ASDs [6]. The most widely used implementation is parent training programs for families with children with ASDs in order to increase their knowledge about the condition, to suggest behavioral intervention strategies to manage the children's inadequate behaviors in everyday life, and to recommend psychotherapy for parents to ameliorate their emotional burden and to reduce their stress levels. In various studies, the objective of telehealth has been to make parents competent, as well as to ensure that they are able to perform a functional analysis of their children's behavior and to learn functional communication techniques. Such objectives are usually achieved through dedicated remote training with the support of educational videos, web-based programs, and weekly videoconferencing coaching sessions with an operator [3,9–12]. The results show that, in the case of direct training with a behavioral analyst, parents become competent and increase their ability to perform a functional analysis and to use functional communication techniques. Thus, telematic tools become effective, acceptable, and usable for the parents [3,6,9,12–17]. The application of these techniques by parents makes it possible to reduce the inadequate behavior of children, with a peak reduction greater than 90%, and to improve the children's social communication skills.

2. Materials and Methods

To contribute to the growing research of telehealth applied to ASDs, in this paper, we aimed to investigate the feasibility and efficacy of a tele-assisted parent-mediated intervention for children with ASD in the context of an applied behavior analysis (ABA)-based treatment [9,18]. We compared, in a randomized controlled trial (RCT), the efficacy of the parent-mediated intervention that was delivered via telehealth or in-person approaches. The RCT is registered with ID ISRCTN15312724 at the ISRCTN (International Standard Randomised Controlled Trial Number) primary clinical trial registry—http://www.isrctn.com/ISRCTN15312724. Using tele-interventions, we aim at reducing parental distress due to commute time, strict schedules and unfamiliar environments. Furthermore, we aim to create a higher family engagement in the therapy and foster skills generalization in the home context.

We hypothesize that the parents of children on the autism spectrum randomly assigned to the tele-assisted intervention will perceive (1) a decrease in the severity of disruptive and noncompliant behavior in their children after the intervention and (2) that their children become easier to manage compared to children on the autism spectrum who undergo the intervention without telehealth assistance, and that he/she will show (3) lower parental distress and (4) improvements in the parent–child functional interaction.

The tele-assisted intervention was designed and implemented through a web platform, providing video conference tools and ABA assignments for parents that included cues, prompts, and reinforcements. The tele-assisted intervention was planned by chartered ABA psychotherapists, well-experienced in parent coaching and treatment, who delivered the intervention to both groups. The psychotherapists were teamed with bioengineers who implemented the intervention protocol via a web platform. The web platform was developed within the G Suite, a suite of cloud computing, productivity, and collaboration tools, software, and products developed by Google (https://gsuite.google.com).

2.1. Applied Behavior Analysis Therapy for Autism Spectrum Disorders

The ABA method studies particular dynamic interactions between the organism and its environment, and this method has been adapted to improve challenging behaviors in children with ASDs [18,19]. ABA therapy for autism is usually administered with a high intensity and used to achieve specific, measurable goals [19]. In this field, ABA is based on behaviorist theories that state that simple and complex behavior can be taught through a system of rewards and consequences. Most of the time, this therapy is intended to "extinguish" undesirable behaviors and to teach desired behaviors and skills.

ABA focuses on a behavioral approach, making it possible to simultaneously improve behavioral, cognitive, social, and communicative skills [19,20]. This system uses "reinforcement" (i.e., rewards) to motivate children with autism to learn new skills, as well as multiple trials that start with a prompt (i.e., antecedent) to execute the desired behavior. ABA therapy starts with an evaluation to determine a child's challenges and strengths in the areas of behavior, cognition, communication, and social interactions. Then, the ABA therapist sets appropriate goals for the child and recommends a particular number of hours of therapy per week.

The basic structure of an ABA intervention is a set of repeated behavioral trials consisting of an antecedent, behavior, and consequence in discrete trial training (DTT) implementation, while in natural environment teaching (NET), the motivators are selected by the preferences of the children during natural social interactions, while any attempt at compliance is rewarded [21].

Overall, systematic reviews [18,19,21,22] have demonstrated that ABA interventions show promising evidence in terms of efficacy and are a viable intervention for individuals on the autism spectrum, both in telehealth and in-person [9,23], although the variability of the study designs, the heterogeneity of the participants' clinical presentation, and the methodological limitations reduce the generalizability of study findings.

ABA protocols in children and adults on the autism spectrum are individually delivered, with the involvement of family members or in a group-based format. While individual ABA protocols ensure a better personalization of the therapy objectives and strategies to the specific needs and skills of the single subject, group-based ABA interventions take advantage of the influence of social interaction, promoting experience-sharing, improving self-acceptance, and supporting insights of both personal strengths and impairments.

2.2. Inclusion Criteria

The inclusion criteria were as follows: (1) parents of children aged between 30 months and 10 years; (2) a clinical diagnosis of an ASD for the children of the recruited families based on the Diagnostic and Statistical Manual of Mental Disorders-Fifth Edition (DSM-5) criteria from a licensed clinical child neuropsychiatrist; (3) DSM-5 severity scores from moderate (level 2) to severe (level 3) in both the social communication and the restricted interests and repetitive behaviors domains; (4) not being on psychiatric medication; (5) not receiving any other intervention directly related to behavioral skills during the trial.

All children had a previous diagnosis that was further confirmed through the assessment and the consensus of the experienced professionals on the research team (i.e., a child neuropsychiatrist and a clinical psychologist).

2.3. Participants

Families were recruited as part of an ongoing research program and were tested at our clinical facilities. We enrolled $N = 88$ parents of 44 children with ASDs, aged 30 months–10 years. A first screening based on inclusion criteria was implemented, and $n = 74$ parents of children with ASDs were eligible; $n = 36$ (30:6 male/female) children fully met the entry criteria and their parents were enrolled in the present study (Figure 1).

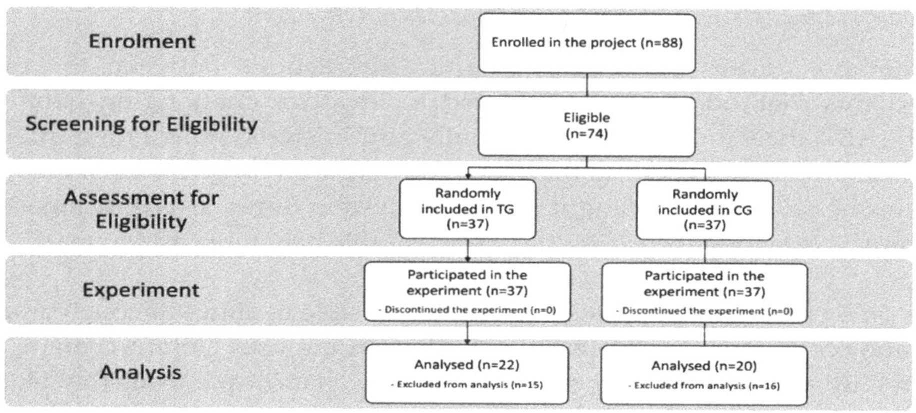

Figure 1. Subject recruitment, assignment, and assessment procedures.

Parents were randomly assigned to the tele-assisted group (TG) or to the control group (CG), applying exactly the same protocol without telehealth assistance. A randomized block design was used to ensure that intervention groups were balanced with respect to gender, age, and developmental quotient (DQ). Finally, another 30 parents were excluded due to missing data. There were no dropouts during the interventions. Data were complete for $N = 20$ parents (9:11 males/females) of $N = 11$ children (9:2 males/females; mean age in months = 69.6; standard deviation (SD) = 32.9; mean DQ = 68.8; SD = 21.4) in the CG and for $N = 22$ parents (10:12 males/females) of $N = 12$ children (10:2 males/females; mean age in months = 69.1; SD = 22.5; mean DQ = 63.8; SD = 16.9) in the experimental group (Table 1).

Table 1. Demographic and clinical characteristics of the sample.

Preintervention Variables			CG (n = 20)		TG (n = 22)		Comparison between Groups				
			M	*SD*	*M*	*SD*	*M*	*SE*	*t*	d.f. *	*p*-Value
Child Demographic	Age in months		69.6	32.9	69.1	22.5	0.509	8.79	0.058	33.1	0.945
	DQ		68.8	21.4	63.8	16.9	4.93	5.99	0.822	36.1	0.416
Outcome Variables	*PSI/SF*	PD	30.1	9.31	31.8	10.5	−1.77	3.05	−579	40.0	0.566
		P–CDI	28.6	9.41	29.4	7.09	−0.809	2.59	−0.312	35.2	0.757
		DC	38.2	6.79	40.0	8.50	0.245	2.36	0.104	39.4	0.918
		Total	96.9	13.8	99.2	11.7	−2.33	3.97	−0.588	37.6	0.560
	HSQ-ASD	SI	3.10	1.69	3.68	1.50	−0.577	0.495	−1.17	40.0	0.251
		DS	2.48	1.41	2.46	1.60	0.026	0.465	0.056	40.0	0.956
		Total	2.67	1.34	2.92	1.42	−0.258	0.427	−0.604	40.0	0.549

Developmental Quotient (DQ); Mean (*M*); Standard Deviation (*SD*); Standard Error (*SE*); Parental Stress Index/Short Form (PSI/SF); Home Situation Questionnaire-ASD Version (HSQ-ASD); Parental Distress (PD); Parent–Child Dysfunctional Interaction (P–CDI); Difficult Child (DC); * equal variance not assumed.

All of the above-mentioned children were attending mainstream public schools for 27 h a week, with a special teacher for 10–12 h. All children were Italian.

All children were scored at or above the clinical cut-off on the Autism Diagnostic Observation Schedule, Second Edition (ADOS-2), module three. The child psychologist collected information from parents concerning developmental milestones (including joint attention, social interaction, pretend play, and repetitive behaviors, with an onset prior to 3 years of age) and current behaviors.

2.4. *Intervention Protocols*

The protocol consisted of three consecutive phases. In phase I, all of the enrolled parents received 12 2 h-long plenary sessions of informative parent training about ASD characteristics and ABA/behavioral principles. The intervention protocol then consisted of two consecutive sections of 12 weeks each, i.e., phases II and III. The present study reports the results of the phase III comparison between CG and TG groups.

Phase II lasted 12 weeks. In phase II, all of the enrolled parents received 2 h/week of group behavioral therapy administered in homogeneous groups (based on the developmental age, target behaviors, and ASD level of their children). In this phase, all of the children of the enrolled parents received 1 h/week of one-to-one ABA therapy, where parents were allowed and invited to observe the therapists during treatment sessions.

Phase III lasted 12 weeks. In phase III, the intervention protocol consisted of the administration of 2 h/week of tele-assisted one-to-one behavioral parent training and coaching to participants belonging to the TG, while 2 h/week of in-person one-to-one behavioral parent training and couching was administered to participants belonging to the CG.

All of the therapies were administered by a clinical psychologist with a postmaster's degree in behavioral modification and analysis. Considering the usual ABA protocols last 25–40 h/week, our protocol can be considered to be low intensity. Testing the efficacy of low-intensity protocols, mediated by parents in natural environments, is of the utmost importance to develop more efficient implementations.

2.5. *Ethics*

All subjects gave their informed consent for inclusion before they participated in the study. The study was conducted in accordance with the Declaration of Helsinki, and the protocol was approved by the Ethic Committee of the Research Ethics and Bioethics Committee (http://www.cnr.it/ethics) of the National Research Council of Italy (CNR) (Prot. N. CNR-AMMCEN 54444/2018 01/08/2018). All of the parents of the children who took part in the study gave their consent to participate in this study, signing a written consent form.

2.6. *Outcome Measures*

The outcome measures for all of the TG and CG participants were assessed during the weeks before and after the intervention sessions (week 1 and week 12 of phase III, respectively). The general measures were assessed by direct observations of the parents. The primary outcome measurement tools were the Home Situation Questionnaire (HSQ-ASD) [24] and the Parental Stress Index (PSI/SF) [25,26], both of which are objective measures of the perception and influence of children's behavior on the psychological state of their parents. The investigators who assessed the outcome measures were blinded to intervention allocation. There were no significant differences between the prephase III outcome measures of either group (Table 1).

2.6.1. Home Situation Questionnaire (HSQ-ASD)

The HSQ-ASD is a caregiver-rated scale designed to assess the severity of disruptive and noncompliant behavior in children. Its modified and revised version for ASD consists of 27 items describing different situations or settings that are common for children on the spectrum. Parents are asked to indicate whether their children have problems with compliance in these situations and, if so, to rate the severity on a 0–9 Likert scale, with higher scores indicating greater non-compliance. Factor analysis of the questionnaire yielded two distinctive 12-items subscales: (1) Social Inflexibility (SI) ($\alpha = 0.84$) and (2) Demand-Specific (DS) ($\alpha = 0.89$) [24]. The first subscale comprises items regarding compliance with changes in daily social routines, while the second one is related to demand avoidance for daily living tasks. The two subscales are moderately correlated ($r = 0.51$). The subscale totals' test–retest reliability were all significant with $r = 0.57$ for socially inflexible, $r = 0.58$ for demand specific, and $r = 0.57$ for the combined total. Convergent validity was assessed with previously known scales. HSQ-ASD was correlated with scales measuring problem behaviors and daily living skills, while was not correlated with IQ or communication skills.

2.6.2. Parental Stress Index/Short Form (PSI/SF)

The PSI/SF is a self-assessment questionnaire designed for the early identification of factors that can compromise the normal development of a child. The Italian validation of the test affects only the short form (PSI/SF), which derives directly from the extended form, since it contains all entries with identical words. The test is based on the hypothesis that the stress that a parent experiences is the joint result of certain characteristics of their children, the parents themselves, and a series of situations closely related to their parental role. Data relating to the mother have been added to the short form, including age, marital status, education, and profession. This test investigates three main domains of stressors, namely, those associated with the characteristics of the children, those of the parents, and those of situational-demographic events. The short form is composed of 36 items, divided into three subscales: (1) Parental Distress (PD), which taps into parental feelings; (2) Parent–Child Dysfunctional Interaction (P–CDI), which focuses on the perception of the child as not responding to parental expectations; (3) Difficult Child (DC), which is centered on some of the characteristics of the child that make it easy or difficult to manage. The expected time to complete the questionnaire was between 10 and 15 min [25]. Raw total scores above 90 or 33 on the PD and DC subscales and above 27 on the PCDI subscale are considered clinically elevated. Test–retest reliability coefficients of the total stress score have been reported to be $r = 0.84$, for the PD subscale $r = 0.85$, for the PCDI subscale $r = 0.68$ and for the DC subscale $r = 0.78$. For the internal consistency of the PSI/SF, reports for total stress have been $\alpha = 0.91$, for PD $\alpha = 0.87$, for PCDI $\alpha = 0.80$ and for the DC subscale $\alpha = 0.85$. A subsequent study on parents of ASD children [26] found a similar internal consistency: PD $\alpha = 0.91$, for PCDI $\alpha = 0.85$ and for the DC subscale $\alpha = 0.82$ and $\alpha = 0.91$ for the total score.

2.7. Statistical Analysis

After having controlled for multivariate analysis of covariance (MANCOVA) assumptions of normality using the Shapiro–Wilk test and homogeneity using Box's M test of the equality of covariance matrices, parametric statistics were applied in order to analyze the group effects on the intervention. Levene's test of equality of error variances was performed post hoc.

Total HSQ-ASD and PSI/SF scores were used as primary outcome measures, while the single subscales were used as secondary measures. Group and parental gender were used as factors, while child age and DQ, together with the preintervention variables, were used as covariates. A two-sided test with an alpha level of 0.05 was used, after adjustment using the Šidák correction for multiple comparisons. Sensitivity analysis was performed using G*Power 3.1 for MANOVA with 2 groups and 2 factors and 4 covariates. With a total sample size of 42, we can identify large effects with sizes with $f^2(\text{U}) > 0.631$. To increase the confidence in the results, we computed 95% bias-corrected confidence intervals for our data using a bias-corrected and accelerated (BCa) bootstrap ($n = 1000$).

Finally, to further explore the intervention effects, as an ancillary analysis we also used a paired t-test between pre- and postintervention variables for each group separately.

The raw data for each participant comprising the demographics and assessment, HSQ-ASD and PSI/SF preintervention and postintervention scores (Table S1), as well as the complete statistics for the assumptions (Tables S2–S5), are provided in the Supplementary Materials, together with the complete analysis of covariance (ANCOVA) for the secondary outcomes variables (Tables S6 and S7), in order to provide an analytical picture of the sample distribution and to allow replicability.

SPSS software (v. 26, IBM Corporation, Armonk, NY, USA) was used to run statistical analyses.

3. Results

The demographic and clinical characteristics of the sample are reported in Table 1. No significant differences between the TG and the CG were found with respect to any demographic or clinical variable (Table 1).

The multivariate test found no effect of age, DQ, or parental gender on the outcome variables. There was a statistically significant effect in the outcome variables PSI/SF, $F(2, 33) = 39.9$, $p < 0.001$ (*Wilk's* $\Lambda = 0.293$, $\eta_p^2 = 0.707$) and HSQ-ASD, $F(2, 33) = 3.59$, $p = 0.039$ (*Wilk's* $\Lambda = 0.821$, $\eta_p^2 = 0.179$). There was also a significant effect of the experimental group, $F(2, 33) = 11.7$, $p < 0.001$ (*Wilk's* $\Lambda = 0.586$, $\eta_p^2 = 0.414$) (Table 2). Univariate analyses led to a significant effect of the group on both outcome variables: PSI/SF ($M = 8.28$, standard error (SE) = 1.91; $F(1, 34) = 18.7$, $p < 0.001$, $\eta_p^2 = 0.355$) and HSQ-ASD ($M = 0.742$, $SE = 0.358$; $F(1, 34) = 4.30$, $p = 0.046$, $\eta_p^2 = 0.112$) with a larger decrease in the TG (Table 3).

Table 2. Multivariate tests for primary outcome variables.

Effect	*Wilks'* Λ	F(2, 33)	p-Value	η_p^2	Obs. Power
PSI/SF	0.293	39.9	<0.001 *	0.707	1.00
HSQ-ASD	0.821	3.59	0.039 *	0.179	0.624
Group	0.586	11.7	<0.001 *	0.414	0.990
Parental Gender (PG)	0.976	0.406	0.669	0.024	0.110
Group × PG	0.978	0.378	0.688	0.022	0.106
Intercept	0.830	3.37	0.046 *	0.170	0.596
Age	0.955	0.785	0.464	0.045	0.172
DQ	0.994	0.103	0.902	0.006	0.064

Developmental Quotient (DQ) i.e., Griffiths Mental Development Scales III total score; Parental Stress Index/Short Form (PSI/SF); Home Situation Questionnaire-ASD Version (HSQ-ASD); Design: Intercept + Age + DQ +PSI + HSQ + Group + PG + Group × PG. * $p < 0.001$.

Table 3. Univariate Analysis for primary outcome variables.

Source	Dependent Variable	Hyp. df	df Errors	*MS*	*F*	*p*-Value	η_p^2	Obs. Power
Group	PSI/SF	1	34	686	18.7	<0.001 *	0.355	0.988
	HSQ-ASD	1	34	5.50	4.30	0.046 *	0.112	0.522
Parental Gender	PSI/SF	1	34	30.2	0.824	0.370	0.024	0.143
	HSQ-ASD	1	34	0.010	0.005	0.946	0.000	0.051
Group × PG	PSI/SF	1	34	11.1	0.305	0.586	0.009	0.083
	HSQ-ASD	1	34	0.660	0.517	0.477	0.015	0.108

Mean Square (*MS*). Design: Intercept + Age + DQ +PSI + HSQ + Group + Parental Gender + Group. * Parental Gender.

Extending the analyses to the subscales, we found no interaction among the secondary outcome variables and age, DQ, or parental gender. All subscales had a significant multivariate effect (Table S6). Univariate effects for group differences were significant for PD ($M = 4.93$, $SE = 2.16$; $F(1, 31) = 5.23$, $p = 0.029$, $\eta_p^2 = 0.145$), SI ($M = 4.92$, $SE = 0.386$; $F(1, 31) = 5.69$, $p = 0.023$, $\eta_p^2 = 0.155$), and DS ($M = 1.16$, $SE = 0.383$; $F(1, 31) = 9.23$, $p = 0.005$, $\eta_p^2 = 0.229$), while barely significant for P–CDI ($M = 3.82$, $SE = 1.92$; $F(1, 31) = 3.94$, $p = 0.056$, $\eta_p^2 = 0.113$) and not significant for DC ($M = 0.173$, $SE = 2.63$; $F(1, 31) = 0.004$, $p = 0.\ 948$, $\eta_p^2 < 0.001$).

Finally, we analyzed the two groups separately; as shown in Figure 2 (and Table 4), the TG displayed a significant improvement in PSI/SF, $t(21) = 5.10$, $p = 0.001$, with a decrease in stress of 7%. Conversely, the CG showed no significant change—$t(19) = -1.19$, $p = 0.241$. Likewise, the postintervention total scores of the HSQ-ASD decreased by 20% in the TG (Figure 3). The paired t-test indicated a significant improvement in the TG, $t(21) = 2.32$, $p = 0.035$, but not in the CG, $t(19) = 0.145$, $p = 0.890$. All children in the TG improved. Complete descriptive statistics of outcome variables are reported in the Supplementary Materials (Tables S8 and S9).

The complete raw data (Table S1) and pre- and postphase III results for each participant are reported in the Supplementary Materials (Tables S2–S9).

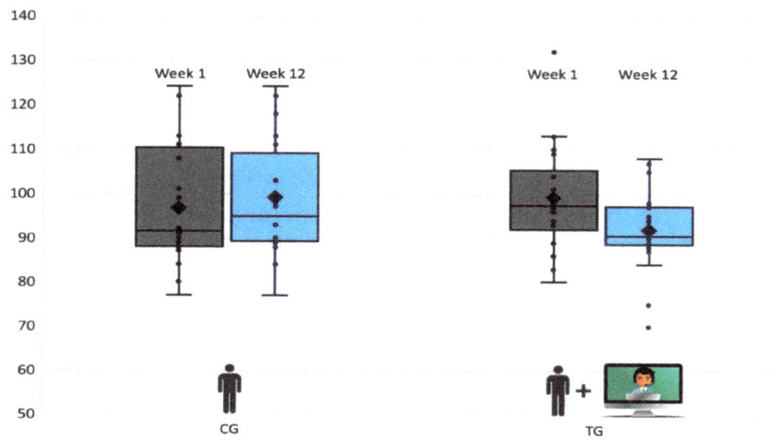

Figure 2. Box-plot of postphase III gains for Control Group (CG) and Tele-assisted Group (TG) in the Parental Stress Index/Short Form (PSI/SF) Test.

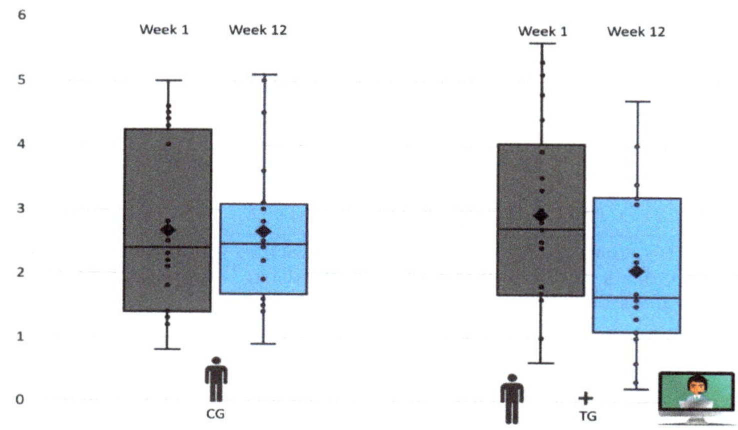

Figure 3. Box-plot of postphase III gains for gains for control group (CG) and tele-assisted group (TG) in the Home Situation Questionnaire-ASD Version (HSQ-ASD) Test.

Table 4. Pre- and postphase III comparison of outcome measures for control group (CG) and tele-assisted group (TG) separately.

Group	Test	Factor	*MD*	*SE*	*t*	df	BCa 95% Difference C.I.			*p*-Value
CG	PSI/SF	PD	−0.450	2.03	−0.225	19	−4.46	-	3.26	0.844
		P–CDI	1.65	2.13	0.777	19	−3.27	-	5.89	0.464
		DC	−3.00	2.34	−1.30	19	−7.45	-	1.79	0.225
		Total	−1.80	1.44	−1.19	19	−4.53	-	0.797	0.241
	HSQ-ASD	SI	0.050	0.172	0.288	19	−0.230	-	0.422	0.778
		DS	0.140	0.227	0.596	19	−0.250	-	0.573	0.542
		Total	0.020	0.133	0.145	19	−0.208	-	0.275	0.890
TG	PSI/SF	PD	3.13	1.75	1.80	21	−0.176	-	6.16	0.090
		P–CDI	3.68	1.22	3.02	21	1.17	-	6.32	0.010 *
		DC	0.227	2.50	0.091	21	−5.39	-	5.26	0.919
		Total	6.95	1.34	5.10	21	4.57	-	9.67	0.001 *
	HSQ-ASD	SI	0.823	0.393	2.06	21	0.036	-	1.53	0.052
		DS	1.03	0.351	2.90	21	0.378	-	1.69	0.012 *
		Total	0.863	0.367	2.32	21	0.137	-	1.57	0.035 *

Mean Difference (*MD*) between pre- and postintervention for each scale; Standard Deviation (*SD*); Standard Error (*SE*); Parental Stress Index/Short Form (PSI/SF); Home Situation Questionnaire-ASD Version (HSQ-ASD); Parental Distress (PD); Parent–Child Dysfunctional Interaction (P–CDI); Difficult Child (DC); Bias Corrected Accelerated Bootstrap (BCa). * $p < 0.05$.

4. Discussion

In this study, the feasibility and efficacy of a tele-assisted ABA intervention program for families with children with ASDs was described and evaluated in a randomized controlled trial. To the best of our knowledge, this study is one of the first to focus on a tele-assisted ABA intervention program [9]. The intervention consisted of informative group parent training, behavioral group therapy, and individual therapy, engaging parents in behavioral interactive play activities with their young children, aged 3–10, with or without the addition of tele-assistance.

We found an effect of the tele-assisted intervention group on the parents' stress levels and perception of the disruptive and noncompliant behavior of their children. This can be inferred by a significant change in the PSI/SF scores in the TG with a mean decrease of 8.28 points (−8.39%), in comparison to the CG and HSQ-ASD scores by the TG with a mean decrease of 0.742 points (−28.1%).

We found an increased ability of parents belonging to the TG to face stress, as highlighted by the PD subscale (−4.93 points; −16.1%), in comparison to the CG, and to cope with their children's inadequate behaviors, as pointed out by a significant decrease in the SI (−0.920 points; −30.1%) and DS (−1.16 points; −49.5%) subscales and as suggested by the barely significant effect of the P–CDI subscale (−3.82 points; −14.2%).

Interestingly, we found no change in the judgment of the difficulties associated with a specific child (DC subscale, as well as if both the parental stress was reduced and the children's behaviors were perceived as improved). This result is not surprising, given that our experimental intervention focused on teaching parents coping and interactional skills to manage challenging behaviors, rather than to change their perception regarding their children's temperament. The strength of this study is also its limitation. Focusing on parental perception allowed us to better understand it, but in order to generalize the results and to assess the therapeutic efficacy of the protocol, future replication should also assess behavioral changes through direct and independent measures.

We had no parents drop out during the trial. All of the parents in the TG demonstrated high interest in the web-based platform and sustained motivation throughout each experimental session. Unfortunately, 40% of the parents did not complete all of the pre- and post-tests and were therefore excluded; thus, increasing the parents' collaboration not only for the therapy sessions, but also to complete the tests would be important for future replications. Participants identified several benefits associated with telehealth including its flexibility, reduction in commute time, access to providers, and more family engagement. Parents and children experiencing the tele-assisted sessions showed the usually demonstrated parent–child interactions at home, especially initiating and sharing play activities. This is in line with the previous literature reporting how effective, acceptable, and usable ubiquitous communication technology is for the parents [27–29]. Moreover, as reported by themselves, all parents in the TG spontaneously practiced the learned lessons at home subsequent to the tele-assisted intervention, just as is usually reported by parents following in-person parent coaching sessions.

Parent–child interactions were not influenced by computer, tablet, or general technology concerns, e.g., internet connection, digital divide, or anxiety regarding their performance when using technology. These qualitative results are in contrast with those reported by Cole et al. who identified access to high speed internet and the opinion that telehealth was not as effective as in-person treatment as their primary barriers [30]. Our hypothesis is that given the specificity of our center, which is highly focused on technology, recruited parents could had a more favorable propensity toward technology, and future study should replicate the results with a more diverse population and aim to validate structured interviews or questionnaires to assess parental propensity to initiate a tele-intervention in an easily replicable fashion.

Furthermore, while ABA interventions are usually time-intensive, we administered a low-dose intervention, suggesting that the additional hour of tele-assistance could be pivotal for the success of the implementation. From informal exchanges with the participants, many parents reported challenges in generalizing and personalizing the techniques learned during the courses and in generalizing the daily life situations the skills learned through observations in the laboratory. The addition of tele-assistance helped the therapists fill the gap, reaching families of children with ASDs in their homes.

This evidence encourages further experimental studies regarding the long-term application of tele-assisted interventions in ASD therapy.

5. Conclusions

The obtained results support the idea that an ABA tele-assistive intervention can be an effective treatment for families with children on the autism spectrum following initial parent training. In line with our hypothesis, we found a significant positive effect of the ABA tele-assistive intervention in terms of parents' stress levels, perception of the disruptive and noncompliant behavior of their children, coping with their children in cases of inadequate behaviors, as well as in the influence on their children's behavior. We expect that further studies with larger samples may replicate these findings. All of the raw data gathered, and the analysis described in this study, are reported in the Supplementary Materials for future comparisons.

Author Contributions: Conceptualization, F.M., D.V. and G.P.; methodology, F.M., L.R., D.V. and G.P.; software, A.P., G.T. and G.P.; validation, F.M., L.R., P.C., C.F., I.C., and R.M.; formal analysis, G.T., A.A.A., D.V. and G.P.; investigation, F.M., P.C., C.F., I.C. and R.M.; resources, F.M., P.C., L.R., D.V. and G.P.; data curation, F.M., P.C., C.F., I.C., R.M. and A.A.A.; writing—original draft preparation, F.M., D.V. and G.P.; writing—review and editing, F.M., D.V. and G.P.; visualization, F.M., D.V. and G.P.; supervision, F.M., D.V. and G.P.; project administration, G.P.; funding acquisition, G.P. All authors have read and agreed to the published version of the manuscript.

Acknowledgments: We acknowledge all the children and their parents for their help and participation. A special thank you to the Soc. Coop. Soc. Occupazione e Solidarietà for its constant support.

References

1. American Psychiatric Association. *The Diagnostic and Statistical Manual of Mental Disorders: DSM-5*; American Psychiatric Publishing: Washington, DC, USA, 2013.
2. Styles, M.; Alsharshani, D.; Samara, M.; Alsharshani, M.; Khattab, A.; Qoronfleh, M.W.; Al-Dewik, N.I. Risk factors, diagnosis, prognosis and treatment of autism. *Front. Biosci. (Landmark. Ed.)* **2020**, *25*, 1682–1717. [PubMed]
3. Alfuraydan, M.; Croxall, J.; Hurt, L.; Kerr, M.; Brophy, S. Use of telehealth for facilitating the diagnostic assessment of Autism Spectrum Disorder (ASD): A scoping review. *PLoS ONE* **2020**, *15*, e0236415. [CrossRef] [PubMed]
4. Solomon, D.; Soares, N. Telehealth Approaches to Care Coordination in Autism Spectrum Disorder. In *Interprofessional Care Coordination for Pediatric. Autism Spectrum Disorder*; McClain, M.B., Shahidullah, J., Mezher, K., Eds.; Springer Nature: Cham, Switzerland, 2020; pp. 289–306.
5. Reichow, B.; Hume, K.; Barton, E.E.; Boyd, B.A. Early intensive behavioral intervention (EIBI) for young children with autism spectrum disorders (ASD). *Cochrane Database Syst. Rev.* **2018**, *5*, CD009260. [CrossRef] [PubMed]
6. Hao, Y.; Franco, J.H.; Sundarrajan, M.; Chen, Y. A Pilot Study Comparing Tele-therapy and In-Person Therapy: Perspectives from Parent-Mediated Intervention for Children with Autism Spectrum Disorders. *J. Autism Dev. Disord.* **2020**. [CrossRef] [PubMed]
7. World Health Organization. *Global Diffusion of eHealth: Making Universal Health Coverage Achievable*; Report of the Third Global Survey on eHealth; World Health Organization: Geneva, Switzerland, 2016.
8. Juárez, A.P.; Weitlauf, A.S.; Nicholson, A.; Pasternak, A.; Broderick, N.; Hine, J.; Stainbrook, A.; Warren, Z. Early identification of ASD through telemedicine: Potential value for underserved populations. *J. Autism Dev. Disord.* **2018**, *48*, 2601–2610. [CrossRef] [PubMed]
9. Ferguson, J.; Craig, E.A.; Dounavi, K. Telehealth as a Model for Providing Behaviour Analytic Interventions to Individuals with Autism Spectrum Disorder: A Systematic Review. *J. Autism Dev. Disord.* **2019**, *49*, 582–616. [CrossRef]
10. Knutsen, J.; Wolfe, A.; Burke, B.L.; Hepburn, S.; Lindgren, S.; Coury, D. A systematic review of telemedicine in autism spectrum disorders. *Rev. J. Autism Dev. Disord.* **2016**, *3*, 330–344. [CrossRef]

11. Lindgren, S.; Wacker, D.P.; Suess, A.; Schieltz, K.; Pelzel, K.; Kopelman, T.; Lee, J.; Romani, P.; Waldron, D. Telehealth and autism: Treating challenging behavior at a lower cost. *Pediatrics* **2016**, *137*, S167–S175. [CrossRef]
12. Parsons, D.; Cordier, R.; Vaz, S.; Lee, H.C. Parent-mediated intervention training delivered remotely for children with autism spectrum disorder living outside of urban areas: Systematic review. *J. Med. Int. Res.* **2017**, *19*, e198. [CrossRef]
13. Machalicek, W.; Lequia, J.; Pinkelman, S.; Knowles, C.; Raulston, T.; Davis, T.; Alresheed, F. Behavioral telehealth consultation with families of children with autism spectrum disorder. *Behav. Interv.* **2016**, *31*, 223–250. [CrossRef]
14. Simacek, J.; Dimian, A.F.; McComas, J.J. Communication intervention for young children with severe neurodevelopmental disabilities via telehealth. *J. Autism Dev. Disord.* **2017**, *477*, 44–67.
15. Suess, A.N.; Wacker, D.P.; Schwartz, J.E.; Lustig, N.; Detrick, J. Preliminary evidence on the use of telehealth in an outpatient behavior clinic. *J. Appl. Behav. Anal.* **2016**, *49*, 686–692. [CrossRef] [PubMed]
16. Salomone, E.; Arduino, G.M. Parental attitudes to a telehealth parent coaching intervention for autism spectrum disorder. *J. Telemed. Telecare* **2017**, *23*, 416–420. [CrossRef] [PubMed]
17. Ingersoll, B.; Wainer, A.L.; Berger, N.I.; Pickard, K.E.; Bonter, N. Comparison of a Self-Directed and Therapist-Assisted Telehealth Parent-Mediated Intervention for Children with ASD: A Pilot RCT. *J. Autism Dev. Disord.* **2016**, *46*, 2275–2284. [CrossRef] [PubMed]
18. Mazza, M.; Pino, M.C.; Vagnetti, R.; Filocamo, A.; Attanasio, M.; Calvarese, A.; Valenti, M. Intensive intervention for adolescents with autism spectrum disorder: Comparison of three rehabilitation treatments. *Int. J. Psychiatry Clin. Pract.* **2020**, 1–9. [CrossRef] [PubMed]
19. Yu, Q.; Li, E.; Li, L.; Liang, W. Efficacy of Interventions Based on Applied Behavior Analysis for Autism Spectrum Disorder: A Meta-Analysis. *Psychiatry Investig.* **2020**, *17*, 432–443. [CrossRef]
20. Leaf, J.B.; Leaf, R.; McEachin, J.; Cihon, J.H.; Ferguson, J.L. Advantages and Challenges of a Home- and Clinic-Based Model of Behavioral Intervention for Individuals Diagnosed with Autism Spectrum Disorder. *J. Autism Dev. Disord.* **2018**, *48*, 2258–2266. [CrossRef]
21. Booth, N.; Keenan, M. Discrete Trial Teaching: A study on the comparison of three training strategies. *Interdiscip. Educ. Psychol.* **2018**, *2*, 3. [CrossRef]
22. Leaf, J.B.; Cihon, J.H.; Ferguson, J.L.; Milne, C.M.; Leaf, R.; McEachin, J. Advances in Our Understanding of Behavioral Intervention: 1980 to 2020 for Individuals Diagnosed with Autism Spectrum Disorder. *J. Autism Dev. Disord.* **2020**. [CrossRef]
23. Tang, J.S.Y.; Falkmer, M.; Chen, N.T.M.; Bölte, S.; Girdler, S. Development and Feasibility of MindChip™: A Social Emotional Telehealth Intervention for Autistic Adults. *J. Autism Dev. Disord.* **2020**. [CrossRef]
24. Chowdhury, M.; Aman, M.G.; Lecavalier, L.; Smith, T.; Johnson, C.; Swiezy, N.; McCracken, J.T.; King, B.; McDougle, C.J.; Bearss, K.; et al. Factor structure and psychometric properties of the revised Home Situations Questionnaire for autism spectrum disorder: The Home Situations Questionnaire-Autism Spectrum Disorder. *Autism* **2016**, *20*, 528–537. [CrossRef] [PubMed]
25. Abidin, R.R. *Parenting Stress Index*, 3rd ed.; Psychological Assessment Resource: Odessa, FL, USA, 1995.
26. Dardas, L.A.; Ahmad, M.M. Psychometric properties of the Parenting Stress Index with parents of children with autistic disorder. *J. Intellect. Disabil. Res.* **2014**, *58*, 560–571. [CrossRef] [PubMed]
27. Baharav, E.; Reiser, C. Using telepractice in parent training in early autism. *Telemed. e-Health* **2010**, *16*, 727–731. [CrossRef] [PubMed]
28. Cason, J.; Behl, D.; Ringwalt, S. Overview of states' use of telehealth for the delivery of early intervention (IDEA Part C) services. *Int. J. Telerehabil.* **2012**, *4*, 39. [CrossRef]
29. Owen, N. Feasibility and acceptability of using telehealth for early intervention parent counselling. *Adv. Ment. Health* **2020**, *18*, 39–49. [CrossRef]
30. Cole, B.; Pickard, K.; Stredler-Brown, A. Report on the use of telehealth in early intervention in Colorado: Strengths and challenges with telehealth as a service delivery method. *Int. J. Telerehabil.* **2019**, *11*, 33. [CrossRef]

9

Genetic Variation and Autism: A Field Synopsis and Systematic Meta-Analysis

Jinhee Lee [1,†], Min Ji Son [2,†], Chei Yun Son [3,†], Gwang Hun Jeong [4,†], Keum Hwa Lee [5,†], Kwang Seob Lee [6], Younhee Ko [7], Jong Yeob Kim [2], Jun Young Lee [8], Joaquim Radua [9,10,11,12], Michael Eisenhut [13], Florence Gressier [14], Ai Koyanagi [15,16,17], Brendon Stubbs [18,19], Marco Solmi [9,20,21], Theodor B. Rais [22], Andreas Kronbichler [23], Elena Dragioti [24], Daniel Fernando Pereira Vasconcelos [25], Felipe Rodolfo Pereira da Silva [25], Kalthoum Tizaoui [26], André Russowsky Brunoni [27,28,29,30], Andre F. Carvalho [31,32], Sarah Cargnin [33], Salvatore Terrazzino [33], Andrew Stickley [34,35], Lee Smith [36], Trevor Thompson [37], Jae Il Shin [5,*] and Paolo Fusar-Poli [9,38,39,*]

1 Department of Psychiatry, Yonsei University Wonju College of Medicine, Wonju 26426, Korea; jinh.lee95@yonsei.ac.kr
2 Yonsei University College of Medicine, Seoul 03722, Korea; minji9144@hanmail.net (M.J.S.); crossing96@yonsei.ac.kr (J.Y.K.)
3 Department of Psychological & Brain Sciences, Washington University in St. Louis, St. Louis, MO 63130, USA; hy321321@naver.com
4 College of Medicine, Gyeongsang National University, Jinju 52727, Korea; gwangh.jeong@gmail.com
5 Department of Pediatrics, Yonsei University College of Medicine, Seoul 03722, Korea; AZSAGM@yuhs.ac
6 Severance Hospital, Yonsei University College of Medicine, Seoul 03722, Korea; kwangseob@yuhs.ac
7 Division of Biomedical Engineering, Hankuk University of Foreign Studies, Gyeonggi-do 17035, Korea; younko@hufs.ac.kr
8 Department of Nephrology, Yonsei University Wonju College of Medicine, Wonju 26426, Korea; junyoung07@yonsei.ac.kr
9 Early Psychosis: Interventions and Clinical-detection (EPIC) Lab, Department of Psychosis Studies, Institute of Psychiatry, Psychology & Neuroscience, King's College London, London SE5 8AB, UK; radua@clinic.cat (J.R.); marco.solmi83@gmail.com (M.S.)
10 Mental Health Networking Biomedical Research Centre (CIBERSAM), 08036 Barcelona, Spain
11 Centre for Psychiatry Research, Department of Clinical Neuroscience, Karolinska Institute, 11330 Stockholm, Sweden
12 Institut d'Investigacions Biomèdiques August Pi i Sunyer (IDIBAPS), 08036 Barcelona, Spain
13 Department of Pediatrics, Luton & Dunstable University Hospital NHS Foundation Trust, Luton LU4ODZ, UK; michael_eisenhut@yahoo.com
14 CESP, Inserm UMR1178, Department of Psychiatry, Assistance Publique-Hôpitaux de Paris, Bicêtre University Hospital, 94275 Le Kremlin Bicêtre, France; florence.gressier@aphp.fr
15 Research and Development Unit, Parc Sanitari Sant Joan de Déu, Universitat de Barcelona, Fundació Sant Joan de Déu, CIBERSAM, 08830 Barcelona, Spain; a.koyanagi@pssjd.org
16 ICREA, Pg. Lluis Companys 23, 08010 Barcelona, Spain
17 Instituto de Salud Carlos III, Centro de Investigación Biomédica en Red de Salud Mental, CIBERSAM, 28029 Madrid, Spain
18 Physiotherapy Department, South London and Maudsley NHS Foundation Trust, London SE5 8AZ, UK; brendon.stubbs@kcl.ac.uk
19 Department of Psychological Medicine, Institute of Psychiatry, Psychology and Neuroscience, King's College London, London SE5 8AF, UK
20 Department of Neurosciences, University of Padua, 90133 Padua, Italy
21 Neurosciences Center, University of Padua, 90133 Padua, Italy
22 Department of Psychiatry, University of Toledo Medical Center, Toledo, OH 43614, USA; Theodor.Rais@utoledo.edu
23 Department of Internal Medicine IV, Medical University Innsbruck, Anichstraße 35, 6020 Innsbruck, Austria; andreas.kronbichler@i-med.ac.at

[24] Pain and Rehabilitation Centre, and Department of Health, Medicine and Caring Sciences, Linköping University, SE-581 85 Linköping, Sweden; elena.dragioti@liu.se
[25] Laboratory of Histological Analysis and Preparation (LAPHIS), Federal University of the Parnaiba Delta, Parnaiba 64202-020, Brazil; vasconcelos@ufpi.edu.br (D.F.P.V.); feliperodolfo.15@hotmail.com (F.R.P.d.S.)
[26] Department of Basic Sciences, Medicine Faculty of Tunis, Tunis El Manar University, 15 Rue Djebel Lakdar, Tunis 1007, Tunisia; kalttizaoui@gmail.com
[27] University Hospital, University of São Paulo, São Paulo CEP 05508-000, Brazil; brunowsky@gmail.com
[28] Service of Interdisciplinary Neuromodulation, Department and Institute of Psychiatry, University of São Paulo Medical School, São Paulo CEP 01246-903, Brazil
[29] Laboratory of Neuroscience and National Institute of Biomarkers in Neuropsychiatry, Department and Institute of Psychiatry, University of São Paulo Medical School, São Paulo CEP 01246-903, Brazil
[30] Department of Psychiatry and Psychotherapy, University Hospital, LMU Munich, 80336 Munich, Germany
[31] Centre for Addiction & Mental Health, Toronto, ON M6J 1H4, Canada; andre.carvalho@camh.ca
[32] Department of Psychiatry, University of Toronto, Toronto, ON M5T 1R8, Canada
[33] Department of Pharmaceutical Sciences and Interdepartmental Research Center of Pharmacogenetics and Pharmacogenomics (CRIFF), University of Piemonte Orientale, 28100 Novara, Italy; sarah.cargnin@uniupo.it (S.C.); salvatore.terrazzino@uniupo.it (S.T.)
[34] The Stockholm Center for Health and Social Change (SCOHOST), Södertörn University, 141 89 Huddinge, Sweden; amstick66@gmail.com
[35] Department of Preventive Intervention for Psychiatric Disorders, National Institute of Mental Health, National Center of Neurology and Psychiatry, 4-1-1 Ogawahigashicho, Kodaira, Tokyo 187-8553, Japan
[36] The Cambridge Centre for Sport and Exercise Sciences, Anglia Ruskin University, Cambridge CB1 1PT, UK; lee.smith@anglia.ac.uk
[37] Department of Psychology, University of Greenwich, London SE10 9LS, UK; T.Thompson@greenwich.ac.uk
[38] OASIS Service, South London and Maudsley NHS Foundation Trust, London SE8 5HA, UK
[39] Department of Brain and Behavioral Sciences, University of Pavia, 27100 Pavia, Italy
* Correspondence: shinji@yuhs.ac (J.I.S.); paolo.fusar-poli@kcl.ac.uk (P.F.-P.)
† These authors contributed equally.

Abstract: This study aimed to verify noteworthy findings between genetic risk factors and autism spectrum disorder (ASD) by employing the false positive report probability (FPRP) and the Bayesian false-discovery probability (BFDP). PubMed and the Genome-Wide Association Studies (GWAS) catalog were searched from inception to 1 August, 2019. We included meta-analyses on genetic factors of ASD of any study design. Overall, twenty-seven meta-analyses articles from literature searches, and four manually added articles from the GWAS catalog were re-analyzed. This showed that five of 31 comparisons for meta-analyses of observational studies, 40 out of 203 comparisons for the GWAS meta-analyses, and 18 out of 20 comparisons for the GWAS catalog, respectively, had noteworthy estimations under both Bayesian approaches. In this study, we found noteworthy genetic comparisons highly related to an increased risk of ASD. Multiple genetic comparisons were shown to be associated with ASD risk; however, genuine associations should be carefully verified and understood.

Keywords: autism spectrum disorder; false positive report probability (FPRP); Bayesian false-discovery probability (BFDP); meta-analysis; Genome-Wide Association Studies (GWAS)

---

1. Introduction

Autism spectrum disorder (ASD) is a brain-based neurodevelopmental disorder characterized by pervasive impairments in reciprocal social communication, social interaction, and restricted and repetitive behaviors or interests, resulting in a substantial burden of individuals, families, and society [1,2]. The repeated reports of recent increase in the prevalence of ASD have raised substantial public concerns. For example, in large, nationwide population-based studies, the estimated ASD prevalence was reported to be 2.47% among U.S. children and adolescents in 2014–2016 [3–5].

Although the full range of etiologies underlying ASD remain largely unexplained, progress has been made in the past decade in identifying some neurobiological and genetic risk factors, and it has been well established that combination of genetic and environmental factors is involved in the etiopathogenesis of autism [1,6]. There is a strong genetic background of ASD, which was demonstrated by the fact that heritability is as high as 80–90% [7,8]. It is possible to estimate the heritability of ASD by taking into the account its covariance within twins, as twins are matched for many characteristics, including in utero and family environment, as well as other developmental aspects [7,9,10].

ASD is polygenic and genetic variants contribute to ASD risk and phenotypic variability. The results of previous studies showed genome-wide genetic links between ASD [11,12]. They indicated that typical variation in social behavior and adaptive functioning and multiple types of genetic risk for ASD influence a continuum of behavioral and developmental traits.

To the best of our knowledge, this is the comprehensive study to summarize the loci that are associated with ASD among the several known loci reported to be related with ASD. We have synthesized all available susceptibility loci for ASD retrieved from meta-analyses regarding the association between the individual polymorphisms and ASD. For the study, we reviewed observational studies, Genome-Wide Association Studies (GWAS) meta-analyses, the combined analysis of GWAS discovery and replication cohorts, the GWAS catalog and GWAS data from GWAS meta-analyses [13]. Furthermore, we applied a Bayesian approaches including false positive report probability (FPRP) and Bayesian false discovery probability (BFDP) to estimate the noteworthiness of the evidence [14,15]. Using these popular Bayesian statistics (i.e., FPRP and BFDP), our study shows that the results of genotype associations between the gene variant and disease were found to be noteworthy (genuine associations). Through these methods, we selected only statistically meaningful values excluding false-positive values and analyzed them again. We aimed to provide an overview to interpret the statistical significance of reported findings and discuss the identified associations in the suggested genetic risk factors for ASD.

2. Materials and Methods

This review was conducted following a registered protocol. The specified methods are available on the PROSPERO database with the registration number CRD42018091704. The Preferred Reporting Items for Systematic Reviews and Meta-Analyses (PRISMA) guidelines of this review are shown in Supplementary Table S1.

2.1. *Experimental Section*

2.1.1. Inclusion and Exclusion Criteria

Studies were included if they satisfied the following conditions: (1) estimated the risk of ASD in humans using meta-analyses in terms of odds ratio (OR) and 95% confidence interval (CI); (2) published in English. Articles were excluded if (1) they did not cover the subject of genetic polymorphism or ASD; (2) did not have individual results for ASD; (3) did not use statistical methods of meta-analysis.

2.1.2. Search Strategy

A PubMed search was performed to extract data from meta-analyses regarding the gene polymorphisms of ASD published until 1 August, 2019. Two of the authors (MJ Son and CY Son) used the search terms (autism AND meta OR meta-analysis) and obtained relevant articles, first, by scanning the titles and abstracts and, second, by reviewing the full-text (Figure 1). During the selection process, all genetic, gen*, and related terms were included in the relevant articles. Any disagreements were resolved by discussion and consensus. In the case of GWAS, the GWAS catalog was additionally used, as well as PubMed, for a more precise search.

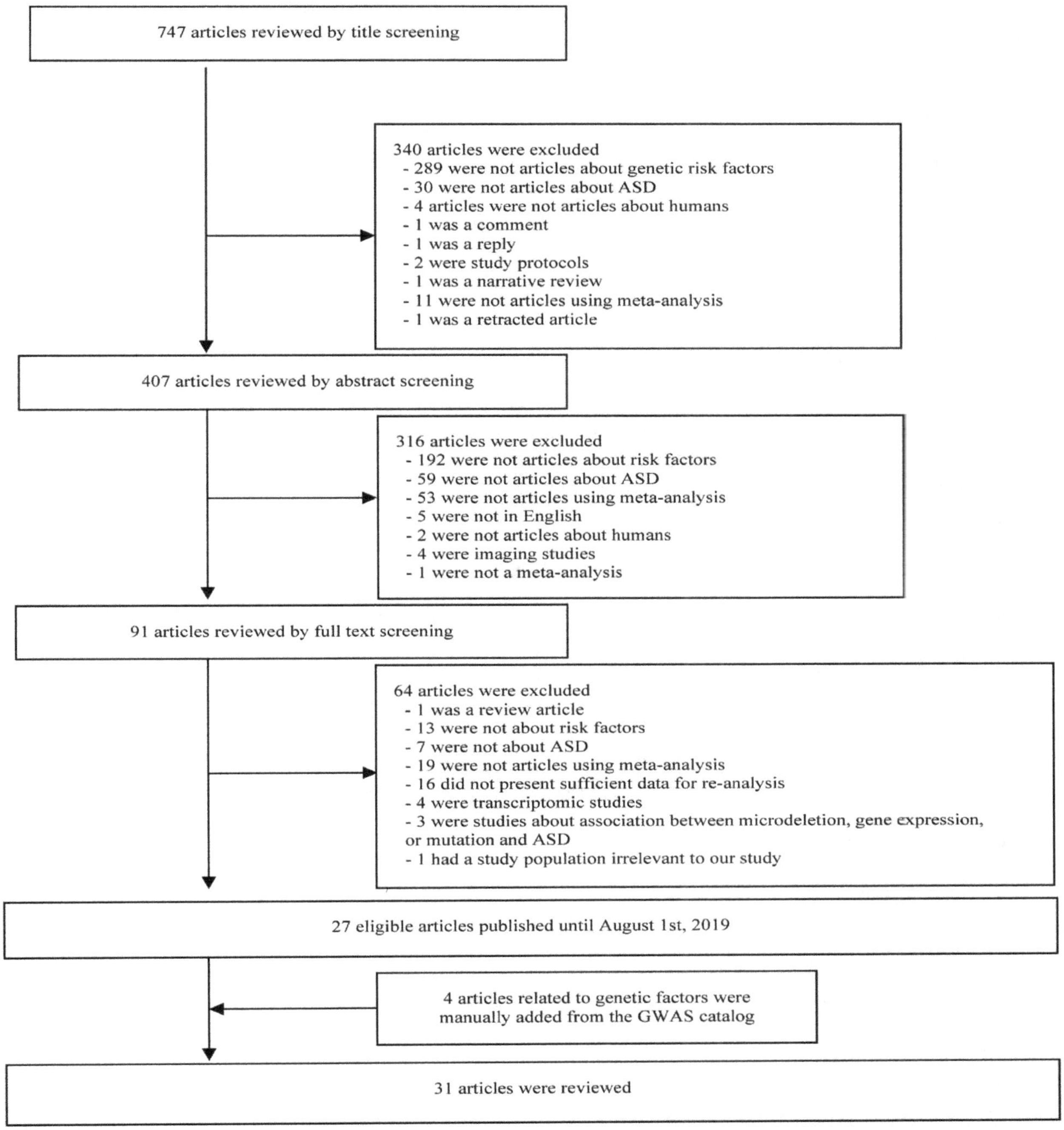

Figure 1. Flow chart of literature search.

2.1.3. Data Extraction

From each article, we extracted the first author, year of publication, the number of individual studies included, the number of cases and controls, and the number of families if a meta-analysis included family-based studies, the type of statistical model (fixed or random) and study design. We also recorded gene name, gene variants, genotypic comparison, OR with 95% CI, and the corresponding p-value. We retrieved all the main data (preferably adjusted), and, for comprehensiveness we additionally extracted subgroup analysis data if the main data were not statistically significant. When data were incomplete, we contacted the corresponding authors for additional information.

Reported association was considered statistically significant if p-value < 0.05 for meta-analyses of observational studies, and $<5 \times 10^{-8}$ for GWAS or meta-analyses of GWAS. Meanwhile, genetic associations with a $5 \times 10^{-8} < p$-value < 0.05 were defined as being of borderline significance in GWAS or meta-analyses of GWAS. In addition, we recorded genetic comparisons with p-value $< 5 \times 10^{-8}$ for our gene network, even when they were not re-analyzable due to insufficient raw data.

2.2. Statistical Analysis

Evaluations of the statistical significance of studies about genetic polymorphisms too often inferred false positives, when the evaluations were solely based on p-value [15]. Therefore, to clarify "noteworthy" association between re-analyzable genetic variants and ASD, we employed the two Bayesian approaches: FPRP and BFDP [15]. We used the Excel spreadsheets created by Wacholder et al. [15] and Wakefield [14] to calculate FPRP and BFDP, respectively. We computed FPRP at two prior probability levels of 10^{-3} and 10^{-6} and used statistical power to detect two OR levels, 1.2 and 1.5, so that readers can make their own judgment about the evidence for each genetic variant. BFDP is similar to FPRP but uses more information than FPRP [14]. Both prior probability levels were chosen as one of the low and very low values of levels, respectively. We computed BFDP at two prior probabilities levels, 10^{-3} and 10^{-6}. We set the thresholds of noteworthiness of FPRP and BFDP to be <0.2 and <0.8, respectively, as recommended by the original papers and highlighted corresponding results in bold type [14,15]. Gene variants were determined to have a noteworthy association with ASD if they satisfied both thresholds.

2.3. Construction of Protein-Protein Interaction (PPI) Network

We collected genetic comparisons either with noteworthy results under both FPRP and BFDP or with p-value $< 5 \times 10^{-8}$ to establish a network of genes using STRING 9.1 (protein-protein interaction network, PPI network) related to ASD [16]. Genetic comparison results, which show genome-wide significance (p-value $< 5 \times 10^{-8}$) or borderline significance (p-value < 0.05) with a noteworthy association under both Bayesian approaches, were included. Any results with a p-value $< 5 \times 10^{-8}$ that were not re-analyzable were also added in the network analysis. PPI networks provide a critical assessment of protein function on ASD including direct (physical) as well as indirect (functional) associations.

3. Results

3.1. Study Characteristics

The initial PubMed literature search yielded 747 articles. Out these, 656 articles were excluded after screening the title and abstract, and 64 articles were omitted after reviewing the full-text. Twenty-seven studies were finally included for the re-analysis of observational studies, GWAS, and meta-analyses of GWAS (Figure 1).

Additionally, 25 articles were searched on the GWAS catalog, but 14 articles did not meet the criteria were excluded. Among the remaining 11 articles, five articles were not re-analyzable due to insufficient raw data. Moreover, five articles were already included in our dataset from the PubMed search. However, we retained three of the non-re-analyzable articles [17–19] since they satisfied the cut-off value of statistical significance for our PPI network (p-value $< 5 \times 10^{-8}$). Out of the remaining six articles, two were already in our dataset from the literature search from PubMed. Finally, four articles from the GWAS catalog were manually added to 27 articles previously screened from PubMed, leading to a total of 31 eligible articles [17–47] being included in the systematic review (Figure 1).

3.2. Re-Analysis of Meta-Analyses

This paper is divided into two parts: (1) the observational studies part, and (2) the GWAS part. In the observational studies, all statistics were collected considering the overlapping, and results of gene variants with/without statistical significance (Table 1, Supplementary Table S2). Even though genetic variants examined in several studies, we excluded the studies if the data were not significant performed by FPRP or BFDP. In the GWAS part, data from previously published meta-analyses and newly added data from the GWAS catalog were re-analyzed.

3.2.1. Re-Analysis of Meta-Analyses of Observational Studies

Among the 31 eligible studies, 19 were meta-analyses of observational studies, which corresponded to 125 genetic comparisons. Thirty one out of 125 genotype comparisons were reported as being statistically significant using the criteria of p-value < 0.05 as listed in Table 1.

Out of the 31 genotype comparisons (Table 1), three (9.7%), and two (6.5%) were verified to be noteworthy (<0.2) using FPRP estimation, at a prior probability of 10^{-3} and 10^{-6} with a statistical power to detect an OR of 1.2; seven (22.6%) and two (6.5%) were verified to be noteworthy (<0.2) using FPRP estimation, at a prior probability of 10^{-3} and 10^{-6} with a statistical power to detect an OR of 1.5. In terms of BFDP, five (16.1%) and two (6.5%) comparisons had noteworthy findings (<0.8) at a prior probability of 10^{-3} and 10^{-6}. Two single nucleotide polymorphisms (SNPs) were found to be noteworthy under FPRP estimation only, and not under BFDP (Comparison T vs. C, SLC25A12/rs2292813 [20]; C vs. T, SLC25A12/rs2292813 [24]). In contrast, none of the SNPs were identified to be noteworthy exclusively under BFDP. Consequently, five out of 31 SNPs were found noteworthy using both FPRP and BFDP (T vs. C, MTHFR C677T; T (minor), MTHFR C677T; Comparison G vs. A, DRD3/rs167771; C vs. G, RELN/rs362691; A (minor), OXTR/rs7632287).

3.2.2. Re-Analysis of Meta-Analyses of GWAS

Seven GWAS meta-analyses and one study with a combined analysis of GWAS discovery and replication added up to 203 genetic comparisons [30–34,46–48] with statistical or borderline significant results. Out of 277 comparisons, 44 had p-value ≥ 0.05 (Table S2), none of which showed noteworthy estimation of FPRP and BFDP with statistical or borderline significant results. From the 203 comparisons, only one (0.5%), MACROD2/rs4141463 A (minor allele), was statistically significant under the genome-wide significance threshold (p-value $< 5 \times 10^{-8}$), while the remaining 202 comparisons (99.5%) satisfied the criteria of borderline significance ($5 \times 10^{-8} < p$-value < 0.05) previously defined.

We examined the 203 genetic comparisons with a genome-wide or borderline significance using both FPRP and BFDP estimation. With FPRP estimation, forty-one (20.2%) and four (2.0%) were assessed to be noteworthy at a prior probability of 10^{-3} and 10^{-6} with statistical power to detect an OR of 1.2. Moreover, fifty-four (26.6%) and eight (3.9%) were identified as noteworthy at a prior probability of 10^{-3} and 10^{-6} with statistical power to detect an OR of 1.5. Overall, forty genetic comparisons (19.7%) were found noteworthy under both Bayesian approaches, which included a single genetic comparison satisfying the conventional significance threshold of p-value < 0.05 (Table 2).

3.2.3. Re-Analysis of Results from the GWAS Catalog and GWAS Datasets Included in the GWAS Meta-Analyses

Genetic comparisons additionally extracted from the GWAS catalog were also re-analyzed (Table 3). Among the 20 included comparisons, two (10.0%) genotype comparisons, MACROD2/rs4141463 and LOCI105370358-LOCI107984602/rs4773054, extracted from the GWAS catalog were reported to be significant with a p-value $< 5 \times 10^{-8}$. The remaining 18 comparisons were of borderline statistical significance (p-value between 0.05 and 5×10^{-8}).

While assessing noteworthiness, five (25.0%) and three (15.0%) were verified as being noteworthy using FPRP estimation, at a prior probability of 10^{-3} and 10^{-6}, respectively, with the statistical power to detect a 1.2 OR. In addition, eighteen (90.0%) and four (25.0%) showed noteworthiness at a prior probability of 10^{-3} and 10^{-6} with the statistical power to detect a 1.5 OR, respectively. In the BFDP estimation, nineteen (95.0%) and two (10.0%) were assessed as being noteworthy at a prior probability of 10^{-3} and 10^{-6}, respectively. Finally, 18 genetic associations (95%) of both significant and borderline statistically significant results were verified as being noteworthy under both the FPRP and BFDP approaches. The total number of associations included two comparisons with genome-wide significance (p-value $< 5 \times 10^{-8}$) and sixteen comparisons with borderline significance (p-value between 0.05 and 5×10^{-8}).

In order to develop the analysis further, we extracted the GWAS data that was both statistically significant and noteworthy under both Bayesian approaches, from the GWAS meta-analysis and GWAS catalog. They were extracted from five articles [30–34], with 70 of the GWAS data being noteworthy under both FPRP and BFDP. Results with noteworthy association are summarized in Table 4.

Table 1. Re-analysis results of gene variants with statistical significance (p-value < 0.05) from observational studies.

Author, Year	Gene/Variant	Comparison	OR (95% CI)	p-Value	Model	No. of Studies	Power OR 1.2	Power OR 1.5	FPRP Values at Prior Probability				BFDP 0.001	BFDP 0.000001
									OR 1.2		OR 1.5			
									0.001	0.000001	0.001	0.000001		
Gene variants with statistically significance (p-value < 0.05), FPRP < 0.2 and BFDP < 0.8 from observational studies														
Rai 2016 [21]	MTHFR C677T	T vs. C	1.37 (1.25, 1.50)	<0.0001	Fixed	Overall (13)	0.002	0.975	0.000	0.005	0.000	0.000	0.000	0.001
Mohammad et al., 2016 [23]	MTHFR C677T	T (minor)	1.47 (1.31, 1.65)	<0.0001	Fixed	Overall (8)	0.000	0.634	0.000	0.179	0.000	0.000	0.000	0.009
Warrier et al., 2015 [24]	DRD3/rs167771	G vs. A	1.822 (1.398, 2.375)	9.08×10^{-6}	Fixed	Overall (2)	0.001	0.075	0.901	1.000	0.108	0.992	0.649	0.999
Warrier et al., 2015 [24]	RELN/rs362691	C vs. G	0.832 (0.763, 0.908)	3.93×10^{-5}	Fixed	Overall (6)	0.486	1.000	0.071	0.987	0.036	0.974	0.584	0.999
LoParo et al., 2015 [26]	OXTR/rs7632287	A (minor)	1.43 (1.23, 1.68)	0.000005	Random	Caucasian (2)	0.016	0.720	0.451	0.999	0.018	0.950	0.432	0.999
Gene variants with statistically significance (p-value < 0.05), FPRP > 0.2 or BFDP > 0.8 from observational studies														
Liu et al., 2015 [20]	SLC25A12/rs2056202	T vs. C	0.809 (0.713, 0.917)	0.001	Fixed	Overall (8)	0.321	0.999	0.740	1.000	0.478	0.999	0.957	1.000
Liu et al., 2015 [20]	SLC25A12/rs2292813	T vs. C	0.752 (0.649,0.871)	<0.001	Fixed	Overall (7)	0.085	0.946	0.626	0.999	0.131	0.993	0.831	1.000
Pu et al., 2013 [22]	MTHFR C677T	TT+CT vs. CC	1.56 (1.12, 2.18)	0.009	Random	Overall (8)	0.062	0.409	0.993	1.000	0.957	1.000	0.995	1.000
Pu et al., 2013 [22]	MTHFR A1298C	CC vs. AA+AC	0.73 (0.56, 0.97)	0.03	Fixed	Overall (5)	0.181	0.734	0.994	1.000	0.976	1.000	0.997	1.000
Warrier et al., 2015 [24]	SLC25A12/rs2292813	C vs. T	1.372 (1.161, 1.621)	1.97×10^{-4}	Fixed	Overall (6)	0.058	0.853	0.777	1.000	0.191	0.996	0.877	1.000
Warrier et al., 2015 [24]	CNTNAP2/rs7794745	A vs. T	0.887 (0.828, 0.950)	1.00×10^{-3}	Fixed	Overall (3)	0.963	1.000	0.389	0.998	0.380	0.998	0.952	1.000
Warrier et al., 2015 [24]	SLC25A12/rs2056202	T vs. C	1.227 (1.079, 1.396)	2.00×10^{-3}	Fixed	Overall (8)	0.368	0.999	0.837	1.000	0.654	0.999	0.976	1.000
Warrier et al., 2015 [24]	OXTR/rs2268491	T vs. C	1.31 (1.092, 1.572)	4.00×10^{-3}	Fixed	Overall (2)	0.173	0.927	0.955	1.000	0.799	1.000	0.987	1.000
Warrier et al., 2015 [24]	EN2/rs1861972	A vs. G	1.125 (1.035, 1.224)	6.00×10^{-3}	Fixed	Overall (8)	0.933	1.000	0.869	1.000	0.861	1.000	0.993	1.000
Warrier et al., 2015 [24]	MTHFR/rs1801133	T vs. C	1.370 (1.079, 1.739)	1.00×10^{-2}	Random	Overall (10)	0.138	0.772	0.986	1.000	0.926	1.000	0.994	1.000
Warrier et al., 2015 [24]	ASMT/rs4446909	G vs. A	1.195 (1.038, 1.375)	1.30×10^{-2}	Fixed	Overall (3)	0.523	0.999	0.961	1.000	0.928	1.000	0.995	1.000
Warrier et al., 2015 [24]	MET/rs38845	A vs. G	1.322 (1.013, 1.724)	1.60×10^{-2}	Random	Overall (3)	0.237	0.824	0.994	1.000	0.979	1.000	0.998	1.000
Warrier et al., 2015 [24]	SLC6A4/rs2020936	T vs. C	1.244 (1.036, 1.492)	1.90×10^{-2}	Fixed	Overall (4)	0.349	0.978	0.982	1.000	0.950	1.000	0.996	1.000
Warrier et al., 2015 [24]	SLC6A4/STin2 VNTR	12 vs. 9/10	1.492 (1.068, 2.083)	1.90×10^{-2}	Fixed	Caucasian (4)	0.100	0.513	0.995	1.000	0.973	1.000	0.997	1.000
Warrier et al., 2015 [24]	STX1A/rs4717806	A vs. T	0.851 (0.741, 0.978)	2.30×10^{-2}	Fixed	Overall (4)	0.616	1.000	0.974	1.000	0.958	1.000	0.997	1.000
Warrier et al., 2015 [24]	RELN/rs736707	T vs. C	1.269 (1.030, 1.563)	2.50×10^{-2}	Random	Overall (7)	0.299	0.942	0.988	1.000	0.964	1.000	0.997	1.000
Warrier et al., 2015 [24]	PON1/rs662	A vs. G	0.794 (0.642, 0.983)	3.40×10^{-2}	Fixed	Overall (2)	0.329	0.946	0.990	1.000	0.973	1.000	0.997	1.000
Warrier et al., 2015 [24]	OXTR/rs237887	G vs. A	1.163 (1.002, 1.349)	4.70×10^{-2}	Fixed	Overall (2)	0.660	1.000	0.986	1.000	0.979	1.000	0.998	1.000
Warrier et al., 2015 [24]	EN2/rs1861973	T vs. C	0.86 (0.791, 0.954)	3.00×10^{-3}	Fixed	TDT (3)	0.724	1.000	0.858	1.000	0.814	1.000	0.989	1.000
Aoki et al., 2016 [25]	SCL25A12/rs2292813	G (risk allele)	1.190 (1.052, 1.346)	0.006	Random	Overall (9)	0.553	1.000	0.911	1.000	0.849	1.000	0.990	1.000
Aoki et al., 2016 [25]	SCL25A12/rs2056202	G (risk allele)	1.206 (1.035, 1.405)	0.016	Random	Overall (10)	0.474	0.997	0.972	1.000	0.942	1.000	0.996	1.000
LoParo et al., 2015 [26]	OXTR/rs237887	G (minor allele)	0.89 (0.79, 0.98)	0.0239	Random	Overall (3)	0.910	1.000	0.951	1.000	0.947	1.000	0.997	1.000
LoParo et al., 2015 [26]	OXTR/rs2268491	T (minor allele)	1.20 (1.05, 1.35)	0.0075	Random	Overall (3)	0.500	1.000	0.828	1.000	0.707	1.000	0.981	1.000
Wang et al., 2014 [27]	RELN/rs362691	R vs. NR	0.69 (0.56, 0.86)	0.001	Fixed	Overall (7)	0.047	0.620	0.954	1.000	0.607	0.999	0.969	1.000
Torrico et al., 2015 [28]	PTCHD1/rs7052177	T (major allele)	0.58 (0.45, 0.76)	6.8×10^{-5}	Fixed	European (4) †	0.004	0.156	0.948	1.000	0.333	0.998	0.890	1.000
Kranz et al., 2016 [29]	OXTR/rs237889	A vs. G	1.12 (1.01, 1.24)	0.0365	Random	Overall (3)	0.908	1.000	0.970	1.000	0.967	1.000	0.998	1.000

Abbreviations: A, Adenine; C, Cytosine; G, Guanine; T, Thymine; R, Risk allele; NR, Non-risk allele; FPRP, false positive rate probability; BFDP, Bayesian false discovery probability; OR, odds ratio; CI, confidence interval; NA, not available; The bold in the table means significant results by FPRP and BFDP. † This article reported only the number of datasets not the number of individual studies included in the meta-analysis. Thus, we wrote the number of datasets in the parenthesis.

Table 2. Re-analysis results of gene variants with genome wide statistical significance (p-value $< 5 \times 10^{-8}$) and borderline statistical significance ($5 \times 10^{-8} \le p$-value < 0.05) in GWAS meta-analyses.

Author, Year	Gene	Variant	Comparison	OR (95% CI)	p-Value	Power OR 1.2	Power OR 1.5	FPRP Values at Prior Probability				BFDP 0.001	BFDP 0.000001
								OR 1.2		OR 1.5			
								0.001	0.000001	0.001	0.000001		
Gene variants with statistically significance (p-value $< 5 \times 10^{-8}$), FPRP < 0.2 and BFDP < 0.8 from meta-analysis of GWAS													
Anney et al., 2010 [30]	MACROD2	rs4141463	A (minor allele)	0.73 (0.66–0.82)	3.7×10^{-8}	0.013	0.937	0.009	0.898	0.000	0.107	0.008	0.891
Gene variants with statistically borderline significance ($5 \times 10^{-8} \le p$-value < 0.05), FPRP < 0.2 and BFDP < 0.8 from meta-analyses of GWAS													
Anney et al., 2017 [31]	ALPK3 NMB SCAND2P SEC11A SLC28A1 WDR73 ZNF592	rs4842996	T vs. C	1.08 (1.05–1.12)	0.00001044	1.000	1.000	0.032	0.971	0.032	0.971	0.688	1.000
	EXOC4	rs6467494	T vs. C	1.07 (1.04–1.09)	0.0000172	1.000	1.000	0.000	0.000	0.000	0.000	0.000	0.000
	NA	rs13233145	A vs. C	1.07 (1.04–1.10)	0.00002906	1.000	1.000	0.002	0.618	0.002	0.618	0.136	0.994
	NA	rs7684366	T vs. C	0.93 (0.90–0.96)	0.00003137	1.000	1.000	0.007	0.882	0.007	0.882	0.373	0.998
	MEGF10	rs73785549	C vs. G	1.15 (1.08–1.21)	0.0001308	0.950	1.000	0.000	0.070	0.000	0.067	0.005	0.835
	ANO4	rs2055471	A vs. T	1.07 (1.03–1.10)	0.0001334	1.000	1.000	0.002	0.618	0.002	0.618	0.136	0.994
	BNC2	rs7860276	A vs. G	1.10 (1.05–1.15)	0.0003196	1.000	1.000	0.026	0.964	0.026	0.964	0.598	0.999
	NA	rs2293280	C vs. G	1.12 (1.06–1.18)	0.0003606	0.995	1.000	0.020	0.954	0.020	0.954	0.514	0.999
	NA	rs16975940	T vs. C	1.07 (1.03–1.10)	0.0004742	1.000	1.000	0.002	0.618	0.002	0.618	0.136	0.994
	NA	rs10169115	C vs. G	1.06 (1.02–1.09)	0.004465	1.000	1.000	0.041	0.977	0.041	0.977	0.778	1.000
	C10orf76 CUEDC2 ELOVL3 FBXL15 GBF1 HPS6 LDB1 MIR146B NFKB2 NOLC1 PITX3 PPRC1 PSD	rs1409313	T vs. C	1.10 (1.06–1.14)	1.467×10^{-6}	1.000	1.000	0.000	0.145	0.000	0.145	0.014	0.936
	ESRRG	rs12725407	C vs. G	1.10 (1.06–1.14)	2.115×10^{-6}	1.000	1.000	0.000	0.145	0.000	0.145	0.014	0.936
	HDAC4 MIR2467 MIR4269	rs2931203	A vs. T	0.92 (0.88–0.95)	4.243×10^{-6}	1.000	1.000	0.000	0.261	0.000	0.261	0.031	0.970
Ma et al., 2009 [32]	NA	rs7704909	C(minor)/T(major)	1.30 (1.15–1.46)	1.53×10^{-5}	0.088	0.992	0.096	0.991	0.009	0.905	0.295	0.998
	NA	rs1896731	C(minor)/T(major)	0.76 (0.67–0.85)	1.90×10^{-5}	0.053	0.989	0.028	0.966	0.002	0.609	0.076	0.988
	NA	rs12518194	G(minor)/A(major)	1.31 (1.16–1.49)	8.34×10^{-6}	0.091	0.980	0.302	0.998	0.039	0.976	0.605	0.999
	NA	rs4307059	C(minor)/T(major)	1.31 (1.16–1.48)	1.29×10^{-5}	0.079	0.985	0.153	0.995	0.014	0.936	0.383	0.998
	NA	rs4327572	T(minor)/C(major)	1.32 (1.17–1.49)	4.05×10^{-6}	0.062	0.981	0.103	0.991	0.007	0.878	0.249	0.997
Anney et al., 2010 [30]	NA	rs4078417	C (minor allele)	1.19 (1.10–1.30)	5.6×10^{-5}	0.574	1.000	0.167	0.995	0.103	0.991	0.795	1.000
	PPP2R5C	rs7142002	G (minor allele)	0.64 (0.53–0.78)	2.9×10^{-6}	0.004	0.343	0.687	1.000	0.028	0.966	0.459	0.999
Kuo et al., 2015 [33]	NAALADL2	rs3914502	A (minor allele)	1.4 (1.2–1.6)	3.5×10^{-6}	0.012	0.844	0.062	0.985	0.001	0.482	0.051	0.982
	NAALADL2	rs2222447	A (minor allele)	0.7 (0.6–0.8)	5.3×10^{-5}	0.005	0.763	0.030	0.969	0.000	0.178	0.013	0.932
	NA	rs12543592	G (minor allele)	0.7 (0.6–0.8)	3.2×10^{-6}	0.005	0.763	0.030	0.969	0.000	0.178	0.013	0.932
	NA	rs7026342	C (minor allele)	1.6 (1.2–2.0)	1.8×10^{-4}	0.006	0.285	0.864	1.000	0.113	0.992	0.749	1.000
	NA	rs7030851	A (minor allele)	1.6 (1.3–2.0)	1.4×10^{-4}	0.006	0.285	0.864	1.000	0.113	0.992	0.749	1.000

Table 2. *Cont.*

Author, Year	Gene	Variant	Comparison	OR (95% CI)	*p*-Value	Power OR 1.2	Power OR 1.5	FPRP Values at Prior Probability				BFDP 0.001	BFDP 0.000001
								OR 1.2		OR 1.5			
								0.001	0.000001	0.001	0.000001		
Anney et al., 2012 [34]	RASSF5	rs11118968	A	0.44 (0.32–0.61)	2.452×10^{-7}	0.000	0.006	0.930	1.000	0.117	0.993	0.504	0.999
	DNER	rs6752370	G	1.62 (1.33–1.96)	8.526×10^{-7}	0.001	0.214	0.407	0.999	0.003	0.764	0.089	0.990
	YEATS2	rs263035	G	1.39 (1.22–1.57)	2.258×10^{-7}	0.009	0.890	0.013	0.928	0.000	0.115	0.009	0.898
	None	rs29456	A	1.65 (1.37–1.99)	1.226×10^{-7}	0.000	0.159	0.272	0.997	0.001	0.504	0.028	0.967
	None	rs1936295	A	1.69 (1.37–2.09)	6.636×10^{-7}	0.001	0.136	0.620	0.999	0.009	0.905	0.179	0.995
	None	rs4761371	A	0.46 (0.34–0.63)	3.914×10^{-7}	0.000	0.010	0.924	1.000	0.111	0.992	0.521	0.999
	None	rs288604	G	1.58 (1.32–1.88)	2.975×10^{-7}	0.001	0.279	0.207	0.996	0.001	0.473	0.032	0.971
	MACROD2	rs6110458	A	1.46 (1.27–1.69)	1.806×10^{-7}	0.004	0.641	0.084	0.989	0.001	0.383	0.033	0.971
	MACROD2 NCRNA00186	rs14135	G	1.49 (1.28–1.74)	1.778×10^{-7}	0.003	0.534	0.130	0.993	0.001	0.467	0.042	0.977
	NCRNA00186 MACROD2	rs1475531	C	1.53 (1.30–1.79)	2.011×10^{-7}	0.001	0.402	0.083	0.989	0.000	0.213	0.013	0.929
	PARD3B	rs4675502	NA	1.28 (1.16–1.41)	4.34×10^{-7}	0.095	0.999	0.006	0.856	0.001	0.362	0.030	0.969
	NA	rs7711337	NA	0.82 (0.76–0.89)	8.25×10^{-7}	0.350	1.000	0.006	0.854	0.002	0.672	0.091	0.990
	NA	rs7834018	NA	0.64 (0.53–0.77)	7.54×10^{-7}	0.003	0.333	0.465	0.999	0.007	0.871	0.186	0.996
	TAF1C	rs4150167	NA	0.51 (0.39–0.66)	2.91×10^{-7}	0.000	0.021	0.764	1.000	0.015	0.937	0.142	0.994
Gene variants with statistically borderline significance ($5 \times 10^{-8} \leq p$-value < 0.05), FPRP > 0.2 or BFDP > 0.2 from meta-analyses of GWAS													
Waltes et al., 2014 [46]	CYFIP1[c]	rs7170637	G > A	0.85 (0.75, 0.96)	0.007	0.625	1.000	0.934	1.000	0.898	1.000	0.993	1.000
	CAMK4[c]	rs25925	C > G	1.31 (1.04, 1.64)	0.021	0.222	0.881	0.988	1.000	0.954	1.000	0.996	1.000
Anney et al., 2017 [31]	NA	rs1436358	T vs. C	0.86 (0.79–0.93)	0.00001473	0.785	1.000	0.168	0.995	0.137	0.994	0.844	1.000
	MACROD2 MACROD2-AS1	rs6079556	A vs. C	0.94 (0.91–0.97)	0.00001731	1.000	1.000	0.102	0.991	0.102	0.991	0.887	1.000
	LINC00535	chr8_94389815_I	I vs. D	0.92 (0.89–0.96)	0.00002102	1.000	1.000	0.109	0.992	0.109	0.992	0.867	1.000
	LINCR-0001 PRSS55	rs4840484	T vs. C	1.07 (1.04–1.11)	0.00002307	1.000	1.000	0.232	0.997	0.232	0.997	0.945	1.000
Anney et al., 2017 (continued)	ADTRP	rs10947543	C vs. G	0.94 (0.91–0.97)	0.000031	1.000	1.000	0.102	0.991	0.102	0.991	0.887	1.000
	LRRC4 MIR593 SND1 SND1-IT1	chr7_127644308_D	D vs. I	0.93 (0.90–0.97)	0.00003235	1.000	1.000	0.422	0.999	0.422	0.999	0.972	1.000
	CCDC93 DDX18 INSIG2	chr2_118616767_D	I vs. D	0.85 (0.78–0.93)	0.00003531	0.667	1.000	0.374	0.998	0.285	0.997	0.921	1.000
	NA	chr14_99235398_I	I vs. D	0.87 (0.81–0.94)	0.00003765	0.862	1.000	0.327	0.998	0.296	0.998	0.930	1.000
	TTBK1	rs2756174	A vs. C	0.94 (0.91–0.97)	0.00005245	1.000	1.000	0.102	0.991	0.102	0.991	0.887	1.000
	HCG4B HLA-A HLA-H	rs115254791	T vs. G	0.94 (0.90–0.97)	0.00005321	1.000	1.000	0.102	0.991	0.102	0.991	0.887	1.000
	MIR2113	rs9482120	A vs. C	0.94 (0.91–0.97)	0.00009513	1.000	1.000	0.102	0.991	0.102	0.991	0.887	1.000
	CRTAP SUSD5	chr3_33191013_D	I vs. D	0.93 (0.89–0.97)	0.0000957	1.000	1.000	0.422	0.999	0.422	0.999	0.972	1.000
	NA	rs9285005	A vs. G	0.91 (0.86–0.96)	0.0001147	0.999	1.000	0.354	0.998	0.354	0.998	0.956	1.000
	LOC100505609	rs73065342	T vs. C	0.89 (0.83–0.95)	0.0001169	0.976	1.000	0.322	0.998	0.317	0.998	0.941	1.000
	DCAF4 DPF3 PAPLN PSEN1 RBM25 ZFYVE1	rs1203311	A vs. C	0.86 (0.79–0.94)	0.0001394	0.756	1.000	0.540	0.999	0.470	0.999	0.960	1.000
	MACROD2	rs192259652	A vs. T	0.91 (0.85–0.96)	0.0001438	0.999	1.000	0.354	0.998	0.354	0.998	0.956	1.000
	FOXP1	rs76188283	T vs. C	1.09 (1.05–1.14)	0.0002093	1.000	1.000	0.142	0.994	0.142	0.994	0.892	1.000
	CCDC38 NTN4 SNRPF	chr12_96221819_D	I vs. D	0.94 (0.91–0.97)	0.0002128	1.000	1.000	0.102	0.991	0.102	0.991	0.887	1.000
	NA	chr3_182308608_I	D vs. I	0.94 (0.90–0.97)	0.0002755	1.000	1.000	0.102	0.991	0.102	0.991	0.887	1.000
	ASTN2 PAPPA PAPPA-AS1	rs7026354	A vs. G	1.05 (1.03–1.08)	0.0003018	1.000	1.000	0.407	0.999	0.407	0.999	0.979	1.000
	NA	rs2368140	A vs. G	0.94 (0.91–0.98)	0.0003049	1.000	1.000	0.783	1.000	0.783	1.000	0.993	1.000
	NA	rs13016472	T vs. C	0.94 (0.91–0.98)	0.0003629	1.000	1.000	0.783	1.000	0.783	1.000	0.993	1.000
	DSCAM	rs62235658	T vs. C	0.92 (0.87–0.97)	0.0004132	1.000	1.000	0.668	1.000	0.668	1.000	0.986	1.000
	NA	rs3113169	C vs. G	0.93 (0.90–0.97)	0.0004234	1.000	1.000	0.422	0.999	0.422	0.999	0.972	1.000

Table 2. *Cont.*

Author, Year	Gene	Variant	Comparison	OR (95% CI)	*p*-Value	Power OR 1.2	Power OR 1.5	FPRP Values at Prior Probability OR 1.2 0.001	OR 1.2 0.000001	OR 1.5 0.001	OR 1.5 0.000001	BFDP 0.001	BFDP 0.000001
	CASKIN2 GGA3 GRB2 LOC100287042 MIF4GD MIR3678 MIR6785 MRPS7 NUP85 SLC25A19 TMEM94 TSEN54	rs12950709	A vs. G	0.92 (0.87–0.97)	0.0004387	1.000	1.000	0.668	1.000	0.668	1.000	0.986	1.000
	CAMP CDC25A CSPG5 DHX30 MAP4 MIR1226 MIR4443 SMARCC1 ZNF589	rs7429990	A vs. C	0.94 (0.91–0.97)	0.0004525	1.000	1.000	0.102	0.991	0.102	0.991	0.887	1.000
	NA	chr8_84959513_D	D vs. I	0.89 (0.83–0.96)	0.0004634	0.956	1.000	0.728	1.000	0.718	1.000	0.985	1.000
	ACTN2	rs4659712	A vs. G	0.95 (0.92–0.98)	0.0004976	1.000	1.000	0.550	0.999	0.550	0.999	0.986	1.000
	ASB4	rs113706540	T vs. C	0.93 (0.88–0.97)	0.0005006	1.000	1.000	0.422	0.999	0.422	0.999	0.972	1.000
	GJD4	rs7897060	C vs. G	0.95 (0.91–0.98)	0.0005789	1.000	1.000	0.550	0.999	0.550	0.999	0.986	1.000
	AK5 DNAJB4 FAM73A FUBP1 GIPC2 MGC27382 NEXN NEXN-AS1 USP33 ZZZ3	rs12126604	T vs. C	0.92 (0.87–0.97)	0.0006161	1.000	1.000	0.668	1.000	0.668	1.000	0.986	1.000
	SEMA6D	rs17387110	T vs. G	0.95 (0.92–0.98)	0.0006996	1.000	1.000	0.550	0.999	0.550	0.999	0.986	1.000
	NA	chr16_62649826_D	D vs. I	0.87 (0.80–0.95)	0.0007369	0.831	1.000	0.697	1.000	0.657	0.999	0.979	1.000
	NA	rs4239875	A vs. G	1.06 (1.03–1.10)	0.0008018	1.000	1.000	0.672	1.000	0.672	1.000	0.990	1.000
	CTNNA3 DNAJC12 HERC4 MYPN POU5F1P5 SIRT1	chr10_69763783_D	I vs. D	0.91 (0.86–0.97)	0.0008401	0.997	1.000	0.792	1.000	0.791	1.000	0.991	1.000
	CLIC5 ENPP4 ENPP5	rs7762549	A vs. G	0.95 (0.92–0.98)	0.00085	1.000	1.000	0.550	0.999	0.550	0.999	0.986	1.000
	NA	chr18_76035713_D	D vs. I	0.93 (0.88–0.97)	0.000884	1.000	1.000	0.422	0.999	0.422	0.999	0.972	1.000
	BRICD5 CASKIN1 DNASE1L2 E4F1 MIR3180-5 MIR4516 MLST8 PGP PKD1 RAB26 SNHG19 SNORD60 TRAF7	rs2078282	A vs. G	0.94 (0.91–0.98)	0.0009187	1.000	1.000	0.783	1.000	0.783	1.000	0.993	1.000
	OPCML	rs7952100	C vs. G	1.06 (1.03–1.10)	0.0009399	1.000	1.000	0.672	1.000	0.672	1.000	0.990	1.000
	LOC101927907 LRRTM4	rs58500924	A vs. G	0.90 (0.84–0.96)	0.0009721	0.990	1.000	0.581	0.999	0.579	0.999	0.977	1.000
	RNGTT	rs35675874	A vs. G	0.94 (0.91–0.98)	0.001031	1.000	1.000	0.783	1.000	0.783	1.000	0.993	1.000
	LOC101928505 LOC101928539	chr5_57079215_I	D vs. I	1.07 (1.03–1.11)	0.001076	1.000	1.000	0.232	0.997	0.232	0.997	0.945	1.000
	DPP4 SLC4A10	rs2909451	T vs. C	0.94 (0.90–0.98)	0.001078	1.000	1.000	0.783	1.000	0.783	1.000	0.993	1.000
	ERAP2 LNPEP	rs55767008	T vs. C	0.89 (0.82–0.96)	0.001182	0.956	1.000	0.728	1.000	0.718	1.000	0.985	1.000
	C2orf15 KIAA1211L LIPT1 LOC101927070 TSGA10	rs10202643	A vs. T	0.95 (0.92–0.98)	0.001269	1.000	1.000	0.550	0.999	0.550	0.999	0.986	1.000
	AUTS2	rs2293507	T vs. G	0.88 (0.81–0.96)	0.001337	0.890	1.000	0.817	1.000	0.799	1.000	0.989	1.000
	NA	rs138457704	A vs. G	1.07 (1.03–1.11)	0.001357	1.000	1.000	0.232	0.997	0.232	0.997	0.945	1.000
	GLDC	rs13288399	C vs. G	0.95 (0.91–0.98)	0.001357	1.000	1.000	0.550	0.999	0.550	0.999	0.986	1.000
	MTFR1 PDE7A	rs1513723	C vs. G	0.95 (0.92–0.98)	0.001447	1.000	1.000	0.550	0.999	0.550	0.999	0.986	1.000
	ASTN2 ASTN2-AS1 PAPPA TRIM32	rs146737360	T vs. G	0.95 (0.92–0.98)	0.001534	1.000	1.000	0.550	0.999	0.550	0.999	0.986	1.000
	NA	chr6_45726254_D	D vs. I	0.90 (0.83–0.96)	0.001606	0.990	1.000	0.581	0.999	0.579	0.999	0.977	1.000
	NA	rs6742513	C vs. G	1.07 (1.03–1.11)	0.001611	1.000	1.000	0.232	0.997	0.232	0.997	0.945	1.000
	NA	rs73204738	A vs. C	0.92 (0.88–0.97)	0.001617	1.000	1.000	0.668	1.000	0.668	1.000	0.986	1.000
	LINC01553	rs11817353	A vs. C	0.95 (0.92–0.98)	0.001678	1.000	1.000	0.550	0.999	0.550	0.999	0.986	1.000

Table 2. *Cont.*

Author, Year	Gene	Variant	Comparison	OR (95% CI)	p-Value	Power OR 1.2	Power OR 1.5	FPRP Values at Prior Probability OR 1.2 0.001	FPRP OR 1.2 0.000001	FPRP OR 1.5 0.001	FPRP OR 1.5 0.000001	BFDP 0.001	BFDP 0.000001
Anney et al., 2017 (continued)	RAD51B	rs2842330	A vs. C	1.10 (1.04–1.16)	0.001845	0.999	1.000	0.303	0.998	0.303	0.998	0.946	1.000
	RBFOX1	rs12930616	C vs. G	1.05 (1.02–1.09)	0.001985	1.000	1.000	0.913	1.000	0.913	1.000	0.998	1.000
	GRID2	rs6811974	T vs. C	0.95 (0.93–0.98)	0.001995	1.000	1.000	0.550	0.999	0.550	0.999	0.986	1.000
	NA	rs7135621	T vs. C	0.96 (0.93–0.98)	0.002059	1.000	1.000	0.094	0.991	0.094	0.991	0.915	1.000
	GFER NOXO1 NPW RNF151 RPS2 SNHG9 SNORA78 SYNGR3 TBL3 ZNF598	rs55742253	T vs. C	0.93 (0.88–0.98)	0.002075	1.000	1.000	0.868	1.000	0.868	1.000	0.995	1.000
	PTPRB	rs10784860	T vs. C	0.95 (0.91–0.98)	0.002211	1.000	1.000	0.550	0.999	0.550	0.999	0.986	1.000
	LOC101927768	rs9387201	C vs. G	1.09 (1.03–1.14)	0.002427	1.000	1.000	0.142	0.994	0.142	0.994	0.892	1.000
	BTBD11 LOC101929162 PRDM4 PWP1	rs4964602	T vs. G	0.95 (0.91–0.98)	0.00256	1.000	1.000	0.550	0.999	0.550	0.999	0.986	1.000
	NA	rs1376888	T vs. C	1.05 (1.02–1.08)	0.002668	1.000	1.000	0.407	0.999	0.407	0.999	0.979	1.000
	KLHL29	rs10182178	A vs. G	1.05 (1.02–1.08)	0.003508	1.000	1.000	0.407	0.999	0.407	0.999	0.979	1.000
	UBE2H	rs78661858	A vs. G	0.91 (0.85–0.97)	0.003665	0.997	1.000	0.792	1.000	0.791	1.000	0.991	1.000
	VAPA	rs29063	A vs. G	1.04 (1.01–1.07)	0.004075	1.000	1.000	0.873	1.000	0.873	1.000	0.997	1.000
	NA	rs190401890	A vs. T	1.12 (1.04–1.20)	0.004114	0.975	1.000	0.568	0.999	0.562	0.999	0.975	1.000
	LOC102723427	rs192668887	T vs. C	0.91 (0.84–0.97)	0.004205	0.997	1.000	0.792	1.000	0.791	1.000	0.991	1.000
	SLC12A7	rs73031119	A vs. C	0.91 (0.84–0.97)	0.004399	0.997	1.000	0.792	1.000	0.791	1.000	0.991	1.000
	ADGRL2	rs75695875	A vs. G	0.93 (0.87–0.98)	0.004715	1.000	1.000	0.868	1.000	0.868	1.000	0.995	1.000
	NA	rs1943999	C vs. G	0.96 (0.92–0.99)	0.004915	1.000	1.000	0.903	1.000	0.903	1.000	0.998	1.000
	DNAH6	rs2222734	A vs. G	0.92 (0.87–0.98)	0.005058	0.999	1.000	0.906	1.000	0.906	1.000	0.996	1.000
	OR8A1 OR8B12	rs2226753	T vs. C	0.96 (0.93–0.99)	0.005074	1.000	1.000	0.903	1.000	0.903	1.000	0.998	1.000
	TUSC5	rs35713482	A vs. G	1.05 (1.01–1.08)	0.005154	1.000	1.000	0.407	0.999	0.407	0.999	0.979	1.000
	C5orf15 VDAC1	rs67120295	T vs. C	1.06 (1.02–1.10)	0.005745	1.000	1.000	0.672	1.000	0.672	1.000	0.990	1.000
	NA	rs76010911	A vs. G	1.11 (1.04–1.19)	0.006255	0.986	1.000	0.769	1.000	0.767	1.000	0.989	1.000
	MTMR9 SLC35G5 TDH	rs6601581	T vs. C	1.06 (1.02–1.11)	0.006463	1.000	1.000	0.930	1.000	0.930	1.000	0.998	1.000
	HSDL2 MIR3134 PTBP3 SUSD1	rs7024761	A vs. G	1.05 (1.02–1.09)	0.00648	1.000	1.000	0.913	1.000	0.913	1.000	0.998	1.000
	CRTC3 GABARAPL3 IQGAP1 ZNF774	rs2601187	A vs. G	1.05 (1.01–1.08)	0.006859	1.000	1.000	0.407	0.999	0.407	0.999	0.979	1.000
	LOC101927189 LRRC1	rs4715431	A vs. G	1.04 (1.01–1.08)	0.007007	1.000	1.000	0.977	1.000	0.977	1.000	0.999	1.000
	NA	rs646680	A vs. G	0.95 (0.92–0.99)	0.00723	1.000	1.000	0.937	1.000	0.937	1.000	0.998	1.000
	CCNE1	rs12609867	A vs. G	0.95 (0.91–0.99)	0.00743	1.000	1.000	0.937	1.000	0.937	1.000	0.998	1.000
	NOS1AP OLFML2B	rs75192393	T vs. C	1.07 (1.02–1.12)	0.007697	1.000	1.000	0.787	1.000	0.787	1.000	0.993	1.000
	KDM4A KDM4A-AS1 LOC101929592 MIR6079 PTPRF ST3GAL3	rs79857083	T vs. C	1.04 (1.01–1.08)	0.007758	1.000	1.000	0.977	1.000	0.977	1.000	0.999	1.000
	NA	rs142968358	T vs. G	1.04 (1.01–1.07)	0.007789	1.000	1.000	0.873	1.000	0.873	1.000	0.997	1.000
	C3orf30 IGSF11 IGSF11-AS1 UPK1B	rs1102586	A vs. G	1.06 (1.02–1.10)	0.007844	1.000	1.000	0.672	1.000	0.672	1.000	0.990	1.000
	NA	chr11_98107192_D	D vs. I	1.04 (1.01–1.08)	0.00785	1.000	1.000	0.977	1.000	0.977	1.000	0.999	1.000
	C9orf135	rs76014157	A vs. G	0.90 (0.82–0.98)	0.007946	0.962	1.000	0.941	1.000	0.939	1.000	0.997	1.000
	NA	rs6437449	A vs. G	1.07 (1.02–1.11)	0.008708	1.000	1.000	0.232	0.997	0.232	0.997	0.945	1.000
	MYO5A	chr15_52811815_D	I vs. D	0.90 (0.81–0.98)	0.008799	0.962	1.000	0.941	1.000	0.939	1.000	0.997	1.000
	NA	rs9466619	A vs. G	0.95 (0.92–0.99)	0.009071	1.000	1.000	0.937	1.000	0.937	1.000	0.998	1.000

Table 2. *Cont.*

Author, Year	Gene	Variant	Comparison	OR (95% CI)	*p*-Value	Power OR 1.2	Power OR 1.5	FPRP Values at Prior Probability				BFDP 0.001	BFDP 0.000001
								OR 1.2		OR 1.5			
								0.001	0.000001	0.001	0.000001		
Anney et al., 2017 (continued)	NA	rs6117854	A vs. G	0.96 (0.93–0.99)	0.01012	1.000	1.000	0.903	1.000	0.903	1.000	0.998	1.000
	C7orf33	rs6955951	A vs. T	1.04 (1.01–1.07)	0.01015	1.000	1.000	0.873	1.000	0.873	1.000	0.997	1.000
	LHX6	rs72767788	A vs. C	0.95 (0.91–0.99)	0.01093	1.000	1.000	0.937	1.000	0.937	1.000	0.998	1.000
	NA	rs2028664	A vs. C	1.04 (1.01–1.07)	0.01095	1.000	1.000	0.873	1.000	0.873	1.000	0.997	1.000
	ELAVL2	rs180861134	A vs. T	1.05 (1.01–1.09)	0.01104	1.000	1.000	0.913	1.000	0.913	1.000	0.998	1.000
	RASGEF1C	rs12659560	T vs. C	1.04 (1.01–1.07)	0.0112	1.000	1.000	0.873	1.000	0.873	1.000	0.997	1.000
	MIR548AZ SYNE2	rs2150291	T vs. C	1.05 (1.01–1.09)	0.0113	1.000	1.000	0.913	1.000	0.913	1.000	0.998	1.000
	WDFY4	rs118059975	A vs. C	0.95 (0.91–0.99)	0.01146	1.000	1.000	0.937	1.000	0.937	1.000	0.998	1.000
	LINC01525 MAN1A2	rs3820500	A vs. G	1.04 (1.01–1.07)	0.0116	1.000	1.000	0.873	1.000	0.873	1.000	0.997	1.000
	GALNT10	rs17629195	T vs. C	1.04 (1.01–1.07)	0.012	1.000	1.000	0.873	1.000	0.873	1.000	0.997	1.000
	MIR597 TNKS	rs78853604	T vs. C	1.05 (1.01–1.08)	0.01256	1.000	1.000	0.407	0.999	0.407	0.999	0.979	1.000
	EXT1	rs7835763	A vs. T	1.04 (1.01–1.08)	0.01283	1.000	1.000	0.977	1.000	0.977	1.000	0.999	1.000
	NA	rs4652928	A vs. G	0.96 (0.92–0.99)	0.01384	1.000	1.000	0.903	1.000	0.903	1.000	0.998	1.000
	PDE1C	rs11976985	T vs. C	0.95 (0.92–0.99)	0.0141	1.000	1.000	0.937	1.000	0.937	1.000	0.998	1.000
	BAX FTL GYS1	rs2230267	T vs. C	1.04 (1.01–1.07)	0.01429	1.000	1.000	0.873	1.000	0.873	1.000	0.997	1.000
	GRID2	rs6854329	C vs. G	0.92 (0.86–0.99)	0.01486	0.996	1.000	0.963	1.000	0.963	1.000	0.998	1.000
	NA	rs1926229	C vs. G	1.05 (1.01–1.08)	0.01496	1.000	1.000	0.407	0.999	0.407	0.999	0.979	1.000
	NA	rs261351	T vs. C	0.96 (0.93–0.99)	0.01498	1.000	1.000	0.903	1.000	0.903	1.000	0.998	1.000
	RAPGEF2	rs4440173	A vs. G	1.04 (1.01–1.07)	0.01564	1.000	1.000	0.873	1.000	0.873	1.000	0.997	1.000
	MIR4650-1 MIR4650-2 POM121 SBDSP1 SPDYE7P TYW1B	rs4392770	T vs. C	1.05 (1.01–1.09)	0.01564	1.000	1.000	0.913	1.000	0.913	1.000	0.998	1.000
	NA	rs138493916	C vs. G	1.08 (1.02–1.14)	0.01783	1.000	1.000	0.840	1.000	0.840	1.000	0.994	1.000
	NA	rs615512	A vs. G	1.08 (1.02–1.14)	0.01811	1.000	1.000	0.840	1.000	0.840	1.000	0.994	1.000
	EP400 EP400NL PUS1 SNORA49	rs11608890	T vs. G	0.94 (0.88–0.99)	0.0187	1.000	1.000	0.951	1.000	0.951	1.000	0.998	1.000
	DIAPH3	chr13_60161890_I	I vs. D	1.05 (1.01–1.09)	0.01984	1.000	1.000	0.913	1.000	0.913	1.000	0.998	1.000
	ADAM12	rs1674923	T vs. C	0.96 (0.93–0.99)	0.0203	1.000	1.000	0.903	1.000	0.903	1.000	0.998	1.000
	ATP2B2 GHRL GHRLOS IRAK2 LINC00852 MIR378B MIR885 SEC13 TATDN2	rs7619385	A vs. G	1.04 (1.01–1.07)	0.02102	1.000	1.000	0.873	1.000	0.873	1.000	0.997	1.000
	UNC13C	rs75099274	A vs. G	1.08 (1.01–1.14)	0.02123	1.000	1.000	0.840	1.000	0.840	1.000	0.994	1.000
	ZSWIM6	rs10053166	A vs. G	0.95 (0.90–0.99)	0.02226	1.000	1.000	0.937	1.000	0.937	1.000	0.998	1.000
	HIVEP3	rs2786484	T vs. C	0.93 (0.86–0.99)	0.0237	1.000	1.000	0.958	1.000	0.958	1.000	0.998	1.000
	FJX1 TRIM44	rs76847144	T vs. C	0.93 (0.86–0.99)	0.02643	1.000	1.000	0.958	1.000	0.958	1.000	0.998	1.000
	WBSCR17	rs148521358	C vs. G	0.94 (0.88–0.99)	0.02731	1.000	1.000	0.951	1.000	0.951	1.000	0.998	1.000
	MIR3134 SUSD1	rs2564899	T vs. C	0.97 (0.94–1.00)	0.02735	1.000	1.000	0.980	1.000	0.980	1.000	0.999	1.000
	NA	chr8_138837351_I	I vs. D	1.05 (1.01–1.09)	0.0284	1.000	1.000	0.913	1.000	0.913	1.000	0.998	1.000
	LINC01393 MDFIC	rs7799732	A vs. G	1.03 (1.00–1.06)	0.03114	1.000	1.000	0.978	1.000	0.978	1.000	0.999	1.000
	TBX18 TBX18-AS1	rs76397051	A vs. G	1.05 (1.01–1.10)	0.034	1.000	1.000	0.975	1.000	0.975	1.000	0.999	1.000
	NA	rs171794	T vs. C	1.06 (1.01–1.12)	0.03587	1.000	1.000	0.974	1.000	0.974	1.000	0.999	1.000
	GDA	rs4327921	A vs. G	0.97 (0.94–1.00)	0.03938	1.000	1.000	0.980	1.000	0.980	1.000	0.999	1.000
	NA	rs2167341	T vs. G	1.05 (1.00–1.10)	0.04203	1.000	1.000	0.975	1.000	0.975	1.000	0.999	1.000

Table 2. *Cont.*

Author, Year	Gene	Variant	Comparison	OR (95% CI)	*p*-Value	Power OR 1.2	Power OR 1.5	FPRP Values at Prior Probability OR 1.2 0.001	FPRP OR 1.2 0.000001	FPRP OR 1.5 0.001	FPRP OR 1.5 0.000001	BFDP 0.001	BFDP 0.000001
	EVA1C	rs62216215	A vs. C	1.04 (1.00–1.08)	0.04598	1.000	1.000	0.977	1.000	0.977	1.000	0.999	1.000
	LINC01036	rs17589281	T vs. C	0.95 (0.89–1.00)	0.04716	1.000	1.000	0.980	1.000	0.980	1.000	0.999	1.000
	LOC283585	rs61979775	T vs. C	0.97 (0.93–1.00)	0.04813	1.000	1.000	0.980	1.000	0.980	1.000	0.999	1.000
	CHMP4A GMPR2 MDP1 NEDD8 NEDD8-MDP1 TM9SF1 TSSK4	rs72694312	T vs. G	1.06 (1.00–1.11)	0.04814	1.000	1.000	0.930	1.000	0.930	1.000	0.998	1.000
Ma et al., 2009 [32]	NA	rs10065041	T(minor)/C(major)	1.21 (1.08–1.36)	3.24×10^{-4}	0.445	1.000	0.757	1.000	0.581	0.999	0.970	1.000
	NA	rs10038113	C(minor)/T(major)	0.75 (0.70–0.90)	3.40×10^{-6}	0.129	0.897	0.939	1.000	0.688	1.000	0.979	1.000
	NA	rs6894838	T(minor)/C(major)	1.26 (1.12–1.42)	8.00×10^{-5}	0.212	0.998	0.416	0.999	0.131	0.993	0.827	1.000
Anney et al., 2010 [30]	HAT1	rs6731562	G (minor allele)	1.25 (1.11–1.41)	2.0×10^{-4}	0.253	0.998	0.527	0.999	0.220	0.996	0.891	1.000
	POU6F2	rs10258862	G (minor allele)	1.09 (1.00–1.18)	4.6×10^{-2}	0.991	1.000	0.971	1.000	0.971	1.000	0.998	1.000
	NA	rs6557675	A (minor allele)	0.84 (0.76–0.93)	1.0×10^{-3}	0.561	1.000	0.583	0.999	0.440	0.999	0.953	1.000
	MYH11	rs17284809	A (minor allele)	0.63 (0.50–0.79)	5.7×10^{-5}	0.008	0.312	0.891	1.000	0.168	0.995	0.821	1.000
	GSG1L	rs205409	G (minor allele)	0.91 (0.84–0.99)	2.8×10^{-2}	0.980	1.000	0.966	1.000	0.966	1.000	0.998	1.000
	TAF1C	rs4150167	A (minor allele)	0.54 (0.40–0.73)	2.1×10^{-5}	0.002	0.085	0.963	1.000	0.420	0.999	0.905	1.000
Kuo et al., 2015 [33]	GLIS1	rs12082358	C (minor allele)	1.3 (1.1–1.5)	2.2×10^{-4}	0.136	0.975	0.705	1.000	0.251	0.997	0.906	1.000
	GLIS1	rs12080993	A (minor allele)	1.3 (1.1–1.5)	1.5×10^{-4}	0.136	0.975	0.705	1.000	0.251	0.997	0.906	1.000
	GPD2	rs3916984	A (minor allele)	1.3 (1.1–1.5)	3.1×10^{-4}	0.136	0.975	0.705	1.000	0.251	0.997	0.906	1.000
	LRP2/BBS5	rs13014164	C (minor allele)	1.7 (1.3–2.3)	8.6×10^{-5}	0.012	0.209	0.980	1.000	0.735	1.000	0.974	1.000
	PDGFRA	rs7697680	G (minor allele)	1.5 (1.2–1.9)	9.2×10^{-4}	0.032	0.500	0.960	1.000	0.607	0.999	0.967	1.000
	FSTL4	rs11741756	A (minor allele)	1.3 (1.1–1.5)	1.2×10^{-2}	0.136	0.975	0.705	1.000	0.251	0.997	0.906	1.000
	NA	rs13211684	G (minor allele)	1.3 (1.1–1.5)	2.5×10^{-3}	0.136	0.975	0.705	1.000	0.251	0.997	0.906	1.000
	NA	rs10966205	T (minor allele)	1.3 (1.2–1.5)	2.9×10^{-5}	0.136	0.975	0.705	1.000	0.251	0.997	0.906	1.000
	C10orf68	rs10763893	A (minor allele)	1.6 (1.2–2.2)	6.1×10^{-4}	0.038	0.346	0.990	1.000	0.917	1.000	0.992	1.000
	NA	rs12366025	A (minor allele)	1.3 (1.1–1.6)	3.8×10^{-3}	0.225	0.912	0.983	1.000	0.936	1.000	0.995	1.000
	NA	rs11030597	G (minor allele)	1.3 (1.1–1.6)	4.1×10^{-3}	0.225	0.912	0.983	1.000	0.936	1.000	0.995	1.000
	NA	rs7933990	A (minor allele)	1.3 (1.1–1.6)	2.5×10^{-3}	0.225	0.912	0.983	1.000	0.936	1.000	0.995	1.000
	NA	rs11030606	A (minor allele)	1.3 (1.1–1.6)	5.6×10^{-3}	0.225	0.912	0.983	1.000	0.936	1.000	0.995	1.000
	MACROD2	rs17263514	A (minor allele)	1.2 (1.0–1.4)	1.4×10^{-2}	0.500	0.998	0.976	1.000	0.953	1.000	0.996	1.000
	BCAS1/CYP24A1	rs12479663	C (minor allele)	1.5 (1.3–1.9)	4.0×10^{-5}	0.032	0.500	0.960	1.000	0.607	0.999	0.967	1.000

Abbreviations: A, Adenine; C, Cytosine; G, Guanine; T, Thymine; D, Deletion; I, Insertion; R, Risk allele; NR, Non-risk allele; FPRP, false positive rate probability; BFDP, Bayesian false discovery probability; OR, odds ratio; CI, confidence interval; NA, not available.

Table 3. Re-analysis results of gene variants with genome wide statistical significance (p-value $< 5 \times 10^{-8}$) and borderline statistical significance ($5 \times 10^{-8} \leq p$-value < 0.05) in the genome-wide association studies (GWAS) catalog.

Author, Year	Gene	Variant	Comparison	OR (95% CI)	p-Value	Power OR 1.2	Power OR 1.5	FPRP Values at Prior Probability				BFDP 0.001	BFDP 0.000001
								OR 1.2		OR 1.5			
								0.001	0.000001	0.001	0.000001		
Gene variants with statistically significance (p-value < 5 × 10⁻⁸), FPRP < 0.2 and BFDP < 0.8 from GWAS catalog													
Anney et al., 2010 [30]	MACROD2	rs4141463	NA	1.37 (1.22–1.52)	4.00×10^{-8}	0.006	0.956	0.000	0.316	0.000	0.003	0.000	0.208
Chaste et al., 2014 [35]	AL163541.1	rs4773054	NA	2.66 (1.83–3.86)	5.00×10^{-8}	0.000	0.001	0.949	1.000	0.169	0.995	0.526	0.999
Gene variants with statistically borderline significance (5 × 10⁻⁸ ≤ p-value < 0.05), FPRP < 0.2 and BFDP < 0.8 from GWAS catalog													
Anney et al., 2010 [30]	PPP2R5C	rs7142002	NA	1.56 (1.28–1.89)	3.00×10^{-6}	0.004	0.344	0.602	0.999	0.016	0.942	0.338	0.998
Anney et al., 2012 [34]	TAF1C	rs4150167	NA	1.96 (1.52–2.56)	3.00×10^{-7}	0.000	0.025	0.832	1.000	0.031	0.969	0.269	0.997
Anney et al., 2012 [34]	PARD3B	rs4675502	NA	1.28 (1.16–1.41)	4.00×10^{-7}	0.095	0.999	0.006	0.856	0.001	0.362	0.030	0.969
Anney et al., 2012 [34]	AC113414.1	rs7711337	NA	1.22 (1.12–1.32)	8.00×10^{-7}	0.340	1.000	0.002	0.689	0.001	0.429	0.038	0.975
Anney et al., 2012 [34]	AC009446.1, EYA1	rs7834018	NA	1.56 (1.3–1.89)	8.00×10^{-7}	0.004	0.344	0.602	0.999	0.016	0.942	0.338	0.998
Anney et al., 2017 [31]	AL133270.1, AL139093.1	rs142968358	T (risk allele)	1.1 (1.06–1.14)	1.00×10^{-6}	1.000	1.000	0.000	0.145	0.000	0.145	0.014	0.936
Anney et al., 2017 [31]	EXT1	rs7835763	A (risk allele)	1.1 (1.06–1.14)	2.00×10^{-6}	1.000	1.000	0.000	0.145	0.000	0.145	0.014	0.936
Chaste et al., 2014 [35]	INHCAP	rs1867503	NA	1.55 (1.30–1.84)	4.00×10^{-7}	0.002	0.354	0.241	0.997	0.002	0.608	0.058	0.984
Chaste et al., 2014 [35]	CUEDC2	rs1409313	NA	1.75 (1.40–2.18)	4.00×10^{-7}	0.000	0.085	0.610	0.999	0.007	0.876	0.121	0.993
Chaste et al., 2014 [35]	CTU2	rs11641365	NA	2.06 (1.54–2.76)	3.00×10^{-7}	0.000	0.017	0.897	1.000	0.071	0.987	0.433	0.999
Chaste et al., 2014 [35]	AC067752.1, AC024598.1, ZNF365	rs93895	NA	1.91 (1.48–2.47)	2.00×10^{-7}	0.000	0.033	0.804	1.000	0.024	0.961	0.241	0.997
Kuo et al., 2015 [33]	LINC01151, AC108136.1	rs12543592	G (risk allele)	1.43 (1.25–1.67)	3.00×10^{-6}	0.013	0.727	0.318	0.998	0.008	0.895	0.275	0.997
Kuo et al., 2015 [33]	NAALADL2	rs3914502	A (risk allele)	1.4 (1.20–1.60)	4.00×10^{-6}	0.012	0.844	0.062	0.985	0.001	0.482	0.051	0.982
Kuo et al., 2015 [33]	OR2M4	rs10888329	NA	1.82 (1.39–2.33)	8.00×10^{-6}	0.000	0.062	0.809	1.000	0.031	0.970	0.338	0.998
Kuo et al., 2015 [33]	SGSM2	rs2447097	A (risk allele)	1.53 (1.27–1.85)	9.00×10^{-6}	0.006	0.419	0.652	0.999	0.026	0.965	0.467	0.999
Ma et al., 2009 [32]	Intergenic (RNU6-374P - MSNP1)	rs10038113	T (risk allele)	1.33 (1.11–1.43]	3.00×10^{-6}	0.003	0.999	0.000	0.000	0.000	0.000	0.000	0.000
Gene variants with statistically borderline significance (5 × 10⁻⁸ ≤ p-value < 0.05), FPRP > 0.2 or BFDP > 0.8 from GWAS catalog													
Chaste et al., 2014 [35]	AL163541.1	rs4773054	NA	2.9 (1.91–4.39)	7.00×10^{-8}	0.000	0.001	0.970	1.000	0.345	0.998	0.741	1.000
Anney et al., 2017 [31]	HLA-A, AL671277.1	rs115254791	G (risk allele)	1.0869565 (1.05–1.14)	4.00×10^{-6}	1.000	1.000	0.376	0.998	0.376	0.998	0.963	1.000

Abbreviations: A, Adenine; G; Guanine; T, Thymine; FPRP, false positive rate probability; BFDP, Bayesian false discovery probability; OR, odds ratio; CI, confidence interval; F, fixed effects model; R, random effects model; NA, not available; ASD, autism spectrum disorder.

Table 4. Re-analysis results of gene variants with genome wide statistical significance (p-value < 5×10^{-8}) and borderline statistical significance ($5 \times 10^{-8} \leq p$-value < 0.05) in the GWAS datasets included in GWAS meta-analyses (results of FPRP < 0.2 and BFDP < 0.8).

Author, Year	Trait	Gene(s)	Variant	Comparison	OR (95% CI)	p-Value	Power OR 1.2	Power OR 1.5	FPRP Values at Prior Probability				BFDP 0.001	BFDP 0.000001
									OR 1.2		OR 1.5			
									0.001	0.000001	0.001	0.000001		
Anney et al., 2012 [34]	ASD (European)	ERBB4	rs1879532	A	2.02 (1.57–2.59)	1.55×10^{-8}	0.000	0.009	0.595	0.999	0.003	0.757	0.026	0.964
Anney et al., 2012 [34]	Autism (European)	None	rs289932	A	0.49 (0.38–0.64)	5.04×10^{-8}	0.000	0.012	0.772	1.000	0.014	0.932	0.114	0.992
Anney et al., 2012 [34]	ASD	TMEM132B	rs16919315	A	0.53 (0.42–0.67)	5.12×10^{-8}	0.000	0.028	0.589	0.999	0.004	0.800	0.049	0.981
Anney et al., 2012 [34]	Autism (European)	ERBB4	rs1879532	A	1.72 (1.39–2.11)	1.66×10^{-7}	0.000	0.095	0.416	0.999	0.002	0.676	0.044	0.979
Anney et al., 2010 [30]	Autism	NA	rs6557675	A (minor allele)	0.61 (0.51–0.71)	2.20×10^{-7}	0.000	0.126	0.006	0.861	0.000	0.001	0.000	0.048
Anney et al., 2012 [34]	Autism (European)	None	rs289858	A	0.52 (0.40–0.67)	2.81×10^{-7}	0.000	0.027	0.762	1.000	0.015	0.940	0.161	0.995
Anney et al., 2012 [34]	ASD	SYNE2	rs2150291	A	1.72 (1.40–2.13)	2.83×10^{-7}	0.000	0.105	0.579	0.999	0.006	0.864	0.119	0.993
Anney et al., 2012 [34]	ASD (European)	RPH3AL	rs7207517	A	1.97 (1.51–2.57)	3.05×10^{-7}	0.000	0.022	0.817	1.000	0.025	0.963	0.226	0.997
Anney et al., 2012 [34]	Autism (European)	None	rs4761371	A	0.46 (0.34–0.63)	3.91×10^{-7}	0.000	0.010	0.924	1.000	0.111	0.992	0.521	0.999
Anney et al., 2012 [34]	ASD (European)	PRAMEF12	rs1812242	A	1.44 (1.25–1.66)	4.29×10^{-7}	0.006	0.713	0.077	0.988	0.001	0.411	0.038	0.975
Anney et al., 2012 [34]	ASD	None	rs10904487	G	0.63 (0.52–0.75)	4.29×10^{-7}	0.001	0.262	0.198	0.996	0.001	0.440	0.028	0.966
Anney et al., 2012 [34]	Autism (European)	None	rs289932	A	0.67 (0.57–0.79)	5.42×10^{-7}	0.005	0.524	0.286	0.998	0.004	0.784	0.135	0.994
Anney et al., 2010 [30]	Autism	MACROD2	rs4141463	A (minor allele)	0.62 (0.52–0.73)	5.50×10^{-7}	0.000	0.192	0.047	0.980	0.000	0.048	0.002	0.655
Anney et al., 2012 [34]	Autism	None	rs9608521	A	1.46 (1.25–1.69)	7.62×10^{-7}	0.004	0.641	0.084	0.989	0.001	0.383	0.033	0.971
Anney et al., 2012 [34]	ASD	None	rs1408744	A	0.65 (0.54–0.77)	8.06×10^{-7}	0.002	0.385	0.235	0.997	0.002	0.618	0.062	0.985
Anney et al., 2017 [31]	ASD	LINC00535	chr8_94389815_I	I vs. D	1.14 (1.09–1.19)	9.47×10^{-7}	0.990	1.000	0.000	0.002	0.000	0.002	0.686	1.000
Anney et al., 2012 [34]	ASD (European)	PC	rs7122539	A	0.60 (0.49–0.74)	9.64×10^{-7}	0.001	0.162	0.628	0.999	0.011	0.917	0.213	0.996
Anney et al., 2010 [30]	Autism	MACROD2	rs4814324	A (minor allele)	1.58 (1.34–1.86)	9.80×10^{-7}	0.000	0.266	0.076	0.988	0.000	0.128	0.006	0.859
Anney et al., 2010 [30]	Autism	MACROD2	rs6079544	A (minor allele)	1.57 (1.33–1.84)	1.20×10^{-6}	0.000	0.287	0.053	0.982	0.000	0.081	0.004	0.797
Anney et al., 2017 [31]	ASD	EXOC4	rs6467494	T vs. C	1.12 (1.07–1.16)	1.43×10^{-6}	1.000	1.000	0.000	0.000	0.000	0.000	0.197	0.996
Anney et al., 2010 [30]	Autism	MACROD2	rs6079536	A (minor allele)	0.64 (0.54–0.75)	1.60×10^{-6}	0.001	0.307	0.059	0.984	0.000	0.102	0.005	0.837
Anney et al., 2010 [30]	ASD	MYH11	rs17284809	A (minor allele)	0.52 (0.39–0.69)	1.70×10^{-6}	0.001	0.043	0.915	1.000	0.121	0.993	0.636	0.999
Anney et al., 2010 [30]	Autism	MACROD2	rs6079553	A (minor allele)	1.55 (1.31–1.82)	2.10×10^{-6}	0.001	0.344	0.090	0.990	0.000	0.204	0.011	0.920
Anney et al., 2010 [30]	Autism	MACROD2	rs6074798	A (minor allele)	1.56 (1.32–1.84)	2.10×10^{-6}	0.001	0.321	0.123	0.993	0.000	0.287	0.017	0.945
Anney et al., 2017 [31]	ASD	OPCML	rs7952100	C vs.G	1.14 (1.09–1.19)	2.49×10^{-6}	0.990	1.000	0.000	0.002	0.000	0.002	0.686	1.000
Anney et al., 2010 [30]	Autism	MACROD2	rs10446030	G (minor allele)	1.54 (1.30–1.81)	3.20×10^{-6}	0.001	0.375	0.116	0.992	0.000	0.301	0.019	0.951
Kuo et al., 2015 [33]	ASD	STYK1	rs16922945	C (minor allele)	1.86 (1.43–2.43)	3.43×10^{-6}	0.001	0.057	0.891	1.000	0.085	0.989	0.572	0.999
Anney et al., 2010 [30]	ASD	POU5F2	rs10258862	G (minor allele)	1.41 (1.23–1.61)	3.70×10^{-6}	0.009	0.820	0.043	0.978	0.000	0.319	0.027	0.966
Anney et al., 2010 [30]	Autism	MACROD2	rs6079540	A (minor allele)	0.65 (0.55–0.77)	3.70×10^{-6}	0.002	0.385	0.235	0.997	0.002	0.618	0.062	0.985
Anney et al., 2010 [30]	Autism	MACROD2	rs6074787	A (minor allele)	1.53 (1.30–1.80)	4.10×10^{-6}	0.002	0.406	0.147	0.994	0.001	0.418	0.031	0.970
Anney et al., 2010 [30]	ASD	MACROD2	rs6074798	A (minor allele)	1.38 (1.22–1.56)	4.80×10^{-6}	0.013	0.909	0.020	0.954	0.000	0.224	0.018	0.948
Anney et al., 2010 [30]	Autism	MACROD2	rs980319	G (minor allele)	1.52 (1.29–1.79)	5.10×10^{-6}	0.002	0.437	0.184	0.996	0.001	0.543	0.050	0.981

Table 4. *Cont.*

Author, Year	Trait	Gene(s)	Variant	Comparison	OR (95% CI)	p-Value	Power OR 1.2	Power OR 1.5	FPRP Values at Prior Probability OR 1.2 0.001	OR 1.2 0.000001	OR 1.5 0.001	OR 1.5 0.000001	BFDP 0.001	BFDP 0.000001
Anney et al., 2010 [30]	Autism	MACROD2	rs6079537	G (minor allele)	1.52 (1.29–1.79)	6.00×10^{-6}	0.002	0.437	0.184	0.996	0.001	0.543	0.050	0.981
Kuo et al., 2015 [33]	ASD	NA	rs10966205	A (minor allele)	1.52 (1.27–1.83)	6.25×10^{-6}	0.006	0.444	0.609	0.999	0.022	0.957	0.426	0.999
Kuo et al., 2015 [33]	ASD	OR2M4	rs10888329	T (minor allele)	0.55 (0.43–0.72)	8.05×10^{-6}	0.001	0.081	0.916	1.000	0.144	0.994	0.718	1.000
Anney et al., 2010 [30]	ASD	MACROD2	rs6079536	A (minor allele)	0.73 (0.65–0.83)	8.50×10^{-6}	0.022	0.917	0.067	0.986	0.002	0.628	0.084	0.989
Anney et al., 2010 [30]	ASD	NA	rs6557675	A (minor allele)	0.72 (0.63–0.82)	8.70×10^{-6}	0.014	0.877	0.051	0.982	0.001	0.457	0.047	0.980
Kuo et al., 2015 [33]	ASD	NA	rs7933990	A (minor allele)	1.72 (1.35–2.19)	9.40×10^{-6}	0.002	0.133	0.861	1.000	0.075	0.988	0.606	0.999
Kuo et al., 2015 [33]	ASD	MNT	rs2447097	A (minor allele)	1.53 (1.27–1.85)	9.45×10^{-6}	0.006	0.419	0.652	0.999	0.026	0.965	0.467	0.999
Anney et al., 2010 [30]	ASD	GSG1L	rs205409	G (minor allele)	0.72 (0.64–0.82)	9.60×10^{-6}	0.014	0.877	0.051	0.982	0.001	0.457	0.047	0.980
Kuo et al., 2015 [33]	ASD	OR2M4	rs6672981	C (minor allele)	0.55 (0.42–0.72)	9.64×10^{-6}	0.001	0.081	0.916	1.000	0.144	0.994	0.718	1.000
Kuo et al., 2015 [33]	ASD	OR2M4	rs4397683	C (minor allele)	0.55 (0.42–0.72)	9.86×10^{-6}	0.001	0.081	0.916	1.000	0.144	0.994	0.718	1.000
Anney et al., 2010 [30]	ASD	MACROD2	rs980319	G (minor allele)	1.36 (1.20–1.54)	1.00×10^{-5}	0.024	0.939	0.049	0.981	0.001	0.570	0.068	0.987
Kuo et al., 2015 [33]	ASD	BCAS1/CYP24A1	rs12479663	G (minor allele)	1.81 (1.38–2.36)	1.08×10^{-5}	0.001	0.083	0.907	1.000	0.124	0.993	0.687	1.000
Anney et al., 2010 [30]	ASD	MACROD2	rs4814324	A (minor allele)	1.36 (1.20–1.54)	1.10×10^{-5}	0.024	0.939	0.049	0.981	0.001	0.570	0.068	0.987
Kuo et al., 2015 [33]	ASD	KRR1	rs3741496	C (minor allele)	1.49 (1.24–1.78)	1.15×10^{-5}	0.009	0.529	0.565	0.999	0.020	0.954	0.430	0.999
Kuo et al., 2015 [33]	ASD	OR2M4	rs4642918	C (minor allele)	0.56 (0.43–0.73)	1.24×10^{-5}	0.002	0.099	0.917	1.000	0.155	0.995	0.745	1.000
Anney et al., 2010 [30]	ASD	MACROD2	rs6079544	A (minor allele)	1.35 (1.20–1.53)	1.30×10^{-5}	0.033	0.951	0.074	0.988	0.003	0.733	0.124	0.993
Kuo et al., 2015 [33]	ASD	NA	rs13211684	G (minor allele)	1.56 (1.28–1.91)	1.36×10^{-5}	0.006	0.352	0.750	1.000	0.045	0.979	0.572	0.999
Kuo et al., 2015 [33]	ASD	MNT	rs2447095	A (minor allele)	1.52 (1.26–1.84)	1.45×10^{-5}	0.008	0.446	0.695	1.000	0.038	0.975	0.552	0.999
Kuo et al., 2015 [33]	ASD	NA	rs12543592	G (minor allele)	0.67 (0.56–0.81)	1.63×10^{-5}	0.012	0.521	0.744	1.000	0.063	0.985	0.678	1.000
Anney et al., 2010 [30]	ASD	MACROD2	rs6079553	A (minor allele)	1.35 (1.19–1.52)	1.70×10^{-5}	0.026	0.959	0.027	0.965	0.001	0.424	0.041	0.977
Kuo et al., 2015 [33]	ASD	KRR1	rs1051446	C (minor allele)	1.47 (1.23–1.76)	1.77×10^{-5}	0.014	0.587	0.669	1.000	0.045	0.979	0.614	0.999
Anney et al., 2010 [30]	ASD	NA	rs4078417	C (minor allele)	1.38 (1.21–1.57)	1.90×10^{-5}	0.017	0.897	0.055	0.983	0.001	0.524	0.059	0.984
Anney et al., 2010 [30]	ASD	MACROD2	rs10446030	G (minor allele)	1.34 (1.19–1.52)	2.20×10^{-5}	0.043	0.960	0.110	0.992	0.006	0.847	0.210	0.996
Kuo et al., 2015 [33]	ASD	GPD2	rs3916984	T (minor allele)	0.62 (0.49–0.77)	2.25×10^{-5}	0.004	0.256	0.804	1.000	0.056	0.984	0.595	0.999
Kuo et al., 2015 [33]	ASD	NA	rs12366025	T (minor allele)	1.67 (1.31–2.11)	2.49×10^{-5}	0.003	0.184	0.860	1.000	0.086	0.989	0.662	0.999
Ma et al., 2009 [32]	Autism	NA	rs10038113	C(minor)/T(major)	0.67 (0.56–0.81)	2.75×10^{-5}	0.012	0.521	0.744	1.000	0.063	0.985	0.678	1.000
Anney et al., 2010 [30]	ASD	MACROD2	rs6079540	A (minor allele)	0.75 (0.66–0.84)	2.90×10^{-5}	0.034	0.979	0.019	0.950	0.001	0.399	0.037	0.975
Anney et al., 2010 [30]	Autism	HAT1	rs6731562	G (minor allele)	1.51 (1.27–1.81)	3.30×10^{-5}	0.006	0.471	0.562	0.999	0.017	0.946	0.383	0.998
Anney et al., 2010 [30]	ASD	MACROD2	rs6074787	A (minor allele)	1.33 (1.18–1.50)	3.40×10^{-5}	0.047	0.975	0.067	0.986	0.003	0.776	0.147	0.994
Kuo et al., 2015 [33]	ASD	GLIS1	rs12080933	A (minor allele)	1.48 (1.23–1.78)	3.57×10^{-5}	0.013	0.557	0.707	1.000	0.053	0.983	0.648	0.999
Kuo et al., 2015 [33]	ASD	FSTL4	rs11741756	T (minor allele)	1.67 (1.31–2.13)	3.64×10^{-5}	0.004	0.194	0.903	1.000	0.157	0.995	0.785	1.000
Kuo et al., 2015 [33]	ASD	STYK1	rs7953930	G (minor allele)	1.65 (1.30–2.09)	3.83×10^{-5}	0.004	0.215	0.888	1.000	0.133	0.994	0.761	1.000
Anney et al., 2010 [30]	Autism	NA	rs4078417	C (minor allele)	1.50 (1.26–1.79)	4.10×10^{-5}	0.007	0.500	0.509	0.999	0.014	0.933	0.339	0.998
Anney et al., 2010 [30]	ASD	MACROD2	rs4141463	A (minor allele)	0.75 (0.66–0.85)	4.30×10^{-5}	0.049	0.967	0.118	0.993	0.007	0.873	0.243	0.997
Kuo et al., 2015 [33]	ASD	OR2M3	rs11204613	G (minor allele)	0.58 (0.45–0.75)	4.60×10^{-5}	0.003	0.144	0.920	1.000	0.185	0.996	0.799	1.000
Anney et al., 2010 [30]	ASD	MACROD2	rs6079537	G (minor allele)	1.32 (1.17–1.49)	5.40×10^{-5}	0.062	0.981	0.103	0.991	0.007	0.878	0.249	0.997
Anney et al., 2010 [30]	Autism	GSG1L	rs205409	G (minor allele)	0.69 (0.58–0.81)	1.10×10^{-4}	0.011	0.663	0.353	0.998	0.009	0.896	0.271	0.997
Anney et al., 2010 [30]	Autism	POU5F2	rs10258862	G (minor allele)	1.43 (1.21–1.71)	1.80×10^{-4}	0.027	0.700	0.764	1.000	0.112	0.992	0.799	1.000

Abbreviations: ASD, Autism spectrum disorders; A, Adenine; C, Cytosine; G, Guanine; T, Thymine; D, Deletion; I, Insertion; FPRP, false positive rate probability; BFDP, Bayesian false discovery probability; OR, odds ratio; CI, confidence interval; GWAS, Genome-Wide Association Studies; NA, not available.

3.3. Protein-Protein Interaction (PPI) Network

We established PPI networks related to the risk of ASD by filtering genes noteworthy under both FPRP and BFDP or genes with a p-value $< 5 \times 10^{-8}$. We included the results of both re-analyzed and non-re-analyzable genetic comparisons from meta-analyses of observational studies and GWAS, GWAS included in meta-analyses of GWAS, and the GWAS catalog. The statistically significant results of non-re-analyzable studies are presented in the Supplement Table S3.

The major genes that included a strong genetic connection were the myc-associated factor X (MAX) network transcriptional repressor (MNT), oxytocin receptor (OXTR), nucleolar and coiled-body phosphoprotein (NOLC1), peroxisome proliferator-activated receptor gamma related coactivator-related 1 (PPRC1), pyruvate carboxylase (PC), methylenetetrahydrofolate reductase (MTHFR), multiple epidermal growth factor like domains 10 (MEGF10), nuclear factor kappa B subunit 2 (NFKB2), histone deacetylase 4 (HDAC4), etc. (Figure 2 and Table 5).

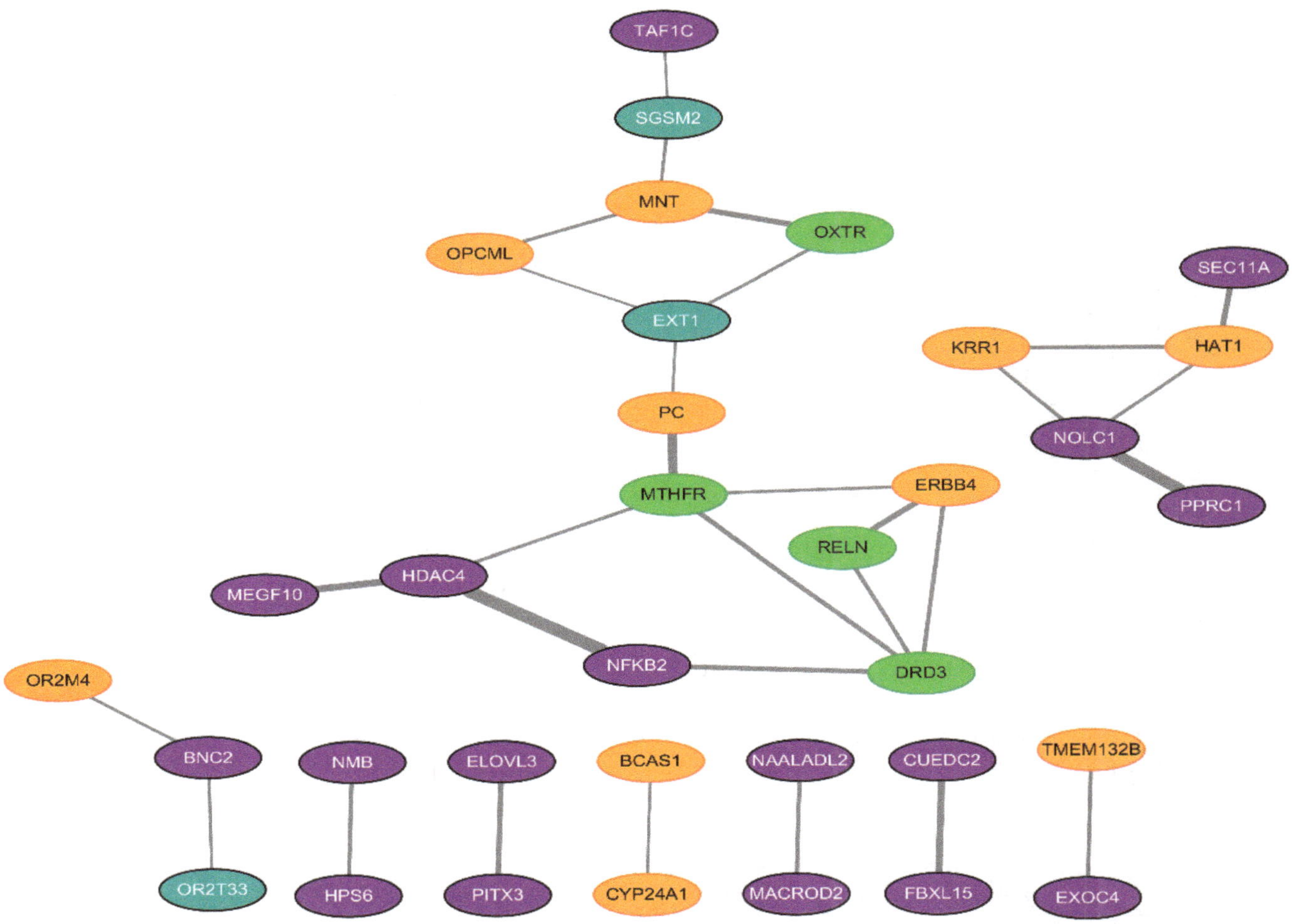

Figure 2. Protein-protein interaction network of ASD. There were 34 distinct genes with about 30 genetic connections among them. The thickness of the line connecting genes represents the score of PPI interaction using STRING9.1 and the color of each gene represents the source of the data; orange, GWAS data: green, GWAS catalog: purple, meta-analysis of GWAS: light green, meta-analysis of observational studies.

Table 5. Lists of genes involved in the PPI network.

Gene	Function of the Encoding Proteins
OXTR	Receptor for oxytocin associated with social recognition and emotion processing
MTHFR	Influences susceptibility to neural tube defect by changing folate metabolism
RELN	Control cell positioning and neural migration during brain development
DRD3	D3 subtype of the five dopamine receptors; localized to the limbic areas of the brain
MNT	Protein member of the Myc/Max/Mad network; transcriptional repressor and an antagonist of Myc-dependent transcriptional activation and cell growth
OPCML	Member of the IgLON subfamily in the immunoglobulin protein superfamily of proteins; localized in the plasma membrane; accessory role in opioid receptor function
PC	Pyruvate carboxylase; gluconeogenesis, lipogenesis, insulin secretion and synthesis of neurotransmitter glutamate
ERBB4	Tyr protein kinase family and the epidermal growth factor receptor subfamily; binds to and is activated by neuregulins, and induces mitogenesis and differentiation
OR2M4	Members of a large family of GPCR; olfactory receptors initiating a neuronal response that triggers the perception of a smell
BCAS1	Oncogene; highly expressed in three amplified breast cancer cell lines and in one breast tumor without amplification at 20q13.2.
CYP24A1	Cytochrome P450 superfamily of enzymes; drug metabolism and synthesis of cholesterol, steroids and other lipids
TMEM132B	The function remains poorly understood despite their mutations associated with non-syndromic hearing loss, panic disorder, and cancer
KRR1	Nucleolar protein; 18S rRNA synthesis and 40S ribosomal assembly
HAT1	Type B histone acetyltransferase; rapid acetylation of newly synthesized cytoplasmic histones; replication-dependent chromatin assembly
SGSM2	GTPase activator; regulators of membrane trafficking
EXT1	Endoplasmic reticulum-resident type II transmembrane glycosyltransferase; involved in the chain elongation step of heparan sulfate biosynthesis
OR2T33	Members of a large family of GPCR; share a 7-transmembrane domain structure with many neurotransmitter and hormone receptors
TAF1C	Binds to the core promoter of ribosomal RNA genes to position the polymerase properly; acts as a channel for regulatory signals
HDAC4	Class II of the histone deacetylase/acuc/apha family; represses transcription when tethered to a promoter
MEGF10	Member of the multiple epidermal growth factor-like domains protein family; cell adhesion, motility and proliferation; critical mediator of apoptotic cell phagocytosis; amyloid-beta peptide uptake in brain
NFKB2	Subunit of the transcription factor complex nuclear factor-kappa-B; central activator of genes involved in inflammation and immune function
BNC2	Conserved zinc finger protein; skin color saturation
NMB	Member of the bombesin-like family of neuropeptides; negatively regulate eating behavior; regulate colonic smooth muscle contraction
HPS6	Organelle biogenesis associated with melanosomes, platelet dense granules, and lysosomes
ELOVL3	GNS1/SUR4 family; elongation of long chain fatty acids to provide precursors for synthesis of sphingolipids and ceramides
PITX3	Member of the RIEG/PITX homeobox family; transcription factors; lens formation during eye development
NAALADL2	Not well-known, but diseases associated with NAALADL2 include Chromosome 6Pter-P24 Deletion Syndrome and Cornelia De Lange Syndrome.
MACROD2	Deacetylase removing ADP-ribose from mono-ADP-ribosylated proteins; translocate from the nucleus to the cytoplasm upon DNA damage

Table 5. *Cont.*

Gene	Function of the Encoding Proteins
CUEDC2	CUE domain-containing protein; down-regulate ESR1 protein levels through progesterone-induced and degradation of receptors
FBXL15	Substrate recognition component of SCF E3 ubiquitin-protein ligase complex; mediates the ubiquitination and subsequent proteasomal degradation of SMURF1
EXOC4	Component of the exocyst complex; targeting exocytic vesicles to specific docking sites on the plasma membrane
NOLC1	Nucleolar protein; act as a regulator of RNA polymerase I; neural crest specification; nucleologenesis
PPRC1	Similar to PPAR-gamma coactivator 1; activate mitochondrial biogenesis through NRF1 in response to proliferative signals
SEC11A	Member of the peptidase S26B family; subunit of the signal peptidase complex; cell migration and invasion, gastric cancer and lymph node metastasis

Abbreviations: OXTR, Oxytocin Receptor; MTHFR, Methylene tetrahydrofolate reductase; RELN, reelin, DRD3, Dopamine Receptor D3; MNT, Myc-associated factor X (MAX) Network Transcriptional Repressor; OPCML, opioid binding protein/cell adhesion molecule-like; PC, Pyruvate carboxylase; ERBB4, Erb-B2 Receptor Tyrosine Kinase 4; OR2M4, olfactory receptor family 2 subfamily M member 4; GPCR, G protein-coupled receptor; BCAS1, Breast Carcinoma Amplified Sequence 1; CYP24A1, Cytochrome P450 Family 24 Subfamily A Member 1; TMEM132B, transmembrane protein 132B; KRR1, KRR1 small subunit processome component homolog; HAT1, histone acetyltransferase 1; SGSM2, small G protein signaling modulator 2; EXT1, Exostosin-1; OR2T33, Olfactory receptor 2T33; TAF1C, TATA-Box Binding Protein Associated Factor, RNA Polymerase I Subunit C; HDAC4, Histone deacetylase 4; MEGF10, Multiple Epidermal Growth Factor Like Domains 10; NFKB2, Nuclear Factor Kappa B Subunit 2; BNC2, basonuclin-2; NMB, Neuromedin B; HPS6, Hermansky–Pudlak syndrome 6; ELOVL3, Elongation Of Very Long Chain Fatty Acids Protein 3, PITX3, Pituitary homeobox 3; NAALADL2, N-Acetylated Alpha-Linked Acidic Dipeptidase Like 2; MACROD2, Mono-ADP Ribosylhydrolase 2; CUEDC2, CUE domain containing 2; FBXL15, F-Box And Leucine Rich Repeat Protein 15; EXOC4, Exocyst Complex Component 4; NOLC1, Nucleolar And Coiled-Body Phosphoprotein 1; PPRC1, peroxisome proliferator-activated receptor gamma, coactivator-related 1; SEC11A, SEC11 Homolog A, Signal Peptidase Complex Subunit.

4. Discussion

To our knowledge, this study is the first study of ASD genetic risk factors, which assessed the levels of evidence of the published meta-analyses showing the association between susceptible loci and ASD. Overall, genetic comparisons with noteworthy results were confirmed as risk factors for ASD. The genetic comparisons highly related to an increased risk of ASD might reflect the implication in neurodevelopment and specific synaptogenesis of ASD.

According to the PPI network, composed of noteworthy results obtained when using both Bayesian approaches, multiple genes were included as a risk factor for ASD. Investigating the lists genes as a risk factor, promising candidates encoded the protein associated with neural development and specification, and also with neurotransmitters and its receptors. These genes were RELN and DRD3 from observational studies, and PC, OPCML, ERBB4, OR2M4, MEGF10, OR2T33, NMB, and NOLC1, from GWAS. In line with our findings, previous reports have supported that the migration and proliferation of neuronal cells is essential to understanding neurodevelopmental disorders such as ASD or schizophrenia [49,50]. In addition, apart from anatomical approaches, genes correlated with neuropeptides and receptors, such as those in the brain or hippocampus, also explain the pathophysiology of the disease at a molecular level [51]. The list of genes included is presented in Table 5.

The present comprehensive re-analyses shows that, although a large number of studies have suggested numerous possible genetic risk factors for ASD, truly significant results are small and a partial part of whole results. For instance, we detected false positive results in 26 out of 31 (83.9%) meta-analyses of observational studies and 163 out of 203 (80.3%) in meta-analyses of GWAS, respectively. However, only a small portion of genetic comparisons with a p-value < 0.05 exhibited noteworthy associations with ASD under both Bayesian approaches (Tables 1–4).

Moreover, we also detected that genetic comparisons with borderline statistical significance ($5 \times 10^{-8} < p\text{-value} < 0.05$) accounted for 53 out of 126 (42%) noteworthy comparisons from GWAS or meta-analyses of GWAS. These genetic comparisons might have been neglected if the p-value alone was considered to determine noteworthiness. Using the two Bayesian approaches as we did, or relaxing the current GWAS threshold as Panagiotou et al. suggests, might enable better interpretation of GWAS results [48].

Based on the observational studies, out of 31 statistically significant genotype comparisons, five (16.1%) were found noteworthy under both FPRP and BFDP: T vs. C, MTHFR C677T; T (minor), MTHFR C677T; G vs. A, DRD3/rs167771; C vs. G, RELN/rs362691; A (minor), OXTR/rs7632287. From the meta-analyses of GWAS, we could confirm that 34 distinct genes are noteworthy under both Bayesian approaches with about 30 genetic connections. However, the fact that all three comparisons with a p-value $< 5 \times 10^{-8}$—rs1879532 (Table S3), rs4773054 (Table 2), rs4141463 (Table 2)—displayed noteworthiness may indicate that the stringent threshold of $p < 5 \times 10^{-8}$ is a good tool for verification of the true noteworthiness of genetic risk factors.

There are several limitations in our review. First, we did not include studies that have not been meta-analyzed, or meta-analyses that had insufficient data in our review. Secondly, we only included the single findings of a meta-analysis with the lowest p-value per genetic variant. Therefore, we could not consider potentially meaningful subgroup analyses for different ethnicity, location, gender, and type of genotype comparison (i.e., random or fixed) when selecting a certain outcome. We focused on whether the individual genotype variant was truly associated with ASD or not, regardless of the specific type of the genotype comparison or ethnicity.

Our study has several strengths and implications. For example, to our knowledge, this is the first study that simultaneously analyzed a sizeable amount of data about genetic factors including not only GWAS but also the GWAS catalog. Despite the known high heritability of ASD and abundant research in ASD that has focused on the underlying genetic causes, the literature on genetic risk factors for ASD has not fully reached a consensus. This comprehensive review of genetic associations linked to ASD may improve understanding of the strengths and limitations of each form of research, and advance better and novel approaches for examining ASD in the field of genetic research. The findings of this study could provide mechanisms that may be explored for the development of novel neurotherapeutic agents both for the prevention and treatment of ASD.

5. Conclusions

In conclusion, we synthesized published meta-analyses on risk factors of ASD to acquire noteworthy findings and false positive results by adopting two Bayesian approaches for genetic factors. We attempted to synthesize all meta-analyses on genetic polymorphisms linked to ASD and found noteworthy genetic factors highly related to an increased risk of ASD. We also investigated their validity by discovering false positive results under Bayesian methods. To verify results obtained from genetic analyses, both approaches may have advantages, especially for interpretation of results obtained from observational studies. We found noteworthy results from GWAS, not only with p-value ranging between 0.05 and 5×10^{-8}, but also from genetic variants within borderline significance rage which were almost half of the genetic variants. This finding speculates that the genetic variants with borderline significance needs to be further analyzed to determine what associations are genuine.

Author Contributions: J.L., M.J.S., J.I.S. and P.F.-P. designed the study. J.L., M.J.S., C.Y.S., G.H.J., K.H.L., K.S.L. and J.I.S. collected the data and M.J.S., G.H.J., K.H.L. and Y.K. did the analysis. J.L., M.J.S., C.Y.S., G.H.J., K.H.L., K.S.L., Y.K., J.Y.K., J.Y.L., J.R., M.E., F.G., A.K. (Ai Koyanagi), B.S., M.S., T.B.R., A.K. (Andreas Kronbichler), E.D., D.F.P.V., F.R.P.d.S., K.T., A.R.B., A.F.C., S.C., S.T., A.S., L.S., T.T., J.I.S., and P.F.-P. wrote the first draft of the manuscript and gave critical comments on manuscript draft. All authors have read and agreed to the published version of the manuscript.

References

1. Lyall, K.; Croen, L.; Daniels, J.; Fallin, M.D.; Ladd-Acosta, C.; Lee, B.K.; Park, B.Y.; Snyder, N.W.; Schendel, D.; Volk, H.; et al. The changing epidemiology of autism spectrum disorders. *Annu. Rev. Public Health* **2017**, *38*, 81–102. [CrossRef] [PubMed]
2. American Psychiatric Association. *Diagnostic and Statistical Manual of Mental Disorders (dsm-5®)*, 5th ed.; American Psychiatric Pub.: Arlington, VA, USA, 2013.
3. Xu, G.; Strathearn, L.; Liu, B.; Bao, W. Prevalence of autism spectrum disorder among us children and adolescents, 2014–2016. *JAMA* **2018**, *319*, 81–82. [CrossRef] [PubMed]
4. Zablotsky, B.; Black, L.I.; Maenner, M.J.; Schieve, L.A.; Blumberg, S.J. Estimated prevalence of autism and other developmental disabilities following questionnaire changes in the 2014 national health interview survey. *Natl. Health Stat. Rep.* **2015**, *87*, 1–20.
5. Christensen, D.L.; Baio, J.; Van Naarden Braun, K.; Bilder, D.; Charles, J.; Constantino, J.N.; Daniels, J.; Durkin, M.S.; Fitzgerald, R.T.; Kurzius-Spencer, M.; et al. Prevalence and characteristics of autism spectrum disorder among children aged 8 years—Autism and developmental disabilities monitoring network, 11 sites, united states, 2012. *MMWR Surveill. Summ.* **2016**, *65*, 1–23. [CrossRef]
6. Kim, J.Y.; Son, M.J.; Son, C.Y.; Radua, J.; Eisenhut, M.; Gressier, F.; Koyanagi, A.; Carvalho, A.F.; Stubbs, B.; Solmi, M.; et al. Environmental risk factors and biomarkers for autism spectrum disorder: An umbrella review of the evidence. *Lancet Psychiatry* **2019**, *6*, 590–600. [CrossRef]
7. Ronald, A.; Hoekstra, R.A. Autism spectrum disorders and autistic traits: A decade of new twin studies. *Am. J. Med. Genet. B Neuropsychiatr. Genet.* **2011**, *156B*, 255–274. [CrossRef]
8. Bai, D.; Yip, B.H.K.; Windham, G.C.; Sourander, A.; Francis, R.; Yoffe, R.; Glasson, E.; Mahjani, B.; Suominen, A.; Leonard, H.; et al. Association of genetic and environmental factors with autism in a 5-country cohort. *JAMA Psychiatry* **2019**. [CrossRef]
9. MacGregor, A.J.; Snieder, H.; Schork, N.J.; Spector, T.D. Twins: Novel uses to study complex traits and genetic diseases. *Trends Genet* **2000**, *16*, 131–134. [CrossRef]
10. Modabbernia, A.; Velthorst, E.; Reichenberg, A. Environmental risk factors for autism: An evidence-based review of systematic reviews and meta-analyses. *Mol. Autism.* **2017**, *8*, 13. [CrossRef]
11. Robinson, E.B.; St Pourcain, B.; Anttila, V.; Kosmicki, J.A.; Bulik-Sullivan, B.; Grove, J.; Maller, J.; Samocha, K.E.; Sanders, S.J.; Ripke, S.; et al. Genetic risk for autism spectrum disorders and neuropsychiatric variation in the general population. *Nat. Genet.* **2016**, *48*, 552–555. [CrossRef]

12. State, M.W.; Levitt, P. The conundrums of understanding genetic risks for autism spectrum disorders. *Nat. Neurosci.* **2011**, *14*, 1499–1506. [CrossRef] [PubMed]
13. MacArthur, J.; Bowler, E.; Cerezo, M.; Gil, L.; Hall, P.; Hastings, E.; Junkins, H.; McMahon, A.; Milano, A.; Morales, J. The new nhgri-ebi catalog of published genome-wide association studies (gwas catalog). *Nucleic Acids Res.* **2016**, *45*, D896–D901. [CrossRef] [PubMed]
14. Wakefield, J. A bayesian measure of the probability of false discovery in genetic epidemiology studies. *Am. J. Hum. Genet.* **2007**, *81*, 208–227. [CrossRef] [PubMed]
15. Wacholder, S.; Chanock, S.; Garcia-Closas, M.; El Ghormli, L.; Rothman, N. Assessing the probability that a positive report is false: An approach for molecular epidemiology studies. *J. Natl. Cancer Inst.* **2004**, *96*, 434–442. [CrossRef] [PubMed]
16. Szklarczyk, D.; Franceschini, A.; Wyder, S.; Forslund, K.; Heller, D.; Huerta-Cepas, J.; Simonovic, M.; Roth, A.; Santos, A.; Tsafou, K.P.; et al. String v10: Protein-protein interaction networks, integrated over the tree of life. *Nucleic Acids Res.* **2015**, *43*, D447–D452. [CrossRef]
17. Wang, K.; Zhang, H.; Ma, D.; Bucan, M.; Glessner, J.T.; Abrahams, B.S.; Salyakina, D.; Imielinski, M.; Bradfield, J.P.; Sleiman, P.M.; et al. Common genetic variants on 5p14.1 associate with autism spectrum disorders. *Nature* **2009**, *459*, 528–533. [CrossRef]
18. Xia, K.; Guo, H.; Hu, Z.; Xun, G.; Zuo, L.; Peng, Y.; Wang, K.; He, Y.; Xiong, Z.; Sun, L.; et al. Common genetic variants on 1p13.2 associate with risk of autism. *Mol. Psychiatry* **2014**, *19*, 1212–1219. [CrossRef]
19. Grove, J.; Ripke, S.; Als, T.D.; Mattheisen, M.; Walters, R.K.; Won, H.; Pallesen, J.; Agerbo, E.; Andreassen, O.A.; Anney, R.; et al. Identification of common genetic risk variants for autism spectrum disorder. *Nat. Genet.* **2019**, *51*, 431–444. [CrossRef]
20. Liu, J.; Yang, A.; Zhang, Q.; Yang, G.; Yang, W.; Lei, H.; Quan, J.; Qu, F.; Wang, M.; Zhang, Z. Association between genetic variants in slc25a12 and risk of autism spectrum disorders: An integrated meta-analysis. *Am. J. Med Genet. Part B Neuropsychiatr. Genet.* **2015**, *168*, 236–246. [CrossRef]
21. Rai, V. Association of methylenetetrahydrofolate reductase (mthfr) gene c677t polymorphism with autism: Evidence of genetic susceptibility. *Metab. Brain Dis.* **2016**, *31*, 727–735. [CrossRef]
22. Pu, D.; Shen, Y.; Wu, J. Association between mthfr gene polymorphisms and the risk of autism spectrum disorders: A meta-analysis. *Autism Res.* **2013**, *6*, 384–392. [CrossRef] [PubMed]
23. Shaik Mohammad, N.; Sai Shruti, P.; Bharathi, V.; Krishna Prasad, C.; Hussain, T.; Alrokayan, S.A.; Naik, U.; Radha Rama Devi, A. Clinical utility of folate pathway genetic polymorphisms in the diagnosis of autism spectrum disorders. *Psychiatr. Genet.* **2016**, *26*, 281–286. [CrossRef] [PubMed]
24. Warrier, V.; Chee, V.; Smith, P.; Chakrabarti, B.; Baron-Cohen, S. A comprehensive meta-analysis of common genetic variants in autism spectrum conditions. *Mol. Autism* **2015**, *6*, 49. [CrossRef] [PubMed]
25. Aoki, Y.; Cortese, S. Mitochondrial aspartate/glutamate carrier slc25a12 and autism spectrum disorder: A meta-analysis. *Mol. Neurobiol.* **2016**, *53*, 1579–1588. [CrossRef]
26. LoParo, D.; Waldman, I.D. The oxytocin receptor gene (oxtr) is associated with autism spectrum disorder: A meta-analysis. *Mol. Psychiatr.* **2015**, *20*, 640–646. [CrossRef]
27. Wang, Z.; Hong, Y.; Zou, L.; Zhong, R.; Zhu, B.; Shen, N.; Chen, W.; Lou, J.; Ke, J.; Zhang, T.; et al. Reelin gene variants and risk of autism spectrum disorders: An integrated meta-analysis. *Am. J. Med. Genet. B Neuropsychiatr. Genet.* **2014**, *165B*, 192–200. [CrossRef]
28. Torrico, B.; Fernandez-Castillo, N.; Hervas, A.; Mila, M.; Salgado, M.; Rueda, I.; Buitelaar, J.K.; Rommelse, N.; Oerlemans, A.M.; Bralten, J.; et al. Contribution of common and rare variants of the ptchd1 gene to autism spectrum disorders and intellectual disability. *Eur. J. Hum. Genet.* **2015**, *23*, 1694–1701. [CrossRef]
29. Kranz, T.M.; Kopp, M.; Waltes, R.; Sachse, M.; Duketis, E.; Jarczok, T.A.; Degenhardt, F.; Gorgen, K.; Meyer, J.; Freitag, C.M.; et al. Meta-analysis and association of two common polymorphisms of the human oxytocin receptor gene in autism spectrum disorder. *Autism Res.* **2016**, *9*, 1036–1045. [CrossRef]
30. Anney, R.; Klei, L.; Pinto, D.; Regan, R.; Conroy, J.; Magalhaes, T.R.; Correia, C.; Abrahams, B.S.; Sykes, N.; Pagnamenta, A.T.; et al. A genome-wide scan for common alleles affecting risk for autism. *Hum. Mol. Genet.* **2010**, *19*, 4072–4082. [CrossRef]
31. The Autism Spectrum Disorders Working Group of The Psychiatric Genomics Consortium. Meta-analysis of gwas of over 16,000 individuals with autism spectrum disorder highlights a novel locus at 10q24.32 and a significant overlap with schizophrenia. *Mol. Autism* **2017**, *8*, 21. [CrossRef]

32. Ma, D.; Salyakina, D.; Jaworski, J.M.; Konidari, I.; Whitehead, P.L.; Andersen, A.N.; Hoffman, J.D.; Slifer, S.H.; Hedges, D.J.; Cukier, H.N.; et al. A genome-wide association study of autism reveals a common novel risk locus at 5p14.1. *Ann. Hum. Genet.* **2009**, *73*, 263–273. [CrossRef] [PubMed]
33. Kuo, P.H.; Chuang, L.C.; Su, M.H.; Chen, C.H.; Chen, C.H.; Wu, J.Y.; Yen, C.J.; Wu, Y.Y.; Liu, S.K.; Chou, M.C.; et al. Genome-wide association study for autism spectrum disorder in taiwanese han population. *PLoS ONE* **2015**, *10*, e0138695. [CrossRef] [PubMed]
34. Anney, R.; Klei, L.; Pinto, D.; Almeida, J.; Bacchelli, E.; Baird, G.; Bolshakova, N.; Bolte, S.; Bolton, P.F.; Bourgeron, T.; et al. Individual common variants exert weak effects on the risk for autism spectrum disorders. *Hum. Mol. Genet.* **2012**, *21*, 4781–4792. [CrossRef] [PubMed]
35. Chaste, P.; Klei, L.; Sanders, S.J.; Hus, V.; Murtha, M.T.; Lowe, J.K.; Willsey, A.J.; Moreno-De-Luca, D.; Timothy, W.Y.; Fombonne, E. A genome-wide association study of autism using the simons simplex collection: Does reducing phenotypic heterogeneity in autism increase genetic homogeneity? *Biol. Psychiatry* **2015**, *77*, 775–784. [CrossRef]
36. Main, P.A.; Angley, M.T.; O'Doherty, C.E.; Thomas, P.; Fenech, M. The potential role of the antioxidant and detoxification properties of glutathione in autism spectrum disorders: A systematic review and meta-analysis. *Nutr. Metab.* **2012**, *9*, 35. [CrossRef]
37. Huang, C.H.; Santangelo, S.L. Autism and serotonin transporter gene polymorphisms: A systematic review and meta-analysis. *Am. J. Med. Genet. B Neuropsychiatr. Genet.* **2008**, *147B*, 903–913. [CrossRef]
38. Curran, S.; Bolton, P.; Rozsnyai, K.; Chiocchetti, A.; Klauck, S.M.; Duketis, E.; Poustka, F.; Schlitt, S.; Freitag, C.M.; Lee, I.; et al. No association between a common single nucleotide polymorphism, rs4141463, in the macrod2 gene and autism spectrum disorder. *Am. J. Med Genet. Part B: Neuropsychiatr. Genet.* **2011**, *156*, 633–639. [CrossRef]
39. Yang, P.Y.; Menga, Y.J.; Li, T.; Huang, Y. Associations of endocrine stress-related gene polymorphisms with risk of autism spectrum disorders: Evidence from an integrated meta-analysis. *Autism Res.* **2017**, *10*, 1722–1736. [CrossRef]
40. Song, R.R.; Zou, L.; Zhong, R.; Zheng, X.W.; Zhu, B.B.; Chen, W.; Liu, L.; Miao, X.P. An integrated meta-analysis of two variants in hoxa1/hoxb1 and their effect on the risk of autism spectrum disorders. *PLoS ONE* **2011**, *6*, e25603. [CrossRef]
41. Chen, N.; Bao, Y.; Xue, Y.; Sun, Y.; Hu, D.; Meng, S.; Lu, L.; Shi, J. Meta-analyses of reln variants in neuropsychiatric disorders. *Behav. Brain Res.* **2017**, *332*, 110–119. [CrossRef]
42. Werling, A.M.; Bobrowski, E.; Taurines, R.; Gundelfinger, R.; Romanos, M.; Grunblatt, E.; Walitza, S. Cntnap2 gene in high functioning autism: No association according to family and meta-analysis approaches. *J. Neural. Transm.* **2016**, *123*, 353–363. [CrossRef] [PubMed]
43. Zhang, T.; Zhang, J.; Wang, Z.; Jia, M.; Lu, T.; Wang, H.; Yue, W.; Zhang, D.; Li, J.; Wang, L. Association between cntnap2 polymorphisms and autism: A family-based study in the chinese han population and a meta-analysis combined with gwas data of psychiatric genomics consortium. *Autism Res.* **2019**, *12*, 553–561. [CrossRef] [PubMed]
44. Noroozi, R.; Taheri, M.; Ghafouri-Fard, S.; Bidel, Z.; Omrani, M.D.; Moghaddam, A.S.; Sarabi, P.; Jarahi, A.M. Meta-analysis of gabrb3 gene polymorphisms and susceptibility to autism spectrum disorder. *J. Mol. Neurosci.* **2018**, *65*, 432–437. [CrossRef] [PubMed]
45. Mahdavi, M.; Kheirollahi, M.; Riahi, R.; Khorvash, F.; Khorrami, M.; Mirsafaie, M. Meta-analysis of the association between gaba receptor polymorphisms and autism spectrum disorder (ASD). *J. Mol. Neurosci.* **2018**, *65*, 1–9. [CrossRef] [PubMed]
46. Waltes, R.; Duketis, E.; Knapp, M.; Anney, R.J.; Huguet, G.; Schlitt, S.; Jarczok, T.A.; Sachse, M.; Kampfer, L.M.; Kleinbock, T.; et al. Common variants in genes of the postsynaptic fmrp signalling pathway are risk factors for autism spectrum disorders. *Hum. Genet.* **2014**, *133*, 781–792. [CrossRef] [PubMed]
47. Torrico, B.; Chiocchetti, A.G.; Bacchelli, E.; Trabetti, E.; Hervas, A.; Franke, B.; Buitelaar, J.K.; Rommelse, N.; Yousaf, A.; Duketis, E.; et al. Lack of replication of previous autism spectrum disorder gwas hits in european populations. *Autism Res.* **2017**, *10*, 202–211. [CrossRef] [PubMed]
48. Panagiotou, O.A.; Ioannidis, J.P.A.; Genome-Wide Significance Project. What should the genome-wide significance threshold be? Empirical replication of borderline genetic associations. *Int. J. Epidemiol.* **2011**, *41*, 273–286. [CrossRef]

49. Skaar, D.A.; Shao, Y.; Haines, J.L.; Stenger, J.E.; Jaworski, J.; Martin, E.R.; DeLong, G.R.; Moore, J.H.; McCauley, J.L.; Sutcliffe, J.S.; et al. Analysis of the reln gene as a genetic risk factor for autism. *Mol. Psychiatry* **2005**, *10*, 563–571. [CrossRef]
50. Glessner, J.T.; Wang, K.; Cai, G.; Korvatska, O.; Kim, C.E.; Wood, S.; Zhang, H.; Estes, A.; Brune, C.W.; Bradfield, J.P.; et al. Autism genome-wide copy number variation reveals ubiquitin and neuronal genes. *Nature* **2009**, *459*, 569–573. [CrossRef]
51. Purcell, A.E.; Jeon, O.H.; Zimmerman, A.W.; Blue, M.E.; Pevsner, J. Postmortem brain abnormalities of the glutamate neurotransmitter system in autism. *Neurology* **2001**, *57*, 1618–1628. [CrossRef]

10

Role of Genetics in the Etiology of Autistic Spectrum Disorder: Towards a Hierarchical Diagnostic Strategy

Cyrille Robert [1,2], Laurent Pasquier [2], David Cohen [3], Mélanie Fradin [2], Roberto Canitano [4], Léna Damaj [2], Sylvie Odent [2] and Sylvie Tordjman [1,5,*]

1 Pôle Hospitalo-Universitaire de Psychiatrie de l'Enfant et de l'Adolescent (PHUPEA), University of Rennes 1 and Centre Hospitalier Guillaume Régnier, 35200 Rennes, France; robertcyrille@live.fr

2 Service de Génétique Clinique, Centre de Référence Maladies Rares Anomalies du Développement (Centre Labellisé pour les Anomalies du Développement de l'Ouest: CLAD Ouest), Hôpital Sud, Centre Hospitalier Universitaire de Rennes, 35200 Rennes, France; laurent.pasquier@chu-rennes.fr (L.P.); Melanie.FRADIN@chu-rennes.fr (M.F.); Lena.DAMAJ@chu-rennes.fr (L.D.); Sylvie.Odent@chu-rennes.fr (S.O.)

3 Hospital-University Department of Child and Adolescent Psychiatry, Pitié-Salpétrière Hospital, Paris 6 University, 75013 Paris, France; david.cohen@psl.aphp.fr

4 Division of Child and Adolescent Neuropsychiatry, University Hospital of Siena, 53100 Siena, Italy; r.canitano@ao-siena.toscana.it

5 Laboratory of Psychology of Perception, University Paris Descartes, 75270 Paris, France

* Correspondence: s.tordjman@yahoo.fr

Academic Editor: Merlin G. Butler

Abstract: Progress in epidemiological, molecular and clinical genetics with the development of new techniques has improved knowledge on genetic syndromes associated with autism spectrum disorder (ASD). The objective of this article is to show the diversity of genetic disorders associated with ASD (based on an extensive review of single-gene disorders, copy number variants, and other chromosomal disorders), and consequently to propose a hierarchical diagnostic strategy with a stepwise evaluation, helping general practitioners/pediatricians and child psychiatrists to collaborate with geneticists and neuropediatricians, in order to search for genetic disorders associated with ASD. The first step is a clinical investigation involving: (i) a child psychiatric and psychological evaluation confirming autism diagnosis from different observational sources and assessing autism severity; (ii) a neuropediatric evaluation examining neurological symptoms and developmental milestones; and (iii) a genetic evaluation searching for dysmorphic features and malformations. The second step involves laboratory and if necessary neuroimaging and EEG studies oriented by clinical results based on clinical genetic and neuropediatric examinations. The identification of genetic disorders associated with ASD has practical implications for diagnostic strategies, early detection or prevention of co-morbidity, specific treatment and follow up, and genetic counseling.

Keywords: autism; genetic disorders; hierarchical diagnostic strategy; child psychiatric and psychological assessment; clinical genetics; neuropediatric evaluation

1. Introduction

Autism Spectrum Disorder (ASD) is considered as a neurodevelopmental disorder defined in the DSM-5 (the Diagnostic and Statistical Manual of Mental Disorders 5th ed.) [1], the most recent diagnostic classification of mental disorders, by social communication deficits associated with repetitive/stereotyped behaviors or interests with early onset (referenced in the DSM-5 as symptoms present at early developmental period and evident in early childhood). According to the historian Normand J. Carrey, the first description of autism can be traced to Itard in his 1828 report on "mutism produced by a lesion of intellectual functions" [2]. In 1943, Leo Kanner [3], American psychiatrist with Austrian origins, borrowed the term *autism* from the Swiss psychiatrist Eugen Bleuler to define a specific syndrome observed in 11 children (the term "autism", derived from the Greek autos which means "oneself", was used for the first time by Eugen Bleuler in 1911 [4] to describe social withdrawal in adult patients with schizophrenia). The Kanner syndrome was characterized by its early onset (from the first year of life) and symptomatology (social withdrawal, sameness, language impairment, stereotyped motor behaviors, and intellectual disability). It is noteworthy that Kanner did not describe autism in individuals with severe intellectual disability and known brain disorders. The same year, the Austrian psychiatrist Hans Asperger [5] distinguished "personalities with autistic tendencies" which differed from the children that Kanner had described, due to the expression of exceptional isolated talents and conserved linguistic abilities. Currently, autism is viewed as an epistatic and multifactorial disorder involving genetic factors and environmental factors (prenatal, neonatal and/or postnatal environmental factors such as gestational diabetes, neonatal hypoxia conditions, exposure to air pollution, parental immigration or sensory/social deficits; for a review, see Tordjman et al., 2014 [6]).

Several literature reviews underline the important role of genetics in the etiology of autism [7–9]. The data come from family and twin studies. Indeed, the concordance rate among monozygotic twins is high (60%–90%) compared to the concordance rate among dizygotic twins (0%–30%) [10,11]. Technological advances in epidemiological and molecular genetics have led recently to new findings in the field of the genetics of neuropsychiatric disorders. These new findings concern also the domain of the genetics of autism and have increased the state of current knowledge on the genetic disorders associated with ASD. Identified genetic causes of ASD can be classified as the cytogenetically visible chromosomal abnormalities, copy number variants (CNVs) (i.e., variations in the number of copies of one segment of DNA, including deletions and duplications), and single-gene disorders [12]. CNVs can have different sizes (small to large deletions or duplications) and therefore concern a variable number of genes according to their size. The number of known genetic disorders associated with ASD has increased with the use of array Comparative Genomic Hybridization (aCGH), also called chromosomal microarrays (CMAs) or high-resolution molecular karyotype, which is one of the most molecular cytogenetic methods used by geneticists. The accuracy of aCGH is 10 to 100 times higher than low-resolution karyotype accuracy and allows detection of small CNVs. Unfortunately, this method does not detect certain genetic anomalies such as balanced chromosome rearrangements (which are rarely involved in developmental disorders) or CNVs present in less than 10% to 20% of cells (somatic mosaicism). CNVs are usually considered to be rare variants but recent techniques have shown that they may be in fact more frequent than expected [13]. In practice, after CNV detection, the geneticist needs to determine the contribution of this variation to the patient's disorder. Most of the time, parental CNVs are also analyzed for family segregation. Among genetic causes of ASD, besides single specific genetic factors, cumulative effects of Single Nucleotide Variants (SNVs: common small variations in the DNA sequence occurring within a population) also have to be taken into consideration. Single-nucleotide polymorphism (SNP) is the term usually used for SNVs occurring in more than 1% of the general population. In the next few years, it will be probably possible to improve the identification and interpretation of SNPs in ASD using new techniques of High Throughput Sequencing, such as targeted sequencing on known genes (gene panel) or Whole Exome/Genome Sequencing. Finally, it should be highlighted that a genetic model of ASD (including cumulative genetic variance) does not exclude the role of environment (including cumulative environmental variance). It is noteworthy that heritability (h^2) is defined as $h^2 = \mathrm{GV}/(\mathrm{GV} + \mathrm{EV})$ where GV is the cumulative genetic variance and EV, the environmental variance [14].

Many susceptibility genes and cytogenetic abnormalities have been reported in ASD and concern almost every chromosome (for a review, see Miles, 2011; available online: http://projects.tcag.ca/autism/) [15]. How can we explain such genetic diversity associated with similar autism cognitive-behavioral phenotypes? Given the current state of knowledge, we can state the hypothesis that the majority of ASD-related genes are involved in brain development and functioning (such as synapse formation and functioning, brain metabolism, chromatin remodeling) [16].

Several studies have reported associations between genetic contribution (such as unbalanced chromosome abnormalities, in particular large chromosomal abnormalities), dysmorphic features and low cognitive functioning [17–19]. Indeed, large chromosomal abnormalities are more often found in children with dysmorphic features, whereas small CNVs and de novo SNPs are more often found in individuals without dysmorphic features. The concept of "syndromic autism" or "complex autism" (autism associated with genetic disorders/genetic syndromes) which qualifies individuals with at least one dysmorphic feature/malformation or severe intellectual disability, is opposed to the concept of "non-syndromic autism" or "simplex"/"pure"/idiopatic autism (isolated autism) which qualifies individuals with moderate intellectual disability to normal cognitive functioning and no other associated signs or symptoms (except the presence of seizures) [19,20]. The prevalence of epilepsy in ASD varies from 5% to 40% (compared to 0.5% to 1% in the general population) according to different variables, including syndromic vs. non-syndromic autism (higher rates of epilepsy are observed in syndromic autism compared to non-syndromic autism) [21–24] and the age of the population (the rate of seizures varies with age and increases especially during the prepubertal period). It is noteworthy that genome-wide association and genetic analyses such as aCGH have revealed hundreds of previously unknown rare mutations and CNVs linked to non-syndromic autism. Some authors [12,19] suggest that syndromic autism (SA), compared to non-syndromic autism (NSA), is associated with a poorer prognosis, a lower male-to-female sex ratio (SA: 3/1; NSA: 6/1), and a lower sibling recurrence risk (SA: 4%–6%; NSA: up to 35%) as well as a lower risk for family history of autism (SA: up to 9%; NSA: up to 20%) given that SA would be more related to accidental mutations than NSA. Similarly, the concept of syndromic intellectual disability (intellectual disability associated with dysmorphism and medical or behavioral signs and symptoms) is widely used as opposed to non-syndromic intellectual disability (intellectual disability without other abnormalities). Intellectual disability and autism spectrum disorder share other similarities given that they are both genetically heterogeneous, and a significant number of genes have been associated with both conditions. It is noteworthy that the concept of non-syndromic autism or non-syndromic intellectual disability depends on technological progress and current state of knowledge. We can foresee, as underlined by Tordjman et al. [25], that individuals with currently and apparently "non-syndromic autism" could become a few years later individuals with "syndromic autism", if new genetic disorders are identified, allowing a better understanding and more efficient identification of discrete clinical symptoms as minor physical anomalies, malformations and associated biological anomalies. For example, individuals with Smith–Magenis syndrome can show in early childhood ASD associated with subtle minor facial dysmorphic features (these discrete dysmorphic features become more evident later), mild or moderate intellectual disability, disrupted sleep patterns and repetitive self-hugging characteristic of this syndrome. The molecular discovery of Smith–Magenis syndrome is relatively recent (1982) and allowed to better know the characteristic behavioral phenotype combined with physical anomalies of Smith–Magenis syndrome (including short stature and scoliosis, not enough specific to help alone to identify the genetic syndrome), orienting towards the search for certain dysmorphic features and the possible identification of this genetic disorder. Thus, some children with Smith–Magenis syndrome could be considered in early childhood, especially before the discovery of Smith–Magenis syndrome in 1982, as individuals with apparently "non-syndromic autism" (they are more viewed as individuals with syndromic autism over their developmental trajectory). Therefore, taking into account this bias, it would be better to consider autism as a behavioral syndrome related either to known genetic disorders or to currently unknown causes.

The objective of this article is to show the diversity of the genetic disorders associated with ASD (including single-gene disorders, CNVs and other chromosomal disorders), and consequently to propose a hierarchical diagnostic strategy with a stepwise evaluation, helping general practitioners/pediatricians and child psychiatrists to collaborate with geneticists and neuropediatricians, in order to search for genetic disorders associated with ASD.

2. Known Genetic Syndromes Associated with Autism Spectrum Disorder

We chose to limit the review of literature to genetic disorders presented in Table 1. Table 1 includes one part on chromosomal disorders and another part on single-gene disorders. The present descriptions focus on autistic traits encountered in each genetic disorder and other symptoms that may be helpful for the diagnosis. Table 1 summarizes these clinical data and indicates the estimated frequency of each genetic disorder in autism and the frequency of autistic traits in each genetic disorder (when available). This table does not present an exhaustive list of genetic disorders associated with ASD. Furthermore, Table 1 includes only genetic syndromes involving a single-gene disorder or a chromosomal rearrangement, and therefore does not include polygenic causes and possible genetic disorders only related to epigenetic mechanisms. It is noteworthy that some studies suggest that the genetic background might play an important role in many ASD individuals, with in particular cumulative genetic effects related to the load of common risk variants [16].

Table 1. Main genetic disorders associated with autistic syndrome.

Genetic Disorder [References]	Estimated Rate (%) of the Disorder in Autism	Estimated Rate (%) of Autism in the Disorder	Degree of Intellectual Disability (ID)	Possible Autistic Behaviors	Other Possible Behaviors	Other Possible Symptoms
Chromosomal Disorders						
Maternal * 15q11–q13 duplication [26–38]	1–2	80–100	Severe	Severe autistic syndrome with severe expressive language impairment	Hyperactivity and aggression	Seizures (75%), hypotonia, genitor/urinary abnormalities
Angelman syndrome * (maternal 15q11-q13 deletion, paternal uniparental disomy, mutations of *UBE3A* that encodes an ubiquitin E3 ligase) [35,39–48]	1	48–80	Severe	No language, stereotypies, sameness	Attention Deficit with Hyperactivity Disorder (ADHD), paroxysmal laughter, tantrums	Facial dysmorphism, microcephaly, seizures (>1 year), ataxia and walking disturbance
Prader–Willi syndrome * (maternal uniparental disomy at 15q11-q13, paternal deletions) [35,49–58] Paternal 15q11-q13 duplication (only few cases reported to be associated with autism): behavioral phenotype similar to Prader–Willi syndrome [58–60]	Not Available (NA)	19–37	Mild to moderate	Motor and verbal stereotypies, rituals	Hyperphagia, obsessive-compulsive traits, temper tantrums	Obesity, growth delay and hypogonadism, facial dysmorphism, Hypotonia
Phelan–McDermid * syndrome (Inherited, de novo deletions at 22q13.3 leading to loss of *SHANK 3*) 22q13.3 duplication [20,61–70]	NA	75–84	Severe	Variable autistic syndrome with social communication impairments, including delayed or absent verbal language	Global developmental delay, atatonia in adolescence and adulthood	Dysmorphic features, hypotonia, gait disturbance, recurring upper respiratory tract infections, gastroesophageal reflux and seizures
16p11.2 duplication 16p11.2 deletion [71–77]	1	33	Severe	Severe autistic syndrome with speech impairment	Gross and fine coordination problems, SCH (Schizophrenia), anxiety, ADHD	Hypotonia (Multiple congenital anomalies are possible with more distal region)
Inverted duplication/deletion 8p21–23 [78,79]	NA	30–57	Variable	Mild to moderate autistic syndrome with absent or delayed verbal language	ADHD	Minor facial dysmorphism, hypotonia, agenesis of the corpus callosum, possible heart defect
Genetic disorder [References]	Estimated rate (%) of the disorder in autism	Estimated rate (%) of autism in the disorder	Degree of intellectual disability (ID)	Autistic behaviors	Other behaviors	Other symptoms
Down syndrome * (trisomy 21) [80–84]	2	5–10	Variable but usually severe when autism	Severe autistic syndrome	-	Facial dysmorphism, heart and intestine malformations
Smith–Magenis syndrome (17p11.2 deletion) [85–88]	<1	80–100	Variable	Self-injurious and stereotyped behaviors, sameness	Tantrums, possible social contact, sleep disturbance	Facial dysmorphism, peripheral neuropathy, hypotonia

Table 1. *Cont.*

Genetic Disorder [References]	Estimated Rate (%) of the Disorder in Autism	Estimated Rate (%) of Autism in the Disorder	Degree of Intellectual Disability (ID)	Possible Autistic Behaviors	Other Possible Behaviors	Other Possible Symptoms
Potocki–Lupski syndrome (17p11.2 duplication) [89]	NA	50–100	Normal to moderate	Decreased eye contact, motor manierisms or posturing, sensory hypersensitivity or preoccupation, repetitive behaviors or interests, lack of appropriate functional or symbolic play and lack of joint attention	Developmental delay, language impairment, and cognitive impairment	hypotonia, poor feeding and failure to thrive in infancy, oral-pharyngeal dysphagia, obstructive and central sleep apnea, structural cardiovascular abnormalities, electroencephalography (EEG), abnormalities, and hypermetropia
2q37 deletion [90–94]	<1	25–35	Mild to moderate	Severe communication impairment, stereotypies	Hypotonia, hyperactivity, Obsessive-Compulsive Disorder (OCD), aggression, sleep disturbance	Facial dysmorphism, microcephaly, growth delay/short stature, intestine and heart malformations, seizure
22q11.21 duplication and 22q11 deletion (DiGeorge/Vélocardio-facial syndrome) [95–100]	NA	<10	Normal to severe ID	Autistic syndrome, Pervasive Developmental Disorder-Not Otherwise Specified PDD-NOS (ICD-10 criteria)	Learning disability, anxiety, ADHD, oppositional-defiant disorder, OCD, motor impairment	Facial dysmorphism, microcephaly, growth delay/short stature, craniofacial abnormalities/cleft palate, heart defect, hypotonia
1q21.1 Copy-Number Variation (CNV) (1q21.1 deletion/ duplication) [101–104]	NA	<30	Normal to mild ID	Autistic syndrome, PDD-NOS (ICD-10 criteria)	Developmental delay, learning disability, anxiety, ADHD, aggression, SCZ and hallucination	Microcephaly (deletion) Macrocephaly (duplication)
Williams-Beuren syndrome * (7q11.23 deletion) and Reciprocal 7q11.23 duplication syndrome [105–117]	<1	<10	Mild to moderate	Autistic syndrome	Overfriendliness, over talkativeness, visual spatial deficit, hyperacusis, feeding and sleep problems	Facial dysmorphism, short stature, heart and endocrine malformations, hypercalcemia
Turner syndrome * (most common monosomy For X chromosome) [37,118,119]	NA	3	Usually normal IQ	Females monosomic for the maternal chromosome X score significantly worse on social adjustment and verbal skills	-	Short stature, skeletal abnormalities, absence of ovarian function, webbed neck, lymphedema in hands and feet, heart defects and kidney problems

Table 1. *Cont.*

Genetic Disorder [References]	Estimated Rate (%) of the Disorder in Autism	Estimated Rate (%) of Autism in the Disorder	Degree of Intellectual Disability (ID)	Possible Autistic Behaviors	Other Possible Behaviors	Other Possible Symptoms
Beckwith–Wiedemann * syndrome (abnormal expression of imprinted genes on chromosome 11p15.5 such as *IGF2* and/or *CDKN1C*) [120–123]	NA	6.8 (replication needed)	Usually normal IQ	Autistic syndrome	-	Pre- and postnatal overgrowth (hemihyperplasia, macroglossia, visceromegaly) and increased risk of embryonal tumors
Isodicentric chromosome 15 or duplication/inversion 15q11 [124,125]	NA	NA	Moderate to severe	Autistic behavior	Developmental delay and intellectual deficit, epilepsy	Early central hypotonia
Ito hypomelanosis [126,127]	NA	NA	Inconstant	Asperger syndrome(high functioning autism) or atypical autism	Psychomotor delay and cognitive deficit	hypopigmented skin lesions along the Blaschko lines, motor delay, seizures, microcephaly or macrocephaly, hypotonia, ophthalmological abnormalities
Single Gene Disorders						
CHARGE syndrome * (*CHD7*, 8q21.1) [128–133]	<1	15–50	Variable but often normal IQ	Variable autistic syndrome	Hyperactivity, obsessive-compulsive traits, tic disorders	Coloboma of the eye, Heart defects, Atresia of the nasal choane, Retardation of growth and/or development, Genital/urinary abnormalities, Ear abnormalities/deafness
Tuberous sclerosis (*TSC1*, 9q34) (*TSC2*, 16p13.3) [134–136]	1–4	25–60	Variable	Severe autistic syndrome	Learning disorder	Ectodermal anomalies, renal lesions, seizures
PTEN macrocephaly syndromes (*PTEN*, 10q23.31) [137–142]	4 in ASD with macro-cephaly	NA	Severe	Autistic syndrome and language delay	=	Progressive macrocephaly, developmental delay, macrosomy, tumors in adulthood
Rett's syndrome * (*MECP2*, Xq28) [117,143–149]	<1 in female	61–100	Severe	Stereotyped hand movements, absence of language, loss of social engagement	Stagnation stage (6–18 months) in girls, then regression stage (12–36 months), pseudostationary t stage (2–10 years), l and late motor t deterioration (>10 years)	Head growth deceleration, progressive motor neuron (gait and truncal apraxia, ataxia, decreasing mobility) and respiratory (hyperventilation, breath holding, apnea) symptoms
San Filippo syndrome # (*SGSH*, 17q25.3) [150–153]	1 replication needed	80–100	Severe	Language impairment, autistic withdrawal, stereotyped behaviors impulsivity, inappropriate affects	Progressive loss of acquisitions	Motor regression, hepatomegaly
Cerebral folate deficiency # (*FOLR1*, 11q13.4) [154–157]	NA	NA	Variable	Autistic syndrome including especially social interaction and language impairment	irritability, movement (such as tremors) and gait disturbances with ataxia, sleep problems	Psychomotor regression, epilepsy, developmental delay, deceleration of head growth, dystonia/hypotonia, visual and hearing deficit
Smith–Lemli–Opitz syndrome # (*DHCR7*, 1q12–13) [158–163]	NA	50	Variable	Self-injurious behaviors, stereotypies ("opisthokinesis") language impairment	Sensory hyper-reactivity, irritability, sleep disturbance	Facial dysmorphism, cleft palate, congenital heart disease, hypospadias, 2–3 toe syndactyly

Table 1. *Cont.*

Genetic Disorder [References]	Estimated Rate (%) of the Disorder in Autism	Estimated Rate (%) of Autism in the Disorder	Degree of Intellectual Disability (ID)	Possible Autistic Behaviors	Other Possible Behaviors	Other Possible Symptoms
Phenylketonuria # (*PAH*, 12q22-q24.1) [20,164,165]	NA	NA	Severe	Self-injurious behavior, lack of social responsiveness	Temper tantrums, hyperactivity	Eczema, hypertonia, seizures, hypo-pigmentation
Adenylosuccinate lyase deficiency # (*ASL*, 22q13.1–13.2) [166–170]	<1	80–100	Variable	Severe autistic syndrome	-	Seizures
Creatine deficiency syndrome # (*GAMT*, 19p13.3) (*CRTR*, Xq28) [171–174]	<1	80–100	Severe	Severe autistic syndrome with poor language	-	Seizures, hypotonia
SHANK 3 (22q13.3) [175–177]	<1	NA	NA	Severe autistic syndrome with no language	-	-
Neurexin family: Neurexin 1 (*NRX1*, 2p16.3) [178–182]	1	NA	Variable	Autistic syndrome	Hyperactivity, depression, learning disability, but also normal behavior	Seizures, hypotonia, facial dysmorphism?
Contactin Associated Protein-like 2 (*CNTNAP2*, 7q35) [183–185]	NA	NA	Variable	Autistic syndrome including verbal language impairment	-	Seizures
Contactin 4 (*CNTN4*, 3p26.2–3p26.3) [186–189]	<1	NA	Variable	Autistic syndrome, PDD-NOS (ICD-10 criteria)	Visual spatial impairment, regression	Facial dysmorphism, developmental delay, hypotonia, ptosis.
Cell adhesion molecule-1 (*CADM1*, 11q22.3–23.2) [190–192]	NA	NA	NA	Autistic syndrome with especially social communication impairment including verbal language deficit	-	-
Protocadherin 10 (*PCDH10*, 4q28) [193]	<1	NA	NA	Autistic syndrome	-	-
Neuroligin family: Neuroligin 3 (*NLG3*, Xq13) Neuroligin 4 (*NLG4*, Xq22.33) [194–196]	<1	NA	Variable	Severe autistic syndrome, PDD-NOS (ICD-10 criteria)	Regression	Tic
Fragile X * (*FMR1*, Xq27.3) [191,196–222]	0–8	0–33	Variable	Poor eye contact , social anxiety, language deficit and stereotypies	Hyperactivity with attention deficit, sensory hyper-reactivity	Facial dysmorphism, macro-orchidism
Neurofibromatosis type 1 [109,223–225]	NA	21–40	inconstant	Restrictive/repetitive behaviors and severe social-communicative impairments	Cognitive deficits and learning difficulties	Café-au-lait spots, iris Lisch nodules, axillary and inguinal freckling, multiple neurofibromas
Sotos syndrome [226,227]	NA	70 (replication needed)	Mild to severe	Self-injurious behavior, physical aggression, and destruction	-	Facial dysmorphism, overgrowth of the body in early life with macrocephaly
Aarskog syndrome [228,229]	NA	NA	-	Variable autistic syndrome	Learning and behavioral disabilities	facial, limbs and genital features, acromelic short stature
Cornelia de Lange syndrome [117,230,231]	NA	43 (replication needed)	Variable	Self-injury, excessive repetitive behaviors and expressive language deficits	Psychomotor delay, language acquisition difficulties	Facial dysmorphism, severe growth delay, abnormal hands and feet, and constant brachymetacarpia of the first metacarpus, various other malformations (heart, kidney, etc.)

Table 1. *Cont.*

Genetic Disorder [References]	Estimated Rate (%) of the Disorder in Autism	Estimated Rate (%) of Autism in the Disorder	Degree of Intellectual Disability (ID)	Possible Autistic Behaviors	Other Possible Behaviors	Other Possible Symptoms
Joubert syndrome [232]	NA	<40	severe intellectual deficit to normal intelligence	Autistic syndrome	-	Facial dysmorphism, abnormal respiratory pattern, nystagmus, hypotonia, ataxia, and delay in achieving motor milestones
Cohen syndrome [117,233–235]	NA	54 (replication needed)	variable	Atypical autism	Often sociable with a cheerful disposition, learning and behavioral problems	Microcephaly, facial dysmorphism, hypotonia, myopia, retinal dystrophy, neutropenia and truncal obesity
Lujan–Fryns syndrome [236]	NA	NA	Mild to moderate	Autistic-like disorder	Behavioral problems, emotional instability, hyperactivity and shyness, schizophrenia	Tall, marfanoid stature, facial dysmorphism, hypernasal voice and generalized hypotonia
Noonan syndrome [237–239]	NA	15 (replication needed)	Mild	ASD	Poor feeding in infancy	Short stature, facial dysmorphism and congenital heart defects
Moebius syndrome [128,240,241]	NA	0–45	Inconstant, mild	ASD	Delayed walk development	Oculofacial paralysis, strabismus
Helsmoortel–Van der Aa syndrome (ADNP-related ID/ASD) [242]	0.17	100	Mild to severe	ASD, behavioral problems, sleep disturbance	Delayed developmental milestones (walking between 19 months and 4.5 years, and speech ranging from sentences to no words)	Facial dysmorphism, hypotonia, seizures, feeding difficulties, visual problems (hypermetropia, strabismus, cortical visual impairment), and cardiac defects
Timothy syndrome (CACNA1C) [243]	NA	50–70 (replication needed)	Inconstant, mild to severe	ASD	Language, motor, and generalized cognitive impairment	Facial dysmorphism, rate-corrected QT (QTc) interval >480 ms, unilateral or bilateral cutaneous syndactyly, heart defects, seizures

Adapted from Tordjman et al. [25]. # These genetic disorders are metabolic disorders (the list is not exhaustive). * The asterisk indicates the existence of epigenetic mechanisms observed in these genetic disorders (the list is not exhaustive).

Interestingly, as underlined by Abrahams and Geschwind [7], the descriptive analysis of Table 1 indicates that each of the many known genes or genomic regions associated with ASD, taken separately, accounts usually and on average for less than 2% of autism cases, suggesting high genetic heterogeneity (the maximum average rate is 5% and concerns the Fragile X syndrome). However, taken all together, these single genetic impairments account at least for 10%–25% of ASD individuals [244] and even 35%–40% in more recent studies [245].

3. Recommended Investigations for the Identification of Genetic Disorders Associated with ASD

Facing such a diversity of genetic disorders associated with ASD (see Table 1), it seems important to clarify, as best as possible with regard to the current state of knowledge, the diagnostic steps towards identification of these genetic disorders. A hierarchical diagnostic strategy with a stepwise evaluation towards identification of genetic disorders associated with autism is proposed and developed in Figure 1.

As it appears in Table 1, the severity of the autistic syndrome is an important variable to take into consideration in the search for genetic disorders associated with ASD. Therefore, the preliminary step in the hierarchical diagnostic strategy is to confirm autism diagnosis and assess autism severity. Furthermore, based on the genetic syndromes listed in Table 1, certain variables are of particular interest such as dysmorphic features, malformations, epilepsy and intellectual disability. It indicates clearly that clinical investigation of behavioral phenotype of autism for identification of genetic disorders associated with ASD requires clinical genetic examination, neuropediatric examination and psychological assessment. In this section, we propose a hierarchal diagnostic strategy with focused investigations for the identification of genetic disorders associated with ASD, based on the history of the individual (including family history and developmental trajectory) and the clinical neurologic and genetic evaluation, but also on up-to-date knowledge and new technology. The first step of the hierarchal diagnostic strategy is a clinical investigation involving: (i) a child psychiatrist's and psychologist's evaluation to confirm autism diagnosis using different observational sources (including an extensive parental interview facilitating the study of family history) and assess autism severity (including behavioral and cognitive assessments); (ii) a neuropediatrician's evaluation to examine neurological symptoms/signs and developmental milestones; and (iii) a geneticist's evaluation to search for dysmorphic features and malformations based on a clinical physical examination. This clinical step is followed by a second step involving laboratory and if necessary neuroimaging or EEG studies oriented by clinical results based on clinical genetic and neuropediatric examinations. These two steps are described below.

3.1. First Step: Clinical Investigation

3.1.1. Autism Diagnosis Using Different Observational Sources and Autism Severity Assessment (Child Psychiatric and Psychological Evaluation)

The preliminary step requires confirming the diagnosis of autism and assessing the severity of autistic behavioral impairments with validated tools used by trained professionals in different observational situations, such as the Autism Diagnostic Interview-Revised [246] (the ADI-R scale is a parental interview) and the Autism Diagnostic Observation Schedule [247] (the ADOS scale allows a direct observation of the individual through a standardized play situation). The psychiatric appreciation of ICD-10 (International Classification of Diseases, World Health Organization, Geneve, Switzerland, 1993) and DSM-5 (American Psychiatric Association, Washington, DC, USA, 2013) diagnostic criteria of autism is also necessary and provides a clinical psychiatric judgment. This approach, combining information from multiple sources based on the clinical psychiatric judgment and the administration of the ADI-R completed by the ADOS improves the confidence in the diagnosis of ASD [248]. Interestingly, the ADI-R scale is validated to assess current behavior but also behavior during the 4–5 years old period (the ADI-R algorithm is based on the 4–5 years old period of life which is supposed to correspond to the most severe period of autistic impairments), allowing to see the evolution between these two periods of life. It happens more frequently than expected that children who fulfill the diagnostic criteria for ASD based on the ADI-R algorithm (parental interview for the 4–5 years old period) do not meet the full diagnostic criteria for ASD based on the ADOS algorithm (direct observation of the child for the current period).

The ADI-R scale is the most common assessment used to conduct an extensive semi-structured parental interview searching for medical and psychiatric family history. This clinical interview should be conducted with empathy and allow a three-generation family tree to be constructed, showing, in particular, family psychiatric history (such as, for example, schizophrenia, depression or bipolar disorder) and ASD behaviors (including delayed language development) within the family (mother's and father's sides). The construction of the pedigree can be very helpful to get specific hypotheses of genetic disorders associated with autism. More generally, higher rates of CNVs are observed in ASD individuals with a family history of psychiatric disorders or developmental disabilities, highlighting the importance to study family history [249]. It is noteworthy that family history is also investigated and analyzed by the neuropediatrician and the geneticist during their evaluation.

Furthermore, the clinician should indicate in the family tree the existence of consanguineous mating, family malformations, deceased infants and spontaneous abortions occurring in the mother but also in relatives (repeated spontaneous abortions are in favor of chromosomal rearrangement [20,250,251]). It is necessary to specify the trimester of pregnancy when spontaneous abortions occurred given that repeated miscarriages at the first trimester of pregnancy are more specifically in favor of genetic anomalies. Reproductive stoppage is rarely evoked but should be investigated because reproductive curtailment following the birth of a child with ASD has been reported [252]. In addition, the birth order of the child with autism has to be noted in the family tree given that a decrease of ASD in later siblings has been observed [253]. The maternal and paternal ages at the time of procreation should be also systematically noted. Indeed, several studies suggest that advanced parental age, in particular for the father, is a risk factor for ASD [254], but there are some discrepancies in the results [253]. Although advanced parental age may be a risk factor, it orients towards genetic testing but does not lead to definitive conclusions.

Finally, a psychological evaluation is necessary in this hierarchical diagnostic strategy to assess the level of cognitive functioning given that intellectual disability and its severity are associated, as indicated previously, with a risk for several genetic disorders in ASD individuals (see Table 1). In addition, the level of cognitive functioning should be taken into consideration and therefore assessed given that severe intellectual disability can introduce an important bias leading to a misdiagnosis of autism. Indeed, ASD is often misdiagnosed in individuals with severe intellectual disability. It should be noted that the diagnosis of autism might be not valid or relevant for genetic disorders associated with severe intellectual disability due to first, the behavioral overlap between severe intellectual disability and autistic behavioral impairments (social communication deficit as well as repeated behaviors or interests), and second, the absence of validity and reliability of autism diagnostic instruments in the context of very low IQ or mental age of less than 24 months [255]. It is noteworthy that the most currently international instruments used for autism diagnosis, such as the ADI-R and the ADOS scales, were not normed in individuals with severe intellectual disability [255]. Cognitive functioning can be assessed, whenever possible with the child, by a psychologist or a neuropsychologist if available, using the age-appropriate Wechsler intelligence scales (Wechsler Preschool and Primary Scale of Intelligence: WPPSI-IV for children between 2 and 7 years old, Wechsler Intelligence Scale for Children: WISC-5 for children between 6 and 16 years old, Wechsler Adult Intelligence Scale: WAIS-IV for individuals above 16 years old) or the Kaufman Assessment Battery for Children (K-ABC) [256]. The Kaufman K-ABC is supposed to be more adapted for nonverbal children but cognitive assessment appears in fact easier to perform using the Wechsler intelligence scales with nonverbal subtests for nonverbal ASD children. Some instruments are of particular interest for intellectual disabled children with ASD such as the Raven's Color Progressive Matrices (CPM) which is a short (20 min) nonverbal intelligence test validated for young children and individuals with intellectual disability [257].

The child psychiatric evaluation and psychological evaluation confirming autism diagnosis from different observational sources and assessing autism severity and intellectual disability are followed by a neuropediatrician's evaluation and a geneticist's evaluation (see Figure 1).

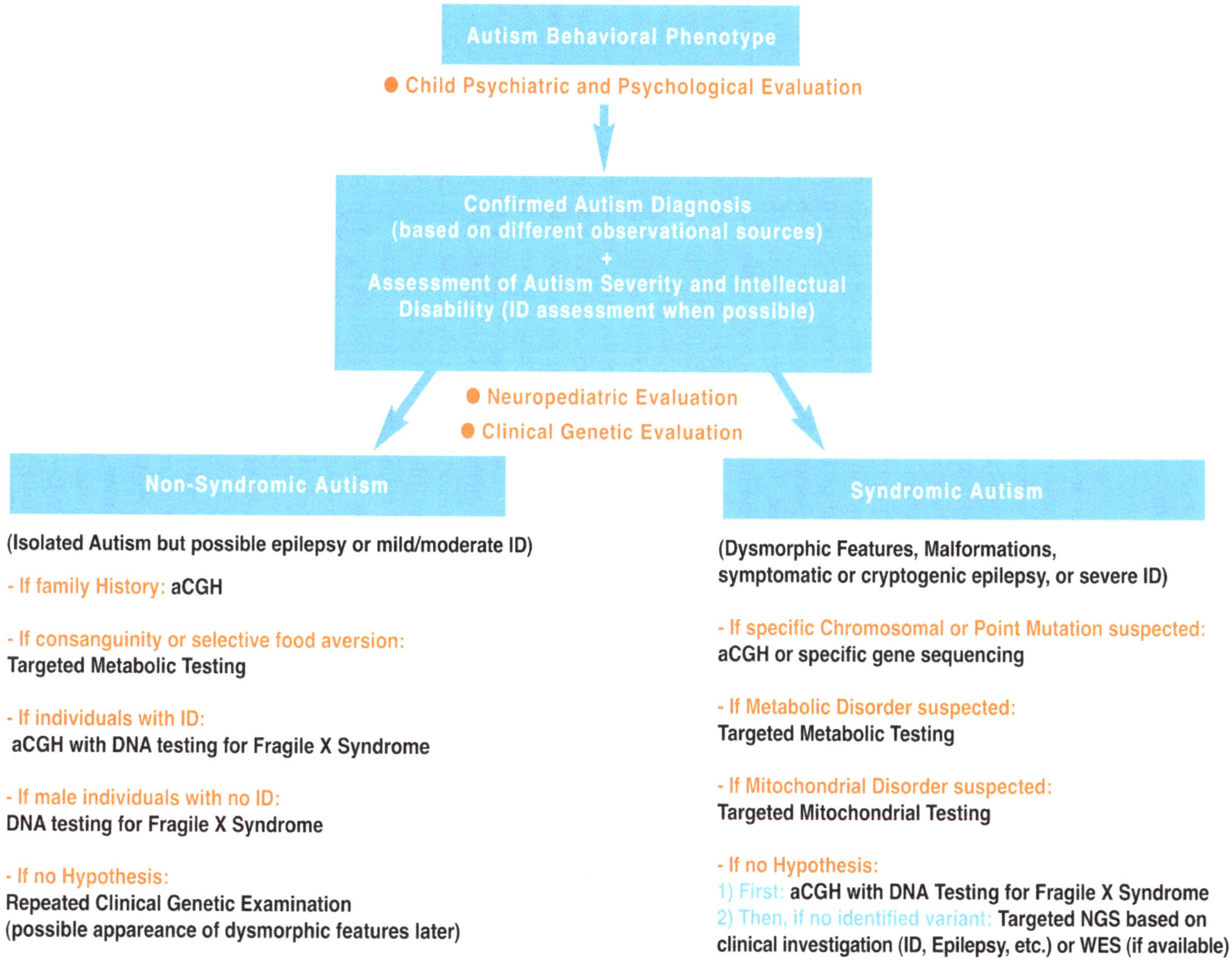
Autism Behavioral Phenotype
Child Psychiatric and Psychological Evaluation
Confirmed Autism Diagnosis
(based on different observational sources)
+
Assessment of Autism Severity and Intellectual Disability (ID assessment when possible)
Neuropediatric Evaluation
Clinical Genetic Evaluation
Non-Syndromic Autism
(Isolated Autism but possible epilepsy or mild/moderate ID)
- If family History: aCGH
- If consanguinity or selective food aversion:
Targeted Metabolic Testing
- If individuals with ID:
aCGH with DNA testing for Fragile X Syndrome
- If male individuals with no ID:
DNA testing for Fragile X Syndrome
- If no Hypothesis:
Repeated Clinical Genetic Examination
(possible appareance of dysmorphic features later)
Syndromic Autism
(Dysmorphic Features, Malformations,
symptomatic or cryptogenic epilepsy, or severe ID)
- If specific Chromosomal or Point Mutation suspected:
aCGH or specific gene sequencing
- If Metabolic Disorder suspected:
Targeted Metabolic Testing
- If Mitochondrial Disorder suspected:
Targeted Mitochondrial Testing
- If no Hypothesis:
1) First: aCGH with DNA Testing for Fragile X Syndrome
2) Then, if no identified variant: Targeted NGS based on
clinical investigation (ID, Epilepsy, etc.) or WES (if available)

Figure 1. Hierarchical diagnostic strategy with a stepwise evaluation towards identification of genetic disorders associated with autism.

3.1.2. Developmental Milestones (Neuropediatric Evaluation)

A neuropediatric examination should be systematically conducted searching for neurological symptoms associated with ASD such as hypotonia, ataxia, abnormal movements or epilepsy. In case of clinical symptoms of epilepsy, the electroencephalogram (EEG) can be a useful tool to detect epileptic brain activity. In complement to this neuropediatric examination, it is necessary to rule out a sensory deficit, such as an auditory or visual deficit, based on ophtamological and ears-nose-throat examination (an audiogram is recommended). In addition, the neuropediatric examination investigates extensively developmental milestones for the following periods (some developmental milestones are often explored also during the child psychiatric evaluation): (i) prenatal period: course of pregnancy, fetal movements, results of ultrasound exams, treatments (in particular, in-utero exposure to thalidomide or valproate, known as teratogenic medications and risk factors for ASD), and other possible prenatal risk factors for ASD (such as gestational diabetes, gestational bleeding or multiple birth [6]); (ii) perinatal period: birth presentation (abnormal presentation in general and breech presentation in particular, have been associated with the development of ASD [258], mode of delivery, clinical status at birth (APGAR, score, weight, body length, and head circumference), premature birth (the risk for autism increased with the severity of preterm birth [259]), conditions related to hypoxia at birth reported as risk factors for ASD (such as umbilical cord complications, meconium aspiration, neonatal anaemia, ABO or Rh incompatibility, hyperbilirubinemia, or birth injury and trauma; for a review, see Gardener et al. [260]), feeding pattern and difficulties, screening tests (hypothyroidism, phenylketonuria), physical examination (apparent dysmorphism and malformations) and neurological examination (neonatal hypotonia); and (iii) postnatal period: psychomotor development, feeding pattern and possible gastrointestinal problems, sleep pattern, epilepsy, sensory dysfunction, language development, early behavioral signs of autism and other atypical behaviors. This clinical evaluation investigates developmental and learning disorders. The study of the height-weight-head circumference growth curve can show a break, decline with regression, or decrease with stagnation. For example, a decrease between 6 and 18 months of head circumference growth should orient the clinician towards the search for Rett syndrome in its first stage (stagnation stage) which occurs before the stage of fast decline of the communication skills (regression stage between 12 and 18 months of age). In addition, a developmental regression should orient the clinician towards the search for metabolic diseases. More generally, neuroimaging is recommended in individuals with ASD and microcephaly [249]. It is noteworthy that parental measures of height-weight-head circumference have also to be considered in order to determine whether the child's height-weight-head circumference measures are really abnormal compared to the parents' ones or whether a parent may be mildly affected, orienting towards a congenital or acquired abnormality.

3.1.3. Physical Examination (Genetic Evaluation)

A clinical genetics evaluation is systematically required and involves an extensive physical examination of the whole body. This physical examination should be conducted by a clinical geneticist trained in dysmorphology searching for dysmorphic features or malformations, and includes photos of the head (face and profile) with a good visibility of the ears, hands (palm and dorsal view) and feet. When clinical geneticists are not easily available, alternative options are to send, as a preliminary step, patients' pictures (face and hands pictures) to a geneticist for a specialized opinion (our group is testing the feasibility and efficiency of such a procedure and is comparing the results obtained based on the analyses of pictures by a group of geneticists to the ones obtained based on the analyses of the same pictures using the genetic search and reference mobile application Face2Gene developed by FDNA: Facial Dysmorphology Novel Analysis). In addition, the skin should be examined with a Wood lamp, in particular when tuberous sclerosis is suspected [251]. Finally, clinical genetics evaluation can greatly benefit, in this strategy of identification of genetic disorders associated with ASD, from examining repeatedly over time the child to follow his/her developmental trajectory and examining at the same time the patient, his/her parents and siblings to compare the findings.

3.2. Second Step: Complementary Investigations (Laboratory Studies)

This secondary investigation includes cytogenetic, molecular analyses, biochemical analyses. Other exams such as neuroimaging and EEG are requested based on the results of the clinical genetic and neuropediatric examinations.

The following hierarchical diagnostic strategy, in line with recent American guidelines [249], can be proposed (see Figure 1).

3.2.1. Non-Syndromic Autism (Isolated ASD)

It should be remembered that non-syndromic autism includes ASD individuals with moderate intellectual disability to normal cognitive functioning (high functioning ASD) and no other associated signs or symptoms (except the possible presence of seizures). To our knowledge, the probability to detect a mutation (CNV or point mutation) is very low in high functioning non-syndromic ASD individuals, and, in this case, we do not recommend molecular analysis. However, in the case of family history of psychiatric disorders or developmental disabilities, it could be of interest to perform aCGH and to collect samples for a research program. In addition, in the case of consanguinity or selective food aversion, it could be useful to perform targeted metabolic testing. In addition, in the case of individuals with intellectual disability or males with no intellectual disability, the search for Fragile X mutation is recommended. If there is no hypothesis, a repeated clinical genetic evaluation over time is proposed given the possible later appearance of dysmorphic features along with the developmental trajectory.

3.2.2. Syndromic Autism (ASD Associated with Dysmorphic Features and/or Malformations and/or Symptomatic or Cryptogenic Epilepsy, and/or Severe Intellectual Disability)

If a specific chromosomal or point mutation is suspected: perform aCGH or specific gene sequencing.

If a metabolic disorder is suspected based on developmental regression (regression observed on the growth curves, including macrocephaly and in particular microcephaly, but also developmental psychomotor regression or neuroregression/neurodegeneration with neurological symptoms), seizures and especially epilepsy (recurrent and refractory seizures), consanguinity and specific dysmorphy or other symptoms described below: perform targeted metabolic testing including measurements of ammonemia and lactatemia, urinary organic acids chromatography, plasmatic amino-acids chromatography, creatine metabolism, iron, vitamin D, glutathione, oxidative stress, and cerebral magnetic resonance spectroscopy combined with standard neuroimaging. A metabolic disease could also be suspected based on certain clinical symptoms, such as digestion-related symptoms (cyclic vomiting, selective eating or gastrointestinal problems), dermatologic and hair changes (rashes, pigmented skin eruptions, hypertrichosis or alopecia), lethargy with hypotonia/extrapyramidal signs (dystonia, abnormal movements), or multiple organ dysfunction (in particular, heart, liver, kidney). In addition, the search for metabolic disorders can be indicated by abnormal biological measures such as anemia or lactic acidosis, and more generally acid/base or electrolyte disturbances. Searching for metabolic disorders is important given the potential availability of treatments such as enzymotherapy for certain metabolic diseases, diet low in phenylalanine for phenylketonuria due to the enzyme phenylalanine hydroxylase deficiency, or supplementation with folinic acid for cerebral folate deficiency. Several metabolic disorders associated with ASD are listed in Table 1 using the superscript #.

If a mitochondrial disorder is suspected based on repeated regressions after three years old, neurological abnormalities (including hypotonia) and multiple organ dysfunction: perform targeted mitochondrial testing including measurement of lactatemia. Abnormal neurologic examination and/or elevated plasma lactate concentration have been indeed found in mitochonfrial diseases [260]. A mitochondrial disorder could be also suspected in case of ASD associated with loss of speech after a febrile illness or immunization with encephalopathy [261]. Finally, it is noteworthy that mitochondrial disease (rare in ASD) has to be differentiated from mitochondrial dysfunction (common in ASD) [262].

If there is no hypothesis of specific syndrome: perform aCGH and molecular diagnosis of Fragile-X syndrome. Without any identified pathogenic variant, we recommend targeted New Generation Sequencing (NGS) on known genes (for example, panels of genes related to intellectual disability or epilepsy based on the clinical examination) or Whole Exome Sequencing (WES) if available.

4. Conclusions

The finality of the hierarchal diagnostic strategy proposed in this article is to identify genetic disorders associated with ASD based on a stepwise evaluation characterized by low invasiveness and cost but high accessibility, feasibility and adaptability of current knowledge and technology to the individual and his/her family. These clinical and laboratory investigations can lead to identify genetic disorders associated with ASD in 35%–40% of individuals [225,262]. The identification of a specific genetic syndrome associated with ASD has practical clinical implications, in terms of diagnostic strategies including early detection and prevention of co-morbidity related to the known medical risks of the genetic disorder, follow up adapted to the genetic disorder with a more precise prognosis, and therapeutic strategies with access to needed services, help provided by specific family associations or specific individualized treatment in some cases. In many cases, identification of genetic disorders does not lead to therapeutic implications but there are a few cases where enzymotherapy, food depletion or supplementation in certain metabolic diseases as well as administration of melatonin associated with acebutolol in Smith–Magenis syndrome have improved considerably the quality of life of patients and their families. It should be noted that sleep problems are frequent in ASD (prevalence of insomnia: 50%–80% [263]) and decreased nocturnal and/or diurnal levels of melatonin (a sleep neurohormone) have been reported in many ASD studies; trial studies support therapeutic benefits of melatonin use in ASD (for a review, see Tordjman et al. [116,264]. Furthermore, the identification of genetic disorders associated with ASD allows unique personalized genetic counseling adapted to each family with regard to the transmission risk to the descendants and the possibility of a prenatal or preimplant diagnosis in the perspective of a future pregnancy. According to the 2013 American guidelines [249], the genetic counselor should note the type of array technology used (e.g., oligonucleotide vs. single-nucleotide polymorphism arrays) and access major databases relevant to this technology in order to provide the best possible and adapted information for the family. Many parents of children with ASD worry about the autism risk for a future pregnancy and knowing that their impaired child has a de novo mutation can be very helpful concerning the decision to have another child. It can be noted that the majority of the found mutations or rearrangements occurs de novo and are therefore not inherited from the parents or relatives [262]. In the same vein, siblings of children with ASD are very often preoccupied by the possible genetic transmission of autism to their future children. This preoccupation is legitimate considering, for instance, that the sisters of a boy with Fragile X Syndrome, even if they express very few or no symptoms, have a risk of 50% to carry the mutation or premutation and therefore a risk of 50% to have a child with Fragile X Syndrome (more severely impaired if it is a male). It is noteworthy that genetic counseling is also offered to families of ASD individuals without identified etiology, using in this case epidemiologic studies, and in particular sibling recurrence-risk updated data [249]. In any case, genetic counseling provides helpful family guidance, and parents of children with ASD are often relieved that biological factors involved in the development of ASD are considered and possibly found when some of them might feel guilty with regard to the role of family environment in ASD. Interestingly, based on our experience and the experience of geneticists or neuropediatricians working with psychoanalysts [265], knowing the underlying genetic cause of a relative's or patient's disorder, far from fixing the family or caregiver representations with regard to genetic determinism, rather creates and stimulates new dynamics within the family as well as the caregiver team centered on the ASD individual and probably related to a better known developmental trajectory with therapeutic perspectives and a parental relief. Finally, given all these implications, it is essential that all individuals (children but also adolescents and adults) with ASD can benefit from a clinical genetic examination and neuropediatric examination searching for associated signs or symptoms helping to identify known genetic disorders.

Acknowledgments: Funds from the Laboratory Psychology of Perception (LPP) were receiving for covering the costs to publish in open access.

Author Contributions: Cyrille Robert and Sylvie Tordjman wrote the manuscript; Sylvie Odent, Laurent Pasquier, David Cohen, Mélanie Fradin, Roberto Canitano and Léna Damaj revised the first draft of the paper; Sylvie Tordjman, Sylvie Odent and Laurent Pasquier modified the article according to the reviewers' comments.

References

1. American Psychiatric Association. *Diagnostic and Statistical Manual of Mental Disorders (DSM-5)*, 5th ed.; American Psychiatric Association: Washington, DC, USA, 2013.
2. Carrey, N.J. Itard's 1828 Memoire on Mutism caused by a lesion of the intellectual functions: A historical analysis. *J. Am. Acad. Child Adolesc. Psychiatry* **1995**, *34*, 1655–1661. [CrossRef] [PubMed]
3. Kanner, L. Austistic disturbances of affective contact. *Nervous Child* **1943**, *32*, 217–253.
4. Bleuler, E. *Dementia Praecox oder Gruppe der Schizophrenien*; Handbuch der Psychiatrie; Deuticke: Leipzig, Germany, 1911.
5. Asperger, H. Die autistischen psychopathen im kindesalter. *Arch. Psychiatry Nervenkrandeiten* **1944**, *117*, 73–136. [CrossRef]
6. Tordjman, S.; Somogyi, E.; Coulon, N.; Kermarrec, S.; Cohen, D.; Bronsard, G.; Bonnot, O.; Weismann-Arcache, C.; Botbol, M.; Lauth, B.; et al. Gene-environment interactions in autism spectrum disorders: Role of epigenetic mechanisms. *Front. Psychiatry* **2014**, *5*, 1–17. [CrossRef] [PubMed]
7. Abrahams, B.S.; Geschwind, D.H. Advances in autism genetics: On the threshold of a new neurobiology. *Nat. Rev. Genet.* **2008**, *9*, 341–355. [CrossRef] [PubMed]
8. Bill, B.R.; Geschwind, D.H. Genetic advances in autism: Heterogeneity and convergence on shared pathways. *Curr. Opin. Genet. Dev.* **2009**, *19*, 271–278. [CrossRef] [PubMed]
9. Muhle, R.; Trentacoste, S.V.; Rapin, I. The genetics of autism. *Pediatrics* **2004**, *113*, 472–486. [CrossRef]
10. Ronald, A.; Hoekstra, R.A. Autism spectrum disorders and autistic traits: A decade of new twin studies. *Am. J. Med. Genet.* **2011**, *156*, 255–274. [CrossRef] [PubMed]
11. Sandin, S.; Lichtenstein, P.; Kuja-Halkola, R.; Larsson, H.; Hultman, C.M.; Reichenberg, A. The familial risk of autism. *JAMA* **2014**, *311*, 1770–1777. [CrossRef] [PubMed]
12. Rosti, R.O.; Sadek, A.A.; Vaux, K.K.; Gleeson, J.G. The genetic landscape of autism spectrum disorders. *Dev. Med. Child Neurol.* **2014**, *56*, 12–18. [CrossRef] [PubMed]
13. Sebat, J.; Lakshmi, B.; Malhotra, D.; Troge, J.; Lese-Martin, C.; Walsh, T. Strong association of de novo copy number mutations with autism. *Science* **2007**, *316*, 445–449. [CrossRef] [PubMed]
14. Hegmann, J.P.; Possidente, B. Estimating genetic correlations from inbred strains. *Behav. Genet.* **1981**, *11*, 103–114. [CrossRef] [PubMed]
15. Miles, J.H. Autism spectrum disorders, a genetics review. *Genet. Med.* **2011**, *13*, 278–294. [CrossRef] [PubMed]
16. Bourgeron, T. From the genetic architecture to synaptic plasticity in autism spectrum disorder. *Nat. Rev. Neurosc.* **2015**, *16*, 551–563. [CrossRef] [PubMed]
17. Miles, J.H.; Hillman, R.E. Value of a clinical morphology examination in autism. *Am. J. Med. Genet.* **2000**, *91*, 245–253. [CrossRef]
18. Jacquemont, M.L.; Sanlaville, D.; Redon, R.; Raoul, O.; Cormier-Daire, V.; Lyonnet, S.; Amiel, J.; Le Merrer, M.; Heron, D.; de Blois, M.C.; et al. Array-based comparative genomic hybridisation identifies high frequency of cryptic chromosomal rearrangements in patients with syndromic autism spectrum disorders. *J. Med. Genet.* **2006**, *43*, 843–849. [CrossRef] [PubMed]
19. Miles, J.H.; Takahashi, T.N.; Bagby, S.; Sahota, P.K.; Vaslow, D.F.; Wang, C.H.; Hillman, R.E.; Farmer, J.E. Essential versus complex autism: Definition of fundamental prognostic subtypes. *Am. J. Med. Genet.* **2005**, *135*, 171–180. [CrossRef] [PubMed]
20. Cohen, D.; Pichard, N.; Tordjman, S.; Baumann, C.; Burglen, L.; Excoffier, E.; Lazar, G.; Mazet, P.; Pinquier, C.; Verloes, A.; et al. Specific genetic disorders and autism: Clinical contribution towards their identification. *J. Autism Dev. Disord.* **2005**, *35*, 103–116. [CrossRef] [PubMed]

21. Amiet, C.; Gourfinkel-An, I.; Bouzamondo, A.; Tordjman, S.; Baulac, M.; Lechat, P.; Cohen, D.J. Epilepsy in autism is associated with intellectual disability and gender: Evidence from a meta-analysis. *Biol. Psychiatry* **2008**, *64*, 577–582. [CrossRef] [PubMed]
22. Amiet, C.; Gourfinkel-An, I.; Lauent, C.; Bodeneau, N.; Genin, B.; Leguern, E.; Tordjman, S.; Cohen, D.J. Does epilepsy in multiplex autism define a different subgroup of clinical characteristics and genetic risk? *Mol. Autism* **2013**, *4*, 47. [CrossRef] [PubMed]
23. Amiet, C.; Gourfinkel-An, I.; Lauent, C.; Carayol, J.; Genin, B.; Leguern, E.; Tordjman, S.; Cohen, D.J. Epilepsy in simplex autism pedigrees is much lower than the rate in multiplex autism pedigrees. *Biol. Psychiatry* **2013**, *74*, 3–4. [CrossRef] [PubMed]
24. Canitano, R. Epilepsy in autism spectrum disorders. *Eur. Child Adolesc. Psychiatry* **2007**, *16*, 61–66. [CrossRef] [PubMed]
25. Tordjman, S.; Cohen, D.; Anderson, G.M.; Canitano, R.; Botbol, M.; Coulon, N.; Roubertoux, P.L. Reframing autism as a behavioral syndrome and not a specific mental disorder: Implications of genetic and phenotypic heterogeneity. *Neurosci. Biobehav. Rev.* **2017**. [CrossRef] [PubMed]
26. Cook, E.H., Jr.; Lindgren, V.; Leventhal, B.L.; Courchesne, R.; Lincoln, A.; Shulman, C.; Lord, C.; Courchesne, E. Autism or atypical autism in maternally but not paternally derived proximal 15q duplication. *Am. J. Hum. Genet.* **1997**, *60*, 928–934. [PubMed]
27. Bolton, P.F.; Dennis, N.R.; Browne, C.E.; Thomas, N.S.; Veltman, M.W.; Thompson, R.J.; Jacobs, P. The phenotypic manifestations of interstitial duplications of proximal 15q with special reference to the autistic spectrum disorders. *Am. J. Hum. Genet.* **2001**, *105*, 675–685. [CrossRef] [PubMed]
28. Cohen, D.; Martel, C.; Wilson, A.; Déchambre, N.; Amy, C.; Duverger, L.; Guile, J.M.; Pipiras, E.; Benzacken, B.; Cavé, H.; et al. Brief report: visual-spatial deficit in a 16-year-old girl with maternally derived duplication of proximal 15q. *J. Autism Dev. Disord.* **2007**, *37*, 1585–1591. [CrossRef] [PubMed]
29. Schroer, R.J.; Phelan, M.C.; Michaelis, R.C.; Crawford, E.C.; Skinner, S.A.; Cuccaro, M.; Simensen, R.J.; Bishop, J.; Skinner, C.; Fender, D.; et al. Autism and maternally derived aberrations of chromosome 15q. *Am. J. Hum. Genet.* **1998**, *76*, 327–336. [CrossRef]
30. Wandstrat, A.E.; Leana-Cox, J.; Jenkins, L.; Schwartz, S. Molecular cytogenetic evidence for a common break-point in the largest inverted duplications for chromosomes 15. *Am. J. Hum. Genet.* **1998**, *62*, 925–936. [CrossRef] [PubMed]
31. Sutcliffe, J.S.; Nurmi, E.L. Genetics of chilhood disorders: XLVII. Autism, Part 6: Duplication and inherited susceptibility of chromosome 15q11–q13 genes in autism. *J. Am. Acad. Child Adolesc. Psychiatry* **2003**, *42*, 253–256. [CrossRef] [PubMed]
32. Jacobsen, J.; King, B.H.; Leventhal, B.L.; Christian, S.L.; Ledbetter, D.H.; Cook, E.H., Jr. Molecular screening for proximal 15q abnormalities in a mentally retard population. *J. Med. Genet.* **1998**, *35*, 534–538. [CrossRef] [PubMed]
33. Steffenburg, S.; Gillberg, C.L.; Seffenburg, U.; Kyllerman, M. Autism in Angelman syndrome: A population-based study. *Pediatr. Neurol.* **1996**, *14*, 131–136. [CrossRef]
34. Peters, S.U.; Beaudet, A.L.; Madduri, N.; Bacino, C.A. Autism in Angelman syndrome: Implications for autism research. *Clin. Genet.* **2004**, *66*, 530–536. [CrossRef] [PubMed]
35. Chamberlain, S.J.; Chen, P.F.; Ng, K.Y.; Bourgois-Rocha, F.; Lemtiri-Chlieh, F.; Levine, E.S.; Lalande, M. Induced pluripotent stem cell models of the genomic imprinting disorders Angelman and Prader-Willi syndromes. *Proc. Natl. Acad. Sci. USA* **2010**, *107*, 17668–17673. [CrossRef] [PubMed]
36. Rangasamy, S.; D'Mello, S.R.; Narayanan, V. Epigenitics, autism spectrum, and neurodevelopmental disorders. *Neurotherapeutics* **2013**, *10*, 742–756. [CrossRef] [PubMed]
37. Grafodatskaya, D.; Chung, B.; Szatmari, P.; Weksberg, R. Autism spectrum disorders and epigenetics. *J. Am. Acad. Child Adolesc. Psychiatry* **2010**, *49*, 794–809. [CrossRef] [PubMed]
38. Dawson, A.J.; Cox, J.; Hovanes, K.; Spriggs, E. PWS/AS MS-MLPA confirms maternal origin of 15q11.2 microduplication. *Case Rep. Genet.* **2015**, *2015*, 474097. [CrossRef] [PubMed]
39. Huang, H.S.; Allen, J.A.; Mabb, A.M. Topoisomerase inhibitors unsilence the dormant allele of Ube3a in neurons. *Nature* **2011**, *481*, 185–189. [CrossRef] [PubMed]
40. Mabb, A.M.; Judson, M.C.; Zylka, M.J.; Philpot, B.D. Angelman syndrome: Insights into genomic imprinting and neurodevelopmental phenotypes. *Trends Neurosci.* **2011**, *34*, 293–303. [CrossRef] [PubMed]

41. Erickson, C.A.; Wink, L.K.; Baindu, B.; Ray, B.; Schaefer, T.L.; Pedapati, E.V.; Lahiri, D.K. Analysis of peripheral amyloid precursor protein in Angelman syndrome. *Am. J. Med. Genet.* **2016**, *170*, 2334–2337. [CrossRef] [PubMed]
42. Li, W.; Yao, A.; Zhi, H.; Kaur, K.; Zhu, Y.; Jia, M.; Wang, Q.; Jin, S.; Zhao, G.; et al. Angelman syndrome protein Ube3a regulates synaptic growth and endocytosis by inhibiting BMP signaling in *Drosophila*. *PLoS Genet.* **2016**, *12*, e1006062. [CrossRef] [PubMed]
43. Meng, L.; Person, R.E.; Beaudet, A.L. Ube3a-ATS is an atypical RNA polymerase II transcript that represses the paternal expression of Ube3a. *Hum. Mol. Genet.* **2012**, *21*, 3001–3012. [CrossRef] [PubMed]
44. Kishino, T.; Lalande, M.; Wasgstaff, J. UBE3A/E6-AP mutations cause Angelman syndrome. *Nat. Genet.* **1997**, *15*, 70–73. [CrossRef] [PubMed]
45. Petit, E.; Hérault, J.; Martineau, J.; Perrot, A.; Barthélémy, C.; Hameury, L.; Sauvage, D.; Lelord, G.; Müh, J.P. Association study with two markers of a human homeogene in infantile autism. *J. Med. Genet.* **1995**, *32*, 269–274. [CrossRef] [PubMed]
46. Clayton-Smith, J. Clinical research on Angelman syndrome in the United Kingdom: Observations on 82 affected individuals. *Am. J. Med. Genet.* **1993**, *46*, 12–15. [CrossRef] [PubMed]
47. Summers, J.A.; Allison, D.B.; Lynch, P.S.; Sandler, L. Behaviour problems in Angelman syndrome. *J. Intellect. Disabil. Res.* **1995**, *39*, 97–106. [CrossRef] [PubMed]
48. Walz, N.C. Parent report of stereotyped behaviors, social interaction, and developmental disturbances in individuals with Angelman syndrome. *J. Autism Dev. Disord.* **2007**, *37*, 940–947. [CrossRef] [PubMed]
49. Dykens, E.M.; Cassidy, S.B. Correlates of maladaptive behavior in children and adults with Prader-Willi syndrome. *Am. J. Med. Genet.* **1995**, *60*, 546–549. [CrossRef] [PubMed]
50. Demb, H.B.; Papola, P. PDD and Prader-Willi syndrome. *J. Am. Acad. Child Adolesc. Psychiatry* **1995**, *34*, 539–540. [CrossRef] [PubMed]
51. Dykens, E.M.; Cassidy, S.B.; King, B.H. Maladaptive behavior differences in Prader-Willi syndrome due to paternal deletion versus maternal uniparental disomy. *Am. J. Ment. Retard.* **1995**, *104*, 67–77. [CrossRef]
52. Veltman, M.W.; Thompson, R.J.; Roberts, S.E.; Thomas, N.S.; Whittington, J.; Bolton, P.F. Prader-Willi syndrome—A study comparing deletion and uniparental disomy cases with reference to autism spectrum disorders. *Eur. Child Adolesc. Psychiatry* **2004**, *13*, 42–50. [CrossRef] [PubMed]
53. Descheemaeker, M.J.; Govers, V.; Vermeulen, P.; Fryns, J.P. Pervasive developmental disorders in Prader-Willi syndrome: The Leuven experience in 59 subjects and controls. *Am. J. Med. Genet.* **2006**, *140*, 1136–1142. [CrossRef] [PubMed]
54. Hogart, A.; Wu, D.; LaSalle, J.M.; Schanen, N.C. The comorbidity of autism with the genomic disorders of chromosome 15q11.2–q13. *Neurobiol. Dis.* **2010**, *38*, 181–191. [CrossRef] [PubMed]
55. Horsthemke, B.; Wagstaff, J. Mechanisms of imprinting of the Prader-Willi/Angelman region. *Am. J. Med. Genet.* **2008**, *146*, 2041–2052. [CrossRef] [PubMed]
56. Buiting, K. Prader-Willi and Angelman syndrome. *Am. J. Med. Genet.* **2010**, *154*, 365–376. [CrossRef] [PubMed]
57. Cassidy, S.B.; Scwartz, S.; Miller, H.; Driscoll, D.J. Prader-Willi syndrome. *Genet. Med.* **2012**, *14*, 10–26. [CrossRef] [PubMed]
58. Bennett, J.A.; Germani, T.; Haqq, A.M.; Zwaigenbaum, L. Autism spectrum disorder in Prader-Willi syndrome: A systematic review. *Am. J. Med. Genet.* **2015**, *167*, 2936–2944. [CrossRef] [PubMed]
59. Veltman, M.W.; Thompson, R.J.; Craig, E.E.; Dennis, N.R.; Roberts, S.E.; Moore, V.; Brown, J.A.; Bolton, P.F. A paternally inherited duplication in the Prader-Willi/Angelman syndrome critical region: A case and family study. *J. Autism Dev. Disord.* **2015**, *35*, 117–127. [CrossRef]
60. Bolton, P.F.; Roobol, M.; Allsopp, L.; Pickles, A. Association between idiopathic infantile macrocephaly and autism spectrum disorders. *Lancet* **2001**, *358*, 726–727. [CrossRef]
61. Roberts, S.E.; Dennis, N.R.; Browne, C.E.; Willatt, L.; Woods, G.; Cross, I.; Jacobs, P.A.; Thomas, S. Characterisation of interstitial duplications and triplications of chromosome 15q11–q13. *Hum. Genet.* **2002**, *110*, 227–234. [CrossRef] [PubMed]

62. Goizet, C.; Excoffier, E.; Taine, L.; Taupiac, E.; El Moneim, A.A.; Arveiler, B.; Bouvard, M.; Lacombe, D. Case with autistic syndrome and chromosome 22q13.3 deletion detected by FISH. *Am. J. Hum. Genet.* **2000**, *96*, 839–844. [CrossRef]
63. Manning, M.A.; Cassidy, S.B.; Clericuzio, C.; Cherry, A.M.; Schwartz, S.; Hudgins, L.; Enns, G.M.; Hoyme, H.E. Terminal 22q deletion syndrome: A newly recognized cause of speech and language disability in the autism spectrum. *Pediatrics* **2004**, *114*, 451–457. [CrossRef] [PubMed]
64. Prasad, C.; Prasad, A.N.; Chodirker, B.N.; Lee, C.; Dawson, A.K.; Jocelyn, L.J.; Chudley, A.E. Genetic evaluation of pervasive developmental disorders: The terminal 22q13 deletion syndrome may represent a recognizable phenotype. *Clin.Genet.* **2000**, *57*, 103–109. [CrossRef] [PubMed]
65. Phelan, M.C.; Rogers, R.C.; Saul, R.A.; Stapleton, G.A.; Sweet, K.; McDermid, H.; Shaw, S.R.; Claytor, J.; Willis, J.; Kelly, D.P. 22q13 Deletion Syndrome. *Am. J. Hum. Genet.* **2001**, *101*, 91–99. [CrossRef]
66. Soorya, L.; Kolevzon, A.; Zweifach, J.; Lim, T.; Dobry, Y.; Schwartz, L.; Frank, Y.; Wang, A.T.; Cai, G.; Parkhomenko, E.; et al. Prospective investigation of autism and genotype-phenotype correlations in 22q13 deletion syndrome and SHANK3 deficiency. *Mol. Autism* **2013**, *4*, 18. [CrossRef] [PubMed]
67. Shcheglovitov, A.; Shcheglovitova, O.; Yazawa, M.; Portmann, T.; Shu, R.; Sebastiano, V.; Krawisz, A.; Froehlich, W.; Bernstein, J.A.; Hallmayer, J.F.; et al. SHANK3 and IGF1 restore synaptic deficits in neurons from 22q13 deletion syndrome patients. *Nature* **2013**, *503*, 267–271. [CrossRef] [PubMed]
68. Phelan, K.; McDermid, H.E. The 22q13.3 deletion syndrome (Phelan-McDermid syndrome). *Mol. Syndromol.* **2012**, *2*, 186–201. [CrossRef] [PubMed]
69. Peca, J.; Feliciano, C.; Ting, J.T.; Wang, W.; Wells, M.F.; Venkatraman, T.N.; Lascola, C.D.; Fu, Z.; Feng, G. SHANK3 mutant mice display autistic-like behaviours and striatal dysfunction. *Nature* **2011**, *472*, 437–442. [CrossRef] [PubMed]
70. Jafri, F.; Fink, J.; Higgins, R.R.; Tervo, R. 22q13.32 deletion and duplication and inversion in the same family: A rare occurrence. *ISRN Pediatr.* **2011**, *2011*, 829825. [CrossRef] [PubMed]
71. Zwanenburg, R.J.; Ruiter, S.A.J.; van Den Heuvel, E.R.; Flapper, B.C.T.; van Ravenswaaij-Arts, C.M.A. Developmental phenotype in Phelan-McDermid (22q13.3 deletion) syndrome: A systematic and prospective study in 34 children. *J. Neurodev. Disord.* **2016**, *8*, 16. [CrossRef] [PubMed]
72. Marshall, C.R.; Noor, A.; Vincent, J.B.; Lionel, A.C.; Feuk, L.; Skaug, J.; Shago, M.; Moessner, R.; Pinto, D.; Ren, Y.; et al. Structural variation of chromosomes in autism spectrum disorder. *Am. J. Hum. Genet.* **2008**, *82*, 477–488. [CrossRef] [PubMed]
73. Hanson, E.; Nasir, R.H.; Fong, A.; Lian, A.; Hundley, R.; Shen, Y.; Wu, B.L.; Holm, I.A.; Miller, D.T. 16p11.2 Study group clinicians cognitive and behavioral characterization of 16p11.2 deletion syndrome. *J. Dev. Behav. Pediatr.* **2010**, *31*, 649–657. [CrossRef] [PubMed]
74. Weiss, L.A.; Shen, Y.; Korn, J.M.; Arking, D.E.; Miller, D.T.; Fossdal, R.; Saemundsen, E.; Stefansson, H.; Ferreira, M.A.; Green, T.; et al. Consortium association between microdeletion and microduplication at 16p11.2 and autism. *New Engl. J. Med.* **2008**, *358*, 667–675. [CrossRef] [PubMed]
75. Kumar, R.A.; KaraMohamed, S.; Sudi, J.; Conrad, D.F.; Brune, C.; Badner, J.A.; Gilliam, T.C.; Nowak, N.J.; Cook, E., Jr.; Dobyns, W.B.; et al. Recurrent 16p11.2 microdeletions in autism. *Hum. Mol. Genet.* **2008**, *17*, 628–638. [CrossRef] [PubMed]
76. Fombonne, E.; Du Mazaubrun, C.; Cans, C.; Grandjean, H. Autism and associated medical disorders in a French epidemiological survey. *J. Am. Child Adolesc. Psychiatry* **1997**, *36*, 1561–1569.
77. Steinman, K.J.; Spence, S.J.; Ramocki, M.B.; Proud, M.B.; Kessler, S.K.; Marco, E.J.; Green Snyder, L.; D'Angelo, D.; Chen, Q.; Chung, W.K.; et al. 16p11.2 Deletion and duplication: Characterizing neurologic phenotypes in a large clinically ascertained cohort. *Am. J. Med. Genet.* **2016**, *9999*, 1–13. [CrossRef] [PubMed]
78. Green Snyder, L.; D'Angelo, D.; Chen, Q.; Bernier, R.; Goin-Kochel, R.P.; Wallace, A.S.; Gerdts, J.; Kanne, S.; Berry, L.; Blaskey, L.; et al. Autism spectrum disorder, developmental and psychiatric features in 16p11.2 duplication. *J. Autism Dev. Disord.* **2016**, *46*, 2734–2748. [CrossRef] [PubMed]
79. Fisch, G.S.; Grossfeld, P.; Falk, R.; Battaglia, A.; Youngblom, J.; Simensen, R. Cognitive-behavioral features of Wolf-Hirschhorn syndrome and other subtelomeric microdeletions. *Am. J. Med. Genet.* **2010**, *154*, 417–426. [CrossRef] [PubMed]
80. Fisch, G.S.; Davis, R.; Youngblom, J.; Gregg, J. Genotype-phenotype association studies of chromosome 8p inverted duplication deletion syndrome. *Behav. Genet.* **2011**, *41*, 373–380. [CrossRef] [PubMed]

81. Bregmen, J.D.; Volkmar, F.R. Autism spectrum disorders in genetic syndromes: Implications for diagnosis, intervention and understanding the wider autism spectrum disorder population. *J. Intellect. Disabil. Res.* **1988**, *53*, 852–873.
82. Mariner, R.; Jackson, A.W.; Levitas, A.; Hagerman, R.J.; Braden, M.; McBogg, P.M.; Smith, A.C.; Berry, R. Autism, mental retardation, and chromosomal abnormalities. *J. Autism Dev. Disord.* **1986**, *16*, 425–440. [CrossRef] [PubMed]
83. Ghaziuddin, M. Autism in down syndrome: Family history correlates. *J. Intellect. Disabil. Res.* **1997**, *41*, 87–91. [CrossRef] [PubMed]
84. Moss, J.; Howlin, P. Autism spectrum disorders in genetic syndromes: Implications for diagnosis, intervention and understanding the wider autism spectrum disorder population. *J. Intellect. Disabil. Res.* **2009**, *53*, 852–873. [CrossRef] [PubMed]
85. Jiang, J.; Jing, Y.; Cost, G.J.; Chiang, J.C.; Kolpa, H.J.; Cotton, A.M.; Carone, D.M.; Carone, B.R.; Shivak, D.A.; Guschin, D.Y.; et al. Translating dosage compensation to trisomy 21. *Nature* **2013**, *500*, 296–300. [CrossRef] [PubMed]
86. Smith, A.C.; McGavran, L.; Robinson, J.; Waldstein, G.; Macfarlane, J.; Zonona, J.; Reiss, J.; Lahr, M.; Allen, L.; Magenis, E. Interstitial deletion of (17) (P11.2p11.2) in nine patients. *Am. J. Hum. Genet.* **1986**, *24*, 393–414. [CrossRef] [PubMed]
87. Vostanis, P.; Harrington, R.; Prendergast, M.; Farndon, P. Case reports of autism with interstitial deletion of chromosome 17 (p11.2 p11.2) and monosomy of chromosome 5 (5pter > 5p15.3). *Psychiatr. Genet.* **1994**, *4*, 109–111. [CrossRef] [PubMed]
88. Laje, G.; Morse, R.; Richter, W.; Ball, J.; Pao, M.; Smith, A.C.M. Autism spectrum features in smith-magenis syndrome. *Am. J. Med. Genet.* **2010**, *154*, 456–462. [CrossRef] [PubMed]
89. Potocki, L.; Bi, W.; Treadwell-Deering, D.; Carvalho, C.M.; Eifert, A.; Friedman, E.M.; Glaze, D.; Krull, K.; Lee, J.A.; Lewis, R.A.; et al. Characterization of Potocki-Lupski syndrome (dup(17) (p11.2p11.2)) and delineation of a dosage-sensitive critical interval that can convey an autism phenotype. *Am. J. Med. Genet.* **2007**, *80*, 633–649. [CrossRef]
90. Ghaziuddin, M.; Burmeister, M. Deletion of chromosome 2q37 and autism: A distinct subtype? *J. Autism Dev. Disord.* **1999**, *29*, 259–263. [CrossRef] [PubMed]
91. Devillard, F.; Guinchat, V.; Moreno-De-Luca, D.; Tabet, A.C.; Gruchy, N.; Guillem, P.; Nguyen Morel, M.A.; Leporrier, N.; Leboyer, M.; Jouk, P.S.; et al. Paracentric inversion of chromosome 2 associated with cryptic duplication of 2q14 and deletion of 2q37 in a patient with autism. *Am. J. Med. Genet.* **2010**, *152*, 2346–2354. [CrossRef] [PubMed]
92. Galasso, C.; Lo-Castro, A.; Lalli, C.; Nardone, A.M.; Gullotta, F.; Curatolo, P. Deletion 2q37: An identifiable clinical syndrome with mental retardation and autism. *J. Child Neurol.* **2008**, *23*, 802–806. [CrossRef] [PubMed]
93. Falk, R.E.; Casas, K.A. Chromosome 2q37 deletion: Clinical and molecular aspects. *Am. J. Med. Genet.* **2007**, *145*, 357–371. [CrossRef] [PubMed]
94. Fisch, G.S.; Falk, R.E.; Carey, J.C.; Imitola, J.; Sederberg, M.; Caravalho, K.S.; South, S. Deletion 2q37 syndrome: Cognitive-Behavioral trajectories and autistic features related to breakpoint and deletion size. *Am. J. Med. Genet.* **2016**, *170*, 2282–2291. [CrossRef] [PubMed]
95. Lo-Castro, A.; Galasso, C.; Cerminara, C.; El-Malhany, N.; Benedetti, S.; Nardone, A.M.; Curatolo, P. Association of syndromic mental retardation and autism with 22q11.2 duplication. *Neuropediatrics* **2009**, *40*, 137–140. [CrossRef] [PubMed]
96. Lo-Castro, A.; Benvenuto, A.; Galasso, C.; Porfirio, C.; Curatolo, P. Autism spectrum disorders associated with chromosomal abnormalities. *Res. Autism Spectr. Disord.* **2010**, *4*, 319–327. [CrossRef]
97. Portnoï, M.F. Microduplication 22q11.2: A new chromosomal syndrome. *Eur. J. Med. Genet.* **2009**, *52*, 88–93. [CrossRef] [PubMed]
98. Baker, K.D.; Skuse, D.H. Adolescents and young adults with 22q11 deletion syndrome: Psychopathology in an at-risk group. *Br. J. Psychiatry* **2005**, *186*, 115–120. [CrossRef] [PubMed]
99. Wenger, T.L.; Miller, J.S.; DePolo, L.M.; de Marchena, A.B.; Clements, C.C.; Emanuel, B.S.; Zackai, E.H.; McDonald-McGinn, D.M.; Schultz, R.T. 22q11.2 duplication syndrome: Elevated rate of autism spectrum disorder and need for medical screening. *Mol. Autism* **2016**, *7*, 27. [CrossRef] [PubMed]

100. Hidding, E.; Swaab, H.; de Sonneville, L.M.J.; van Engeland, H.; Vorstman, J.A.S. The role of COMT and plasma proline in the variable penetrance of autistic spectrum symptoms in 22q11.2 deletion syndrome. *Clin. Genet.* **2016**, *90*, 420–427. [CrossRef] [PubMed]
101. Mefford, H.C.; Sharp, A.J.; Baker, C.; Itsara, A.; Jiang, Z.; Buysse, K.; Huang, S.; Maloney, V.K.; Crolla, J.A.; Baralle, D.; et al. Recurrent rearrangements of chromosome 1q21.1 and variable pediatric phenotypes. *N. Engl. J. Med.* **2008**, *359*, 1685–1699. [CrossRef] [PubMed]
102. Brunetti-Pierri, N.; Berg, J.S.; Scaglia, F.; Belmont, J.; Bacino, C.A.; Sahoo, T.; Lalani, S.R.; Graham, B.; Lee, B.; Shinawi, M.; et al. Recurrent reciprocal 1q21.1 deletions and duplications associated with microcephaly or macrocephaly and developmental and behavioral abnormalities. *Nat. Genet.* **2008**, *40*, 1466–1471. [CrossRef] [PubMed]
103. Bernier, R.; Steinman, K.J.; Reilly, B.; Wallace, A.S.; Sherr, E.H.; Pojman, N.; Mefford, H.C.; Gerdts, J.; Earl, R.; Hanson, E.; et al. Clinical phenotype of the recurrent 1q21.1 copy-number variant. *Gen. Med.* **2016**, *18*, 341–349. [CrossRef] [PubMed]
104. Torres, F.; Barbosa, M.; Maciel, P. Recurrent copy number variations as risk factors for neurodevelopmental disorders: Critical overview and analysis of clinical implications. *J. Med. Genet.* **2016**, *53*, 73–90. [CrossRef] [PubMed]
105. Berg, J.S.; Brunetti-Pierri, N.; Peters, S.U.; Kang, S.H.; Fong, C.T.; Salamone, J.; Freedenberg, D.; Hannig, V.L.; Prock, L.A.; Miller, D.T.; et al. Speech delay and autism spectrum behaviors are frequently associated with duplication of the 7q11.23 Williams-Beuren syndrome region. *Genet. Med.* **2007**, *9*, 427–441. [CrossRef] [PubMed]
106. Depienne, C.; Heron, D.; Betancur, C.; Benyahia, B.; Trouillard, O.; Bouteiller, D.; Verloes, A.; LeGuern, E.; Leboyer, M.; Brice, A. Autism, language delay and mental retardation in a patient with 7q11 duplication. *J. Med. Genet.* **2007**, *44*, 452–458. [CrossRef] [PubMed]
107. Edelmann, L.; Prosnitz, A.; Pardo, S.; Bhatt, J.; Cohen, N.; Lauriat, T.; Ouchanov, L.; González, P.J.; Manghi, E.R.; Bondy, P.; et al. An atypical deletion of the Williams-Beuren syndrome interval implicates genes associated with defective visuospatial processing and autism. *J. Med. Genet.* **2007**, *44*, 136–143. [CrossRef] [PubMed]
108. Gagliardi, C.; Bonaglia, M.C.; Selicorni, A.; Borgatti, R.; Giorda, R. Unusual cognitive and behavioural profile in a Williams syndrome patient with atypical 7q11.23 deletion. *J. Med. Genet.* **2003**, *40*, 526–530. [CrossRef] [PubMed]
109. Lincoln, A.J.; Searcy, Y.M.; Jones, W.; Lord, C. Social interaction behaviors discriminate young children with autism and Williams syndrome. *J. Am. Acad. Child Adolesc. Psychiatry* **2007**, *46*, 323–331. [CrossRef] [PubMed]
110. Sanders, S.J.; Ercan-Sencicek, A.G.; Hus, V.; Luo, R.; Murtha, M.T.; Moreno-de-Luca, D.; Chu, S.H.; Moreau, M.P.; Gupta, A.R.; Thomson, S.A.; et al. Multiple recurrent de novo CNVs, including duplications of the 7q11.23 Williams syndrome region, are strongly associated with autism. *Neuron* **2011**, *70*, 863–885. [CrossRef] [PubMed]
111. Somerville, M.J.; Mervis, C.B.; Young, E.J.; Seo, E.J.; del Campo, M.; Bamforth, S.; Peregrine, E.; Loo, W.; Lilley, M.; Pérez-Jurado, L.A.; et al. Severe expressive-language delay related to duplication of the Williams-Beuren locus. *N. Engl. J. Med.* **2005**, *353*, 1694–1701. [CrossRef] [PubMed]
112. Van der Aa, N.; Rooms, L.; Vandeweyer, G.; van den Ende, J.; Reyniers, E.; Fichera, M.; Romano, C.; Delle Chiaie, B.; Mortier, G.; Menten, B.; et al. Fourteen new cases contribute to the characterization of the 7q11.23 microduplication syndrome. *Eur. J. Hum. Genet.* **2009**, *52*, 94–100. [CrossRef] [PubMed]
113. Makeyev, A.V.; Enkhamandakh, B.; Hong, S.H.; Joshi, P.; Shin, D.G.; Bayarsaihan, D. Diversity and complexity in chromatin recognition by TFII-I transcription factors in pluripotent embryonic stem cells and embryonic tissues. *PLoS ONE* **2012**, *7*, e44443. [CrossRef] [PubMed]
114. Tordjman, S.; Anderson, G.M.; Botbol, M.; Toutain, A.; Sarda, P.; Carlier, M.; Saugier-Veber, P.; Baumann, C.; Cohen, D.; Lagneaux, C.; et al. Autistic disorder in patients with Williams-Beuren syndrome: A reconsideration of the Williams-Beuren syndrome phenotype. *PLoS ONE* **2012**, *7*, e30778. [CrossRef] [PubMed]
115. Tordjman, S.; Anderson, G.M.; Cohen, D.; Kermarrec, S.; Carlier, M.; Touitou, Y.; Saugier-Veber, P.; Lagneaux, C.; Chevreuil, C.; Verloes, A. Presence of autism, hyperserotonemia, and severe expressive language impairment in Williams-Beuren syndrome. *Mol. Autism* **2013**, *4*, 29. [CrossRef] [PubMed]

116. Tordjman, S.; Najjar, I.; Bellissant, E.; Anderson, G.M.; Barburoth, M.; Cohen, D.; Jaafari, N.; Schischmanoff, O.; Fagard, R.; Lagdas, I.; et al. Advances in the research of melatonin in autism spectrum disorders: Literature review and new perspectives. *Int. J. Mol. Sci.* **2013**, *14*, 20508–20542. [CrossRef] [PubMed]
117. Richards, C.; Jones, C.; Groves, L.; Moss, J.; Oliver, C. Prevalence of autism spectrum disorder phenomenology in genetic disorders: A systematic review and meta-analysis. *Lancet Psychiatry* **2015**, *2*, 909–916. [CrossRef]
118. Skuse, D.H.; James, R.S.; Bishop, D.V.; Coppin, B.; Dalton, P.; Aamodt-Leeper, G.; Bacarese-Hamilton, M.; Creswell, C.; McGurk, R.; Jacobs, P.A. Evidence from Turner's syndrome of an imprinted X-linked locus affecting cognitive function. *Nature* **1997**, *387*, 705–708. [CrossRef] [PubMed]
119. Sybert, V.P.; McCauley, E. Turner' syndrome. *N. Engl. J. Med.* **2004**, *351*, 1227–1238. [CrossRef] [PubMed]
120. Kent, L.; Bowdin, S.; Kirby, G.A.; Cooper, W.N.; Maher, E.R. Beckwith Wiedemann syndrome: A behavorial phenotype-genotype study. *Am. Med. Genet.* **2008**, *147*, 1295–1297. [CrossRef] [PubMed]
121. DeBaun, M.R.; Niemitz, E.L.; Feinberg, A.P. Association of in vitro fertilization with Beckwith-Wiedemann syndrome and epigenetic alterations of LIT1 and H19. *Am. J. Hum. Genet.* **2003**, *72*, 156–160. [CrossRef] [PubMed]
122. Smith, A.C.; Choufani, S.; Ferreira, J.C.; Weksberg, R. Growth regulation, imprinted genes, and chromosome 11p15.5. *Pediatr. Res.* **2007**, *61*, 43–47. [CrossRef] [PubMed]
123. Weksberg, R.; Shuman, C.; Beckwith, J.B. Beckwith-Wiedemann syndrome. *Eur. J. Hum. Genet.* **2010**, *18*, 8–14. [CrossRef] [PubMed]
124. Wolpert, C.M.; Menold, M.M.; Bass, M.P.; Qumsiyeh, M.B.; Donnelly, S.L.; Ravan, S.A.; Vance, J.M.; Gilbert, J.R.; Abramson, R.K.; Wright, H.H.; et al. Three probands with autistic disorder and isodicentric chromosome 15. *Am. J. Med. Genet.* **2000**, *96*, 365–372. [CrossRef]
125. Wolpert, C.; Pericak-Vance, M.A.; Abramson, R.K.; Wright, H.H.; Cuccaro, M.L. Autistic symptoms among children and young adults with isodicentric chromosome 15. *Am. J. Med. Genet.* **2000**, *96*, 128–129. [CrossRef]
126. Parisi, L.; di Filippo, T.; Roccella, M. Hypomelanosis of ito: Neurological and psychiatric pictures in developmental age. *Minerva Pediatr.* **2012**, *64*, 65–70. [PubMed]
127. Åkefeldt, A.; Gillberg, C. Hypomelanosis of ito in three cases with autism and autistic-like conditions. *Dev. Med. Child Neurol.* **1991**, *33*, 737–743. [CrossRef] [PubMed]
128. Johansson, M.; Gillberg, C.; Råstam, M. Autism spectrum conditions in individuals with Möbius sequence, CHARGE syndrome and oculo-auriculo-vertebral spectrum: Diagnostic aspects. *Res. Dev. Disabil.* **2010**, *31*, 9–24. [CrossRef] [PubMed]
129. Johansson, M.; Råstam, M.; Billstedt, E.; Danielsson, S.; Strömland, K.; Miller, M.; Gillberg, C. Autism spectrum disorders and underlying brain pathology in CHARGE association. *Dev. Med. Child Neurol.* **2006**, *48*, 40–50. [CrossRef] [PubMed]
130. Smith, I.M.; Nichols, S.L.; Issekutz, K.; Blake, K. Canadian paediatric surveillance program behavioral profiles and symptoms of autism in CHARGE syndrome: Preliminary Canadian epidemiological data. *Am. J. Med. Genet.* **2005**, *133*, 248–256. [CrossRef] [PubMed]
131. Hartshorne, T.S.; Grialou, T.L.; Parker, K.R. Autistic-like behavior in CHARGE syndrome. *Am. J. Med. Genet.* **2005**, *133*, 257–261. [CrossRef] [PubMed]
132. Patten, S.A.; Jacobs-McDaniels, N.L.; Zaouter, C.; Drapeau, P.; Albertson, R.C.; Moldovan, F. Role of Chd7 in zebrafish: A model for CHARGE syndrome. *PLoS ONE* **2012**, *7*, e31650. [CrossRef] [PubMed]
133. Blake, K.D.; Prasad, C. CHARGE syndrome. *Orphanet J. Rare Dis.* **2006**, *1*, 34. [CrossRef] [PubMed]
134. Bolton, P.F.; Park, R.J.; Higgins, J.N.; Griffiths, P.D.; Pickles, A. Neuro-epileptic determinants of autism spectrum disorders in tuberous sclerosis complex. *Brain* **2002**, *125*, 1247–1255. [CrossRef] [PubMed]
135. Curatolo, P.; Bombardieri, R.; Jozwiak, S. Tuberous sclerosis. *Lancet* **2008**, *372*, 657–668. [PubMed]
136. Jeste, S.S.; Varcin, K.J.; Hellemann, G.S.; Gulsrud, A.C.; Bhatt, R.; Kasari, C.; Wu, J.Y.; Sahin, M.; Nelson, C.A. Symptom profiles of autism spectrum disorder in tuberous sclerosis complex. *Neurology* **2016**. [CrossRef] [PubMed]
137. McBride, K.L.; Varga, E.A.; Pastore, M.T.; Prior, T.W.; Manickam, K.; Atkin, J.F.; Herman, G.E. Confirmation study of PTEN mutations among individuals with autism or developmental delays/mental retardation and macrocephaly. *Autism Res.* **2010**, *3*, 137–141. [CrossRef] [PubMed]
138. Lintas, C.; Persico, A.M. Autistic phenotypes and genetic testing: State-of-the-art for the clinical geneticist. *J. Med. Genet.* **2009**, *46*, 1–8. [CrossRef] [PubMed]

139. Buxbaum, J.D.; Cai, G.; Chaste, P.; Nygren, G.; Goldsmith, J.; Reichert, J.; Anckarsäter, H.; Rastam, M.; Smith, C.J.; Silverman, J.M.; et al. Mutation screening of the PTEN gene in patients with autism spectrum disorders and macrocephaly. *Am. J. Med. Genet.* **2007**, *144*, 484–491. [CrossRef] [PubMed]
140. Herman, G.E.; Butter, E.; Enrile, B.; Pastore, M.; Prior, T.W.; Sommer, A. Increasing knowledge of PTEN germline mutations: Two additional patients with autism and macrocephaly. *Am. J. Med. Genet.* **2007**, *143*, 589–593. [CrossRef] [PubMed]
141. Goffin, A.; Hoefsloot, L.H.; Bosgoed, E.; Swillen, A.; Fryns, J.P. PTEN mutation in a family with Cowden syndrome and autism. *Am. J. Med. Genet.* **2001**, *105*, 521–524. [CrossRef] [PubMed]
142. Spinelli, L.; Black, F.M.; Berg, J.N.; Eickholt, B.J.; Leslie, N.R. Functionally distinct groups of inherited PTEN mutations in autism and tumour syndromes. *J. Med. Genet.* **2015**, *52*, 128–134. [CrossRef] [PubMed]
143. Amir, R.E.; Van Den Veyver, I.B.; Wan, M.; Tran, C.Q.; Francke, U.; Zoghbi, H.Y. Rett syndrome is cause by mutations in X-linked MECP2, encoding methil-CpG-binding protein 2. *Nat. Genet.* **1999**, *23*, 185–188. [PubMed]
144. Olsonn, B.; Rett, A. A review of the Rett syndrome with a theory of autism. *Brain Dev.* **1990**, *12*, 11–15. [CrossRef]
145. Young, D.J.; Bebbington, A.; Anderson, A.; Ravine, D.; Ellaway, C.; Kulkarni, A.; de Klerk, N.; Kaufmann, W.E.; Leonard, H. The diagnosis of autism in a female: Could it be Rett syndrome? *Eur. J. Pediatr.* **2008**, *167*, 661–669. [CrossRef] [PubMed]
146. Neul, J.L. The relationship of Rett syndrome and MECP2 disorders to autism. *Dialogues Clin. Neurosci.* **2012**, *14*, 253–262. [PubMed]
147. Gadalla, K.; Bailey, M.E.; Cobb, S.R. MeCP2 and Rett syndrome: Reversibility and potential avenues for therapy. *Biochem. J.* **2011**, *439*, 1–14. [CrossRef] [PubMed]
148. Neul, J.L.; Kaufmann, W.E.; Glaze, D.G.; Christodoulou, J.; Angus, J.; Clarke, A.J.; Bahi-Buisson, N.; Leonard, H.; Bailey, M.E.S.; Schanen, C.; et al. Rett syndrome: Revised diagnostic criteria and nomenclature. *Ann. Neurol.* **2010**, *68*, 944–950. [CrossRef] [PubMed]
149. Ramocki, M.B.; Peters, S.U.; Tavyev, Y.J.; Zhang, F.; Carvalho, C.M.; Schaaf, C.P.; Richman, R.; Fang, P.; Glaze, D.G.; Lupski, J.R.; et al. Autism and other neuropsychiatric symptoms are prevalent in individuals with MeCP2 duplication syndrome. *Ann. Neurol.* **2009**, *66*, 771–782. [CrossRef] [PubMed]
150. Nidiffer, F.D.; Kelly, T.E. Developmental and degenerative patterns associated with cognitive, behavioural and motor difficulties in the Sanfilippo syndrome: An epidemiological study. *J. Ment. Defic. Res.* **1983**, *27*, 185–203. [CrossRef] [PubMed]
151. Wraith, J.E. The mucopolysaccharidoses: A clinical review and guide to management. *Arch. Dis. Child.* **1995**, *72*, 263–267. [CrossRef] [PubMed]
152. Ritvo, E.R.; Mason-Brothers, A.; Freeman, B.J.; Pingree, C.; Jenson, W.R.; McMahon, W.M.; Petersen, P.B.; Jorde, L.B.; Mo, A.; Ritvo, A. The UCLA-university of Utah epidemiologic survey of autism: The etiologic role of rare diseases. *Am. J. Psychiatry* **1990**, *147*, 1614–1621. [PubMed]
153. Shapiro, E.; King, K.; Ahmed, A.; Rudser, K.; Rumsey, R.; Yund, B.; Delaney, K.; Nestrasil, I.; Whitley, C.; Potegal, M. The neurobehavioral phenotype in mucopolysaccharidosis type IIIB: An exploratory study. *Mol. Genet. Metab. Rep.* **2016**, *6*, 41–47. [CrossRef] [PubMed]
154. Ramaekers, V.T.; Blau, N. Cerebral folate deficiency. *Dev. Med. Child Neurol.* **2004**, *46*, 843–851. [CrossRef] [PubMed]
155. Moretti, P.; Scaglia, F. Cerebral folate deficiency with developmental delay, autism, and response to folinic acid. *Neurology* **2005**, *64*, 1088–1090. [CrossRef] [PubMed]
156. Gordon, N. Cerebral folate deficiency. *Dev. Med. Child Neurol.* **2009**, *51*, 180–182. [CrossRef] [PubMed]
157. Raidah, S.A.; Mohammed, W.C. Diagnosis and management of cerebral folate deficiency. *Neurosciences* **2014**, *19*, 312–316.
158. Ryan, A.K.; Bartlett, K.; Clayton, P.; Eaton, S.; Mills, L.; Donnai, D.; Winter, R.M.; Burn, J. Smith-Lemli-Opitz syndrome: A variable clinical and biochemical phenotype. *J. Med. Genet.* **1998**, *35*, 558–565. [CrossRef] [PubMed]
159. Kelley, R.I.; Hennekam, R.C.M. The Smith-Lemli-Opitz syndrome. *J. Med. Genet.* **2000**, *37*, 321–335. [CrossRef] [PubMed]
160. Tierny, E.; Nwokoro, N.A.; Porter, F.D.; Freund, L.S.; Ghuman, J.K.; Kelley, R.I. Behavior phenotype in the RSH/ Smith-Lemli-Opitz syndrome. *Am. J. Med. Genet.* **2001**, *98*, 191–200. [CrossRef]

161. Tierny, E.; Nwokoro, N.A.; Kelley, R.I. Behavior phenotype of RSH/Smith-Lemli-Opitz syndrome. *Ment. Retard. Dev. Disabil. Res. Rev.* **2001**, *98*, 191–200.
162. Tint, G.S.; Irons, M.; Elias, E.R.; Batta, A.K.; Frieden, R.; Chen, T.S.; Salen, G. Defective cholesterol biosynthesis associated with the Smith-Lemli-Opitz syndrome. *N. Engl. J. Med.* **1994**, *330*, 107–113. [CrossRef] [PubMed]
163. Thurm, A.; Tierney, E.; Farmer, C.; Albert, P.; Joseph, L.; Swedo, S.; Bianconi, S.; Bukelis, I.; Wheeler, C.; Sarphare, G.; et al. Development, behavior, and biomarker characterization of Smith-Lemli-Opitz syndrome: An update. *J. Neurodev. Disord.* **2016**, *8*, 12. [CrossRef] [PubMed]
164. Baieli, S.; Pavone, L.; Meli, C.; Fiumara, A.; Coleman, M. Autism and phenylketonuria. *J. Autism Dev. Disord.* **2003**, *33*, 201–204. [CrossRef] [PubMed]
165. Miladi, N.; Larnaout, A.; Kaabachi, N.; Helayem, M.; Ben Hamida, M. Phenylketonuria: An underlying etiology of autistic syndrome report. *J. Child Neurol.* **1992**, *7*, 22–23. [CrossRef] [PubMed]
166. Fon, E.A.; Sarrazin, J.; Meunier, C.; Alarcia, J.; Shevell, M.I.; Philippe, A.; Leboyer, M.; Rouleau, G.A. Adenylosuccinate lyase (ADSL) and infantile autism: Absence of previously reported point mutation. *Am. J. Hum. Genet.* **1995**, *18*, 554–557. [CrossRef] [PubMed]
167. Jaeken, J.; van den Berghe, G. An infantile autistic syndrome characterized by the presence of succinylpurines in body fluids. *Lancet* **1984**, *2*, 1058–1061. [PubMed]
168. Race, V.; Marie, S.; Vincent, M.F.; van der Berghe, G. Clinical, biochemical and molecular genetic correlations in adenylosuccinate lyase deficiency. *Hum. Mol. Genet.* **2000**, *9*, 2159–2163. [CrossRef] [PubMed]
169. Stone, R.L.; Aimi, J.; Barshop, B.A.; Jaeken, J.; van den Berghe, G.; Zalkin, H.; Dixon, J.E. A mutation in adenylosuccinate lyase associated with mental retardation autistic features. *Nat. Genet.* **1992**, *1*, 59–63. [CrossRef] [PubMed]
170. Jinnah, H.A.; Sabina, R.L.; Van Den Berghe, G. Metabolic disorders of purine metabolism affecting the nervous system. *Handb. Clin. Neurol.* **2013**, *113*, 1827–1836. [PubMed]
171. Nasrallah, F.; Feki, M.; Kaabachi, N. Creatine and creatine deficiency syndromes: Biochemical and clinical aspects. *Pediatr. Neurol.* **2010**, *42*, 163–171. [CrossRef] [PubMed]
172. Póo-Argüelles, P.; Arias, A.; Vilaseca, M.A.; Ribes, A.; Artuch, R.; Sans-Fito, A.; Moreno, A.; Jakobs, C.; Salomons, G. X-linked creatine transporter deficiency in two patients with severe mental retardation and autism. *J. Inherit. Metab. Dis.* **2006**, *29*, 220–223. [CrossRef] [PubMed]
173. Schulze, A.; Bauman, M.; Tsai, A.C.; Reynolds, A.; Roberts, W.; Anagnostou, E.; Cameron, J.; Nozzolillo, A.A.; Chen, S.; Kyriakopoulou, L.; et al. Prevalence of creatine deficiency syndromes in children with nonsyndromic autism. *Pediatrics* **2016**. [CrossRef] [PubMed]
174. Campistol, J.; Díez-Juan, M.; Callejón, L.; Fernandez-De Miguel, A.; Casado, M.; Garcia Cazorla, A.; Lozano, R.; Artuch, R. Inborn error metabolic screening in individuals with nonsyndromic autism spectrum disorders. *Dev. Med. Child Neurol.* **2016**, *58*, 842–847. [CrossRef] [PubMed]
175. Durand, C.M.; Betancur, C.; Boeckers, T.M.; Bockmann, J.; Chaste, P.; Fauchereau, F.; Nygren, G.; Rastam, M.; Gillberg, I.C.; Anckarsäter, H.; et al. Mutations in the gene encoding the synaptic scaffolding protein SHANK3 are associated with autism spectrum disorders. *Nat. Genet.* **2007**, *39*, 25–27. [CrossRef] [PubMed]
176. Moessner, R.; Marshall, C.R.; Sutcliffe, J.S.; Skaug, J.; Pinto, D.; Vincent, J.; Zwaigenbaum, L.; Fernandez, B.; Roberts, W.; Szatmari, P.; et al. Contribution of SHANK3 mutations to autism spectrum disorder. *Am. J. Hum. Genet.* **2007**, *81*, 1289–1297. [CrossRef] [PubMed]
177. Guiltmatre, A.; Huquet, G.; Delorme, R.; Bourgeron, T. The emerging role of *SHANK* genes in neuropsychiatric disorders. *Dev. Neurobiol.* **2014**, *74*, 113–122. [CrossRef] [PubMed]
178. Feng, J.; Schroer, R.; Yan, J.; Song, W.; Yang, C.; Bockholt, A.; Cook, E.H., Jr.; Skinner, C.; Schwartz, C.E.; Sommer, S.S. High frequency of neurexin 1β signal peptide structural variants in patients with autism. *Neurosci. Lett.* **2006**, *27*, 10–13. [CrossRef] [PubMed]
179. Ching, M.S.; Shen, Y.; Tan, W.H.; Jeste, S.S.; Morrow, E.M.; Chen, X.; Mukaddes, N.M.; Yoo, S.Y.; Hanson, E.; Hundley, R.; et al. Deletions of NRXN1 (neurexin-1) predispose to a wide spectrum of developmental disorders. *Am. J. Med. Genet.* **2010**, *153*, 937–947. [CrossRef] [PubMed]
180. Autism Genome Project Consortium. Mapping autism risk loci using genetic linkage and chromosomal rearrangements. *Nat. Genet.* **2007**, *39*, 319–328.
181. Viñas-Jornet, M.; Esteba-Castillo, S.; Gabau, E.; Ribas-Vidal, N.; Baena, N.; San, J.; Ruiz, A.; Coll, M.D.; Novell, R.; Guitart, M. A common cognitive, psychiatric and dysmorphic phenotype in carriers of *NRXN1* deletion. *Mol. Genet. Genom. Med.* **2014**, *2*, 512–521. [CrossRef] [PubMed]

182. Dabell, M.P.; Rosenfeld, J.A.; Bader, P.; Escobar, L.F.; El-Khechen, D.; Vallee, S.E.; Dinulos, M.B.P.; Curry, C.; Fisher, J.; Tervo, R.; et al. Investigation of *NRXN1* deletions: Clinical and molecular characterization. *Am. J. Med. Genet.* **2013**, *161*, 717–731. [CrossRef] [PubMed]
183. Alarcon, M.; Abrahams, B.S.; Stone, J.L. Linkage, association, and gene-expression analyses identify *CNTNAP2* as an autism-susceptibility gene. *Am. J. Med. Genet.* **2008**, *82*, 150–159. [CrossRef] [PubMed]
184. Werling, A.M.; Bobrowski, E.; Taurines, R.; Gundelfinger, R.; Romanos, M.; Grünblatt, E.; Walitza, S. *CNTNAP2* gene in high functioning autism: No association according to family and meta-analysis approaches. *J. Neural Transm.* **2016**, *123*, 353–363. [CrossRef] [PubMed]
185. Murdoch, J.D.; Gupta, A.R.; Sanders, S.J.; Walker, M.F.; Keaney, J.; Fernandez, T.V.; Murtha, M.T.; Anyanwu, S.; Ober, G.T.; Raubeson, M.J.; et al. No evidence for association of autism with rare heterozygous point mutations in contactin-associated protein-like 2 (*CNTNAP2*), or in other contactin-associated proteins or contactins. *PLoS Genet.* **2015**, *11*, e1004852. [CrossRef] [PubMed]
186. Bakkaloglu, B.; O'Roak, B.J.; Louvi, A.; Gupta, A.R.; Abelson, J.F.; Morgan, T.M.; Chawarska, K.; Klin, A.; Ercan-Sencicek, A.G.; Stillman, A.A.; et al. Molecular cytogenetic analysis and resequencing of contactin associated protein-like 2 in autism spectrum disorders. *Am. J. Hum. Genet.* **2008**, *82*, 165–173. [CrossRef] [PubMed]
187. Fernandez, T.; Morgan, T.; Davis, N.; Klin, A.; Morris, A.; Farhi, A.; Lifton, R.P.; State, M.W. Disruption of contactin 4 (CNTN4) results in developmental delay and other features of 3p deletion syndrome. *Am. J. Hum. Genet.* **2004**, *74*, 1286–1293. [CrossRef] [PubMed]
188. Roohi, J.; Montagna, C.; Tegay, D.H.; Palmer, L.E.; DeVincent, C.; Pomeroy, J.C.; Christian, S.L.; Nowak, N.; Hatchwell, E. Disruption of contactin 4 in three subjects with autism spectrum disorder. *J. Med. Genet.* **2008**, *46*, 176–182. [CrossRef] [PubMed]
189. Karayannis, T.; Au, E.; Patel, J.C.; Kruglikov, I.; Markx, S.; Delorme, R.; Héron, D.; Salomon, D.; Glessner, J.; Restituito, S.; et al. Cntnap4 differentially contributes to GABAergic and dopaminergic synaptic transmission. *Nature* **2014**, *511*, 236–240. [CrossRef] [PubMed]
190. Zhiling, Y.; Fujita, E.; Tanabe, Y. Mutations in the gene encoding CADM1 are associated with autism spectrum disorder. *Biochem. Biophys. Res. Commun.* **2008**, *377*, 926–929. [CrossRef] [PubMed]
191. Fujita, E.; Tanabe, Y.; Imhof, B.A.; Mamsi, M.Y.; Momoi, T. A complex of synaptic adhesion molecule CADM1, a molecule related to autism spectrum disorder, with MUPP1 in the cerebellum. *J. Neurochem.* **2012**, *123*, 886–894. [CrossRef] [PubMed]
192. Kitagishi, Y.; Minami, A.; Nakanishi, A.; Ogura, Y.; Matsuda, S. Neuron membrane trafficking and protein kinases involved in autism and ADHD. *Int. J. Mol. Sci.* **2015**, *16*, 3095–3115. [CrossRef] [PubMed]
193. Morrow, E.M.; Yoo, S.Y.; Flavell, S.W.; Kim, T.K.; Lin, Y.; Hill, R.S.; Mukaddes, N.M.; Balkhy, S.; Gascon, G.; Hashmi, A.; et al. Identifying autism loci and genes by tracing recent shared ancestry. *Science* **2008**, *321*, 218–223. [CrossRef] [PubMed]
194. Jamain, S.; Quach, H.; Betancur, C.; Rastam, M.; Colineaux, C.; Gillberg, I.C.; Soderstrom, H.; Giros, B.; Leboyer, M.; Gillberg, C.; et al. Mutations of the X-linked genes encodage neuroligins NLGN3 and NLGN4 are associated with autism. *Nat. Genet.* **2003**, *34*, 27–29. [CrossRef] [PubMed]
195. Laumonnier, F.; Bonnet-Brilhault, F.; Gomot, M.; Blanc, R.; David, A.; Moizard, M.P.; Raynaud, M.; Ronce, N.; Lemonnier, E.; Calvas, P.; et al. X-linked mental retardation and autism are associated with a mutation in the *NLGN4* gene, a member of the neuroligin family. *Am. J. Hum. Genet.* **2004**, *74*, 552–557. [CrossRef] [PubMed]
196. Yan, J.; Oliveira, G.; Coutinho, A.; Yang, C.; Feng, J.; Katz, C.; Sram, J.; Bockholt, A.; Jones, I.R.; Craddock, N.; et al. Analysis of the neuroligin 3 and 4 genes in autism and other neuropsychiatric patients. *Mol. Psychiatry* **2005**, *10*, 329–332. [CrossRef] [PubMed]
197. Fisch, G.S. Is autism associated with the fragile X syndrome? *Am. J. Med. Genet.* **1992**, *43*, 47–55. [CrossRef] [PubMed]
198. Fisch, G.S. What is associated with the fragile X syndrome? *Am. J. Med. Genet.* **1993**, *48*, 112–121. [CrossRef] [PubMed]
199. Rogers, S.J.; Wehner, D.E.; Hagerman, R. The behavioral phenotype in fragile X: Symptoms of autism in very young children with fragile X syndrome, idiopathic autism, and other developmental disorders. *J. Dev. Behav. Pediatr.* **2001**, *22*, 409–417. [CrossRef] [PubMed]

200. Bailey, D.B., Jr.; Hatton, D.D.; Skinner, M.; Mesibov, G. Autistic behavior, FMR1 protein, and developmental trajectories in young males with fragile X syndrome. *J. Autism Dev. Disord.* **2001**, *31*, 165–174. [CrossRef] [PubMed]
201. Belmonte, M.K.; Bourgeron, T. Fragile X syndrome and autism at the intersection of genetic and neural netwoks. *Nat. Neurosci.* **2006**, *9*, 1221–1225. [CrossRef] [PubMed]
202. Kau, A.S.; Tierney, E.; Bukelis, I.; Stump, M.H.; Kates, W.R.; Trescher, W.H.; Kaufmann, W.E. Social behavior profile in young males with fragile X syndrome: Characteristics and specificity. *Am. J. Med. Genet.* **2004**, *126*, 9–17. [CrossRef] [PubMed]
203. Loesch, D.Z.; Bui, Q.M.; Dissanayake, C.; Clifford, S.; Gould, E.; Bulhak-Paterson, D.; Tassone, F.; Taylor, A.K.; Hessl, D.; Hagerman, R.; et al. Molecular and cognitive predictors of the continuum of autistic behaviours in fragile X. *Neurosci. Biobehav. Rev.* **2007**, *31*, 315–326. [CrossRef] [PubMed]
204. Clifford, S.; Dissanayake, C.; Bui, Q.M.; Huggins, R.; Taylor, A.K.; Loesch, D.Z. Autism spectrum phenotype in males and females with fragike X full mutation and premutation. *J. Autism Dev. Disord.* **2007**, *337*, 738–747. [CrossRef] [PubMed]
205. Harris, S.W.; Hessl, D.; Goodlin-Jones, B.; Ferranti, J.; Bacalman, S.; Barbato, I.; Tassone, F.; Hagerman, P.J.; Herman, H.; Hagerman, R.J. Autism profiles of males with fragile X syndrome. *Am. J. Ment. Retard.* **2008**, *113*, 427–438. [CrossRef] [PubMed]
206. Dölen, G.; Carpenter, R.L.; Ocain, T.D.; Bear, M.F. Mechanism-based approaches to treating fragile X. *Pharmacol. Ther.* **2010**, *127*, 78–93. [CrossRef] [PubMed]
207. McLennan, Y.; Polussa, J.; Tassone, F.; Hagerman, R. Fragile X syndrome. *Curr. Genom.* **2011**, *12*, 216–224. [CrossRef] [PubMed]
208. Bar-Nur, O.; Caspi, I.; Benvenisty, N. Molecular analysis of FMR 1 reactivation in fragile-X induced pluripotent stem cells and their neuronal derivatives. *J. Mol. Cell. Biol.* **2012**, *4*, 180–183. [CrossRef] [PubMed]
209. Hagerman, R.; Lauterborn, J.; Au, J.; Berry-Kravis, E. Fragile X syndrome and targeted treatment trials. *Results Probl. Cell Differ.* **2012**, *54*, 297–335. [PubMed]
210. Tabolacci, E.; Chiurazzi, P. Epignetics, fragile X syndrome and transcriptional therapy. *Am. J. Med. Genet.* **2013**, *161*, 2797–2808. [CrossRef] [PubMed]
211. De Vries, B.B.; Halley, D.J.; Oostra, B.A.; Niermeijer, C. The fragile X syndrome. *Am. J. Med. Genet.* **1998**, *35*, 579–589. [CrossRef]
212. Tolmie, J. The genetics of mental retardation. *Curr. Opin. Psychiatry* **1998**, *11*, 507–513. [CrossRef]
213. Hagerman, R.J. Fragile X syndrome. *Child Adolesc. Psychiatr. Clin. N. Am.* **1996**, *5*, 895–911. [CrossRef]
214. Hagerman, R.J.; Chudley, A.E.; Knoll, J.H.; Jackson, A.W.; Kemper, M.; Ahmad, R. Autism in fragile X females. *Am. J. Med. Genet.* **1986**, *23*, 375–380. [CrossRef] [PubMed]
215. Hatton, D.D.; Sideris, J.; Skinner, M.; Mankowski, J.; Bailey, D.B., Jr.; Roberts, J.; Mirrett, P. Autistic behavior in children with fragile X syndrome: Prevalence, stability, and the impact of FMRP. *Am. J. Med. Genet.* **2006**, *140*, 1804–1813. [CrossRef] [PubMed]
216. Roberts, J.E.; Tonnsen, B.L.; McCary, L.M.; Caravella, K.E.; Shinkareva, S.V. Brief report: Autism symptoms in infants with fragile X syndrome. *J. Autism Dev. Disord.* **2016**, *46*, 3830–3837. [CrossRef] [PubMed]
217. Einfeld, S.; Molony, H.; Hall, W. Autism is not associated with the fragile X syndrome. *Am. J. Med. Genet.* **1989**, *34*, 187–193. [CrossRef] [PubMed]
218. Reiss, A.L.; Freund, L. Behavioral phenotype of fragile X syndrome; DSM-III-R autistic behavior in male children. *Am. J. Med. Genet.* **1992**, *43*, 35–46. [CrossRef] [PubMed]
219. Todd, R.D.; Hudziak, J.J. Genetics of autism. *Curr. Opin. Psychiatry* **1993**, *6*, 486–488. [CrossRef]
220. Farzin, F.; Perry, H.; Hessl, D.; Loesch, D.; Cohen, J.; Bacalman, S.; Gane, L.; Tassone, F.; Hagerman, P.; Hagerman, R. Autism spectrum disorders and attention-deficit/hyperactivity disorder in boys with the fragile X premutation. *J. Dev. Behav. Pediatr.* **2006**, *27*, 137–144. [CrossRef]
221. Hagerman, R.J.; Berry-Kravis, E.; Kaufmann, W.E.; Ono, M.Y.; Tartaglia, N.; Lachiewicz, A.; Kronk, R.; Delahunty, C.; Hessl, D.; Visootak, J.; et al. Advances in the treatment of fragile X syndrome. *Pediatrics* **2009**, *123*, 378–390. [CrossRef] [PubMed]
222. Hallmayer, J.; Hebert, J.M.; Spiker, D.; Lotspeich, L.; McMahon, W.M.; Petersen, P.B.; Nicholas, P.; Pingree, C.; Lin, A.A.; Cavalli-Sforza, L.L.; et al. Autism and the X chromosome. Multipoint sib-pair analysis. *Arch. Gen. Psychiatry* **1996**, *53*, 985–989. [CrossRef] [PubMed]

223. Constantino, J.N.; Zhang, Y.; Holzhauer, K.; Sant, S.; Long, K.; Vallorani, A.; Malik, L.; Gutmann, D.H. Distribution and Within-Family specificity of quantitative autistic traits in patients with neurofibromatosis type I. *J. Pediatr.* **2015**, *167*, 621–626. [CrossRef] [PubMed]
224. Garg, S.; Plasschaert, E.; Descheemaeker, M.J.; Huson, S.; Borghgraef, M.; Vogels, A.; Evans, D.G.; Legius, E.; Green, J. Autism spectrum disorder profile in neurofibromatosis type I. *J. Autism Dev. Disord.* **2015**, *45*, 1649–1657. [CrossRef] [PubMed]
225. Plasschaert, E.; Descheemaeker, M.J.; Van Eylen, L.; Noens, I.; Steyaert, J.; Legius, E. Prevalence of autism spectrum disorder symptoms in children with neurofibromatosis type 1. *Am. J. Med. Genet.* **2014**, *168*, 72–80. [CrossRef] [PubMed]
226. Timonen-Soivio, L.; Vanhala, R.; Malm, H.; Hinkka-Yli-Salomäki, S.; Gissler, M.; Brown, A.; Sourander, A. Brief report: Syndromes in autistic children in a Finnish birth cohort. *J. Autism Dev. Disord.* **2016**, *46*, 2780–2784. [CrossRef] [PubMed]
227. Sheth, K.; Moss, J.; Hyland, S.; Stinton, C.; Cole, T.; Oliver, C. The behavioral characteristics of Sotos syndrome. *Am. J. Med. Genet.* **2015**, *167*, 2945–2956. [CrossRef] [PubMed]
228. Assumpcao, F.; Santos, R.C.; Rosario, M.; Mercadante, M. Brief report: Autism and Aarskog syndrome. *J. Autism Dev. Disord.* **1999**, *29*, 179–181. [CrossRef] [PubMed]
229. De Wolf, V.; Crepel, A.; Schuit, F.; van Lommel, L.; Ceulemans, B.; Steyaert, J.; Seuntjens, E.; Peeters, H.; Devriendt, K. A complex Xp11.22 deletion in a patient with syndromic autism: Exploration of *FAM120C* as a positional candidate gene for autism. *Am. J. Med. Genet.* **2014**, *164*, 3035–3041. [CrossRef] [PubMed]
230. Parisi, L.; Di Filippo, T.; Roccella, M. Behavioral phenotype and autism spectrum disorders in Cornelia de Lange syndrome. *Ment. Illn.* **2015**, *7*, 5988. [CrossRef] [PubMed]
231. Srivastava, S.; Landy-Schmitt, C.; Clark, B.; Kline, A.D.; Specht, M.; Grados, M.A. Autism traits in children and adolescents with Cornelia de Lange syndrome. *Am. J. Med. Genet.* **2014**, *321*, 1400–1410. [CrossRef] [PubMed]
232. Alvarez Retuerto, A.I.; Cantor, R.M.; Gleeson, J.G.; Ustaszewska, A.; Schackwitz, W.S.; Pennacchio, L.A.; Geschwind, D.H. Association of common variants in the Joubert syndrome gene (*AHI1*) with autism. *Hum. Mol. Genet.* **2008**, *17*, 3887–3896. [CrossRef] [PubMed]
233. Ionita-Laza, I.; Capanu, M.; De Rubeis, S.; McCallum, K.; Buxbaum, J.D. Identification of rare causal variants in sequence-based studies: Methods and applications to *VPS13B*, a gene involved in Cohen syndrome and Autism. *PLoS Genet.* **2014**, *10*, e1004729. [CrossRef] [PubMed]
234. Howlin, P.; Karpf, J.; Turk, J. Behavioural characteristics and autistic features in individuals with Cohen syndrome. *Eur. Child Adolesc. Psychiatry* **2005**, *14*, 57–64. [CrossRef] [PubMed]
235. Chandler, K.E.; Moffett, M.; Clayton-Smith, J.; Baker, G.A. Neuropsychological assessment of a group of UK patients with Cohen syndrome. *Neuropediatrics* **2003**, *34*, 7–13. [CrossRef] [PubMed]
236. Lerma-Carrillo, I.; Molina, J.D.; Cuevas-Duran, T.; Julve-Correcher, C.; Espejo-Saavedra, J.M.; Andrade-Rosa, C.; Lopez-Muñoz, F. Psychopathology in the Lujan-Fryns syndrome: Report of two patients and review. *Am. J. Med. Genet.* **2006**, *140*, 2807–2811. [CrossRef] [PubMed]
237. Alfieri, P.; Piccini, G.; Caciolo, C.; Perrino, F.; Gambardella, M.L.; Mallardi, M.; Cesarini, L.; Leoni, C.; Leone, D.; Fossati, C.; et al. Behavioral profile in RASopathies. *Am. J. Med. Genet.* **2014**, *164*, 934–942. [CrossRef] [PubMed]
238. Adviento, B.; Corbin, I.L.; Widjaja, F.; Desachy, G.; Enrique, N.; Rosser, T.; Risi, S.; Marco, E.J.; Hendren, R.L.; Bearden, C.E.; et al. Autism traits in the RASopathies. *J. Med. Genet.* **2014**, *51*, 10–20. [CrossRef] [PubMed]
239. Ghaziuddin, M.; Bolyard, B.; Alessi, N. Autistic disorder in Noonan syndrome. *J. Intellect. Disabil. Res.* **1994**, *38*, 67–72. [CrossRef] [PubMed]
240. Johansson, M.; Wentz, E.; Fernell, E.; Strömland, K.; Miller, M.T.; Gillberg, C. Autistic spectrum disorders in Moëbius sequence: a comprehensive study of 25 cases. *Dev. Med. Child Neurol.* **2001**, *43*, 338–345. [CrossRef] [PubMed]
241. Briegel, W.; Schimek, M.; Kamp-Becker, I.; Hofmann, C.; Schwab, K.O. Autism spectrum disorders in children and adolescents with Moebius sequence. *Eur. Child Adolesc. Psychiatry.* **2009**, *18*, 515–519. [CrossRef] [PubMed]
242. Helsmoortel, C.; Vulto-van Silfhout, A.T.; Coe, B.P.; Vandeweyer, G.; Rooms, L.; van den Ende, J.; Schuurs-Hoeijmakers, J.H.; Marcelis, C.L.; Willemsen, M.H.; Vissers, L.E.; et al. A SWI/SNF-related autism syndrome caused by de novo mutations in ADNP. *Nat. Genet.* **2014**, *46*, 380–384. [CrossRef] [PubMed]

243. Splawski, I.; Timothy, K.W.; Sharpe, L.M.; Decher, N.; Kumar, P.; Bloise, R.; Napolitano, C.; Schwartz, P.J.; Joseph, R.M.; Condouris, K.; et al. Ca(V)1.2 calcium channel dysfunction causes a multisystem disorder including arrhythmia and autism. *Cell* **2004**, *119*, 19–31. [CrossRef] [PubMed]
244. Huguet, G.; Ey, E.; Bourgeron, T. The genetic landscapes of autism spectrum disorders. *Annu. Rev. Genom. Hum. Genet.* **2013**, *14*, 191–213. [CrossRef] [PubMed]
245. Schaefer, G.B. Clinical genetic aspects of autism spectrum sisorders. *Int. J. Mol. Sci.* **2016**, *17*, 180. [CrossRef] [PubMed]
246. Lord, C.; Rutter, M.; Le Couteur, A. Autism diagnostic interview-revised: A revised version of a diagnostic interview for caregivers of individuals with possible pervasive developmental disorders. *J. Autism Dev. Disord.* **1994**, *24*, 659–685. [CrossRef] [PubMed]
247. Lord, C.; Risi, S.; Lambrecht, L.; Cook, E.; Leventhal, B.; DiValore, P.; Pickles, A.; Rutter, M. The autism diagnostic observation schedule-generic: A standard measures of social and communication deficits associated with the spectrum of autism. *J. Autism Dev. Disord.* **2000**, *30*, 205–223. [CrossRef] [PubMed]
248. Risi, S.; Lord, C.; Gotham, K.; Corsello, C.; Chrysler, C.; Szatmari, P.; Cook, E.H., Jr.; Leventhal, B.L.; Pickles, A. Combining information from multiple sources in the diagnosis of autism spectrum disorders. *J. Am. Acad. Child Adolesc. Psychiatry* **2006**, *45*, 1094–1103. [CrossRef] [PubMed]
249. Schaefer, G.B.; Mendelson, N.J. Clinical genetics evaluation in identifying the etiology of autism spectrum disorders: 2013 guideline revisions. *Genet. Med.* **2013**, *15*, 399–407. [CrossRef] [PubMed]
250. Ponsot, O.; Moutard, M.L.; Villeneuve, N. Orientation Diagnostique en Neurologie Pédiatrique. In *Neurologie Pédiatrique*, 2nd ed.; Flammarion Médecine-Sciences: Paris, France, 1998; pp. 75–87.
251. Simonoff, E.; Bolton, P.; Rutter, M. Mental retardation: Genetics findings, clinical implications and research agenda. *J. Child Psychol. Psychiatry* **1996**, *37*, 259–280. [CrossRef] [PubMed]
252. Hoffmann, T.J.; Windham, G.C.; Anderson, M.; Croen, L.A.; Grether, J.K.; Risch, N. Evidence of reproductive stoppage in families with autism spectrum disorder: A large, population-based cohort study. *JAMA Psychiatry* **2014**, *71*, 943–951. [CrossRef] [PubMed]
253. Ozonoff, S.; Young, G.S.; Carter, A.; Messinger, D.; Yirmiya, N.; Zwaigenbaum, L.; Bryson, S.; Carver, L.J.; Constantino, J.N.; Dobkins, K.; et al. Recurrence risk for autism spectrum disorders: A baby siblings research consortium study. *Pediatrics* **2011**, *128*, 488–495. [CrossRef] [PubMed]
254. Durkin, M.S.; Maenner, M.J.; Newschaffer, C.J.; Lee, L.C.; Cunniff, C.M.; Daniels, J.L.; Kirby, R.S.; Leavitt, L.; Miller, L.; Zahorodny, W.; et al. Advanced parental age and the risk of autism spectrum disorder. *Am. J. Epidemiol.* **2008**, *168*, 1268–1276. [CrossRef] [PubMed]
255. Lord, C. Diagnostic Instruments in Autism Spectrum Disorders. In *Handbook of Autism and Pervasive Developmental Disorders*, 2nd ed.; Cohen, D.J., Volkmar, F.R., Eds.; John, Wiley and Sons Inc.: New York, NY, USA, 1997; pp. 460–483.
256. Anastasi, A. *Psychological Testing*, 6th ed.; Macmillan Publishing Co Inc.: New York, NY, USA, 1988.
257. *Manual for the Raven's Color Progressive Matrices (CPM)*; Les Editions Centre de Psychologie Appliquée (ECPA): Paris, France, 2016.
258. Guinchat, V.; Thorsen, P.; Laurent, C.; Cans, C.; Bodeau, N.; Cohen, D. Pre-peri-and neonatal risk factors for autism. *Acta Obstet. Gynecol. Scand.* **2012**, *91*, 287–300. [CrossRef] [PubMed]
259. Gardener, H.; Spiegelman, D.; Buka, S.L. Perinatal and neonatal risk factors for autism: A comprehensive meta-analysis. *Pediatrics* **2011**, *128*, 344–355. [CrossRef] [PubMed]
260. Weissman, J.R.; Kelley, R.I.; Bauman, M.L.; Cohen, B.H.; Murray, K.F.; Mitchell, R.L.; Kern, R.L.; Natowicz, M.R. Mitochondrial disease in autism spectrum disorder patients: A cohort analysis. *PLoS ONE* **2008**, *3*, e3815. [CrossRef] [PubMed]
261. Rossignol, D.A.; Frye, R.E. Mitochondrial dysfunction in autism spectrum disorders: A systematic review and meta-analysis. *Mol. Psychiatry* **2012**, *17*, 290–314. [CrossRef] [PubMed]
262. Demily, C.; Assouline, M.; Boddaert, N.; Barcia, G.; Besmond, C.; Poisson, A.; Sanlaville, D.; Munnich, A. Genetic approaches in autism spectrum disorders. *Neuropsychiatr. Enfance Adolesc.* **2016**, *64*, 395–401. [CrossRef]
263. Lai, M.C.; Lombardo, M.V.; Baron-Cohen, S. Autism. *Lancet* **2014**, *383*, 896–910. [CrossRef]

264. Tordjman, S.; Anderson, G.M.; Bellissant, E.; Botbol, M.; Charbuy, H.; Camus, F.; Graignic, R.; Kermarrec, S.; Fougerou, C.; Cohen, D.; et al. Day and nighttime excretion of 6-sulphatoxymelatonin in adolescents and young adults with autistic disorder. *Psychoneuroendocrinology* **2012**, *37*, 1990–1997. [CrossRef] [PubMed]
265. Haag, G.; Tordjman, S.; Duprat, A.; Urwand, S.; Jardin, F.; Clement, M.C.; Cukierman, A.; Druon, C.; Maufras du Chatellier, A.; et al. Presentation of a diagnostic grid of the progressive stages of infantile autism as observed in treatment. *Int. J. Psychoanal.* **2005**, *86*, 335–352. [CrossRef] [PubMed]

11

Dysfunctional mTORC1 Signaling: A Convergent Mechanism between Syndromic and Nonsyndromic Forms of Autism Spectrum Disorder?

Juliana Magdalon [1], Sandra M. Sánchez-Sánchez [1,2], Karina Griesi-Oliveira [1] and Andréa L. Sertié [1,*]

1 Hospital Israelita Albert Einstein, Centro de Pesquisa Experimental, São Paulo 05652-900, Brazil; juliana.magdalon@einstein.br (J.M.); sandra.mabel@einstein.br (S.M.S.S.); karina.griesi@einstein.br (K.G.O.)

2 Departamento de Genética e Biologia Evolutiva, Instituto de Biociências, Universidade de São Paulo, São Paulo 05508-090, Brazil

* Correspondence: andrea.sertie@einstein.br

Academic Editor: Merlin G. Butler

Abstract: Whereas autism spectrum disorder (ASD) exhibits striking heterogeneity in genetics and clinical presentation, dysfunction of mechanistic target of rapamycin complex 1 (mTORC1) signaling pathway has been identified as a molecular feature common to several well-characterized syndromes with high prevalence of ASD. Additionally, recent findings have also implicated mTORC1 signaling abnormalities in a subset of nonsyndromic ASD, suggesting that defective mTORC1 pathway may be a potential converging mechanism in ASD pathology across different etiologies. However, the mechanistic evidence for a causal link between aberrant mTORC1 pathway activity and ASD neurobehavioral features varies depending on the ASD form involved. In this review, we first discuss six monogenic ASD-related syndromes, including both classical and potentially novel mTORopathies, highlighting their contribution to our understanding of the neurobiological mechanisms underlying ASD, and then we discuss existing evidence suggesting that aberrant mTORC1 signaling may also play a role in nonsyndromic ASD.

Keywords: mTORC1 signaling pathway; ASD-related syndromes and nonsyndromic/idiopathic ASD; neuronal cell growth; axonal and dendritic morphogenesis; dendritic spine density and maturation; synaptic plasticity; mTORC1-targeted therapies

---

1. Introduction

Autism Spectrum Disorder (ASD) is among the most common developmental neuropsychiatric disorders and affects about 1 in 68 individuals [1]. It is characterized by impairments in two core domains: deficits in social communication and restricted, repetitive pattern of behavior or interests [2]. The presentation of symptoms is variable, ranging from mild to severe, and usually coexists with other psychiatric and medical conditions. There is a strong male bias in ASD, especially among individuals less severely affected (~4 males/1 female affected) [3,4].

ASD may be part of the clinical presentation of well-characterized genetic syndromes, hereinafter referred to as ASD-related syndromes, such as tuberous sclerosis complex (TSC) [5], fragile X syndrome (FXS) [6], Rett syndrome (RTT) [7,8], Angelman syndrome (AS) [9,10], phosphatase and tensin homolog (*PTEN*)-related syndromes [11], neurofibromatosis type 1 (NF1) [12], Timothy syndrome [13], 22q13.3 deletion syndrome [14], among others. These ASD-related syndromes, although representing only 5%–10% of all ASD cases, have contributed greatly to our understanding of ASD pathogenesis [15–17].

On the other hand, for most ASD cases, hereinafter called nonsyndromic ASD (NS-ASD)—even if additional phenotypic traits are present—to distinguish it from the well-defined ASD-related syndromes, the underlying causes remain unknown. Several twin and family studies have provided indisputable evidence for a genetic component underlying NS-ASD with heritability estimates ranging from 38% to 90% depending on the study parameters [18–20]. Recent high-throughput genomic techniques accompanied by large well-characterized cohorts of patients have identified a large number of rare and common variants for further characterization in relation to ASD [20–23], but several rare de novo and highly penetrant protein coding mutations appear to be sufficiently pathogenic to cause NS-ASD by themselves [24–33]. To date, a list of >200 ASD-risk genes categorized as "high confidence", "strong candidate" and "suggestive evidence" can be found at the Simons Foundation Autism Research Initiative [34]. However, none of these genes accounts individually for more than 1%–2% of all cases of NS-ASD and, collectively, these forms of NS-ASD caused by highly penetrant mutations represent approximately 10%–20% of all cases, highlighting the enormous genetic heterogeneity of the disorder [35].

However, in spite of the high clinical and genetic heterogeneity of ASD, shared mechanisms between ASD-related syndromes and NS-ASD are being discovered and several mutated genes seem to converge on key biological pathways to give rise to ASD relevant symptoms [32,33,36–38]. One such pathway is the mechanistic target of rapamycin complex 1 (mTORC1) signaling cascade (Box 1, see below), which is a vital regulator of translation that impacts numerous cellular processes in the developing and mature brain [39,40]. Dysfunctional mTORC1 signaling has been described in several monogenic ASD-related syndromes, such as TSC, *PTEN*-associated ASD (PTEN-ASD), NF1, FXS [41,42], RTT [43] and AS [44,45]. Patient-derived cells and brain tissues as well as rodent models for these syndromes have been used to dissect the consequences of aberrant mTORC1 signaling in brain structure and function, as well as in particular aspects of cognition and behavior. In addition, recent findings suggest that *methyl-CpG binding protein 2* (*MECP2*) duplication syndrome [46] and *cyclin-dependent kinase-like 5* (*CDKL5*)-related syndrome [47] may also be associated with defective mTORC1 cascade activity; however, this needs further mechanistic exploration. Finally, more recently, dysregulation of mTORC1-dependent signaling, both upstream and downstream of its kinase activity, has also been observed in patients and animal models of NS-ASD of both known and unknown etiologies [42,48–55]. Nonetheless, our understanding of the mechanisms by which unbalanced mTORC1 signaling leads to NS-ASD is far less explored and many questions require further clarification, such as: (1) Is there enough evidence in the literature to support altered mTORC1 signaling in NS-ASD pathogenesis? (2) How large is the proportion of NS-ASD cases that show altered mTORC1 signaling? (3) Can the mechanistic insights gained from studying ASD-related syndromes be extrapolated to NS-ASD? (4) Will the putative mTORC1-targeted therapies that have been found to be effective for treating some ASD-related syndromes benefit at least a subgroup of NS-ASD patients?

Herein, we review the main mechanistic and therapeutic insights gained from studying six ASD-related syndromes with evidence for aberrant activation of mTORC1 pathway, and then discuss recent findings potentially linking mTORC1 signaling dysfunction to NS-ASD. A comparison of the main neuropathological features found in patients and rodent models of these ASD forms can be found in Table 1. Importantly, those phenotypes that were rescued by targeting mTORC1 pathway at different levels are also depicted in Table 1. All animal models described herein display ASD-relevant behaviors, except the *cytoplasmic FMR1 interacting protein 1* (*Cyfip1*) transgenic mice, in which ASD traits were not analyzed [52].

Table 1. Main brain functional and morphological features found in patients and/or in vitro human pluripotent stem cells models and/or rodent in vivo and in vitro models of autism spectrum disorder (ASD)-related syndromes and nonsyndromic ASD forms with evidence for aberrant mechanistic target of rapamycin complex 1 (mTORC1) signaling pathway (please see the manuscript text for complete details and references). The phenotypes that were rescued and/or prevented by targeting mTORC1 pathway at different levels are indicated.

Phenotypes	ASD-Related Syndromes						Nonsyndromic or Idiopathic ASD		
	TSC	PTEN	NF1	FXS	AS	RTT	Dup15q	eIF4E-ASD	Idiopathic
mTORC1 signaling	↑	↑	↑	↑	↑	↓	↑	↑	↑/↓
Seizures	Present [*,1]	Present [*,1]	Present	Present	Present	Present	Present	ND	Present
Brain size	↑ [*,1]	↑ [*,1]	↑	↑	↓	↓	↓	ND	↑
Neuron size	↑ [*,1]	↑ [*,1,3]	ND	↑/↓/normal	ND	↓ [*,5,6]	↑ [*,1] (*Cyfip1*)	ND	↓/normal
Neuronal migration	Abnormal [*,1]	Abnormal [*,1]	Abnormal	Abnormal	ND	Abnormal	Abnormal	ND	Abnormal
Neurite arborization	↑ [*,1]	↑ [*,3]	ND	↓/normal	↓	↓ [*,5,6]	↑ [*,1] (*Cyfip1*)	ND	ND
Neurite length	↑/normal	↑	↓	↓	↓	↓	↑/↓ [*,1] (*Cyfip1*)	ND	ND
Spine density	↑ [*,1]/↓ [*,1]/normal	↑ [*,1]	↓	↑/↓/normal	↓ [*,1]	↓	↑ [*] (*Cyfip1*)	↑	↑
Spine length	↑/↓ [*,1]/normal	↑	ND	↑/↓/normal	↓	ND	ND	ND	ND
Immature spine morphology	↓ [*,1]/↑	↑/↓	ND	↑ [*,3,4]	Abnormal [*,1]	↑	↓ (*Cyfip1*)	ND	ND
LTP	↓	↑/↓	↓	↑/↓	↓ [*,1,3]	↓	↓ (*patDp/+*)	↑ [*,7]	↓
mGluR-LTD	↓ [*,1]	↓	ND	↑ [*,3,4]	↑	ND	ND	↑ [*,7]	ND
Protein synthesis	↓ [*,1]/↑ [*,1]	↑	↑ [*,1]	↑ [*,1,2,3,4]	ND	↓ [*,5,6]	ND	↑ [*,7]	↑ [*,8]

↑ = increased; ↓ = decreased; * Phenotypes were rescued by: 1, mTORC1 inhibition (rapamycin); 2, phosphatidylinositide 3-kinase (PI3K) inhibition; 3, ribosomal protein S6 kinase 1 (S6K1) depletion; 4, eukaryotic translation initiation factor (eIF) 4E phosphorylation reduction; 5, insulin-like growth factor 1 (IGF-1) and/or brain-derived neurotrophic factor (BDNF); 6, phosphatase and tensin homolog (PTEN) depletion; 7, 4EGI-1, an inhibitor of eIF4E-eIF4G interaction; 8, p110δ inhibition; *cytoplasmic FMR1 interacting protein 1* (*Cyfip1*) = transgenic mice and/or cultured neuronal cells overexpressing *Cyfip1*; *patDp/+* = model mice for 15q11-13 duplication; ND = not determined; TSC = tuberous sclerosis complex; NF1 = neurofibromatosis type I; FXS = fragile X syndrome; AS = Angelman syndrome; RTT = Rett syndrome; LTP = long-term potentiation; mGluR-LTD = metabotropic glutamate receptor-mediated long-term depression.

2. mTORC1 Signaling Pathway in Monogenic Autism Spectrum Disorder-Related Syndromes

2.1. Tuberous Sclerosis Complex (TSC)

TSC (MIM#191100, #613254), a classical mTORopathy, is caused by loss-of-function mutations in the genes encoding TSC1 or TSC2 [56,57], which, together with TBC1D7 [58], form a complex that acts as a guanosine triphosphate (GTP)ase-activating protein for Ras homolog enriched in brain (RHEB) and negatively regulates mTORC1 [59,60] (Box 1, Figure 1). Therefore, constitutively active mTORC1 signaling constitutes the molecular basis of TSC [61,62]. The prevalence of ASD in TSC has been estimated to be ~36% [63]. Brain pathological features in patients include, in addition to epilepsy [64], benign proliferative lesions and focal malformation of cortical architecture termed cortical tubers, characterized by dysregulated mTORC1 activity, disruption of lamination, hyperexcitable synaptic network, giant cells, astrogliosis, reduced myelination, as well as dysplastic neurons with multiple and longer axons [65–67]. Several animal models with TSC downregulation, including constitutive heterozygous mutant mice and conditional knockout (KO) mice with *Tsc1/2*-deficiency in different cell types, have been used to shed light on the mechanisms by which TSC loss of function leads to brain alterations that, ultimately, converge on the neurocognitive impairments observed in TSC. Consistent brain functional and morphological abnormalities observed in these animals include seizures [68–71], larger brains [69,70,72], deficits in neuronal migration and cortical lamination [68–70,72–74], enlarged and dysplastic neurons [73,75–77] astrogliosis [68–70,73], reduced myelination [72,76], multiple and ectopic axons [78,79], enhanced excitatory network [65,80,81], and disrupted synaptic plasticity in the form of impaired hippocampal long-term potentiation (LTP) [82,83] and metabotropic glutamate receptor-mediated long-term depression (mGluR-LTD) [80,84] (Table 1). Notwithstanding, some conflicting results exist regarding normal/increased neurite length [78,79], reduced/normal/increased dendritic spine density and length [51,75,76,80,85,86] and increased spine head width/immature shape [75,85] (Table 1), possibly due to the use of different animal models or experimental conditions. Importantly, while it is still unknown whether increased neurite length and reduced LTP are dependent exclusively on mTORC1 overactivation, the majority of the other brain alterations in rodent models were partially or completely rescued or prevented by the mTORC1 inhibitor rapamycin [51,69,70,72,75,76,78,81,84,86] (Table 1), including astrogliosis, reduced myelination and ASD-relevant behaviors (not described in Table 1), even when treatment is begun in adulthood [77,87,88], demonstrating that they are dependent on mTORC1 overactivation. Notably, it was shown that cell-autonomous and non-cell autonomous mechanisms still not understood drive astrogliosis in *Tsc1*-deficient mice [68–70,73], and that neuron-specific deletion of *Tsc1* impairs oligodentrocyte maturation and myelination through a non-cell autonomously manner [89]. Interestingly, it was suggested that TSC2 deficiency affects neuronal migration through an abnormal crosstalk between mTORC1 and Reelin-Disabled 1 (Dab1) signaling pathways [74], and leads to increased spine density due to diminished postnatal mTORC1-mediated autophagy and spine pruning [51]. Paralleling these findings, it was shown that *Tsc1/2*-deficient neurons present mTORC1-dependent deficits in mitophagy, leading to mitochondria accumulation in cell soma and depletion from axon and pre-synaptic sites [79], which might also contribute to synaptic transmission dysfunction due to lack of adenosine triphosphate (ATP) [90,91]. On the other hand, an in vitro study has shown that *Tsc2*-deficient neurons have increased autophagy through 5′ adenosine monophosphate (AMP)-activated protein kinase (AMPK) stimulation [92], which could potentially explain the controversial results regarding dendritic spine density observed in different studies. In addition, recent reports revealed mTORC1-dependent alterations in hippocampal protein synthesis in TSC mouse models, including decreased expression of synaptic proteins, such as the plasticity-related Arc protein required for mGluR-LTD [84], which could contribute to the impaired synaptic plasticity, but increased expression of stress-responsive proteins and anti-inflammatory cytokines [86], which may suggest an attempt to deal with the oxidative stress and inflammation that are frequently observed in the brain of individuals with ASD [93].

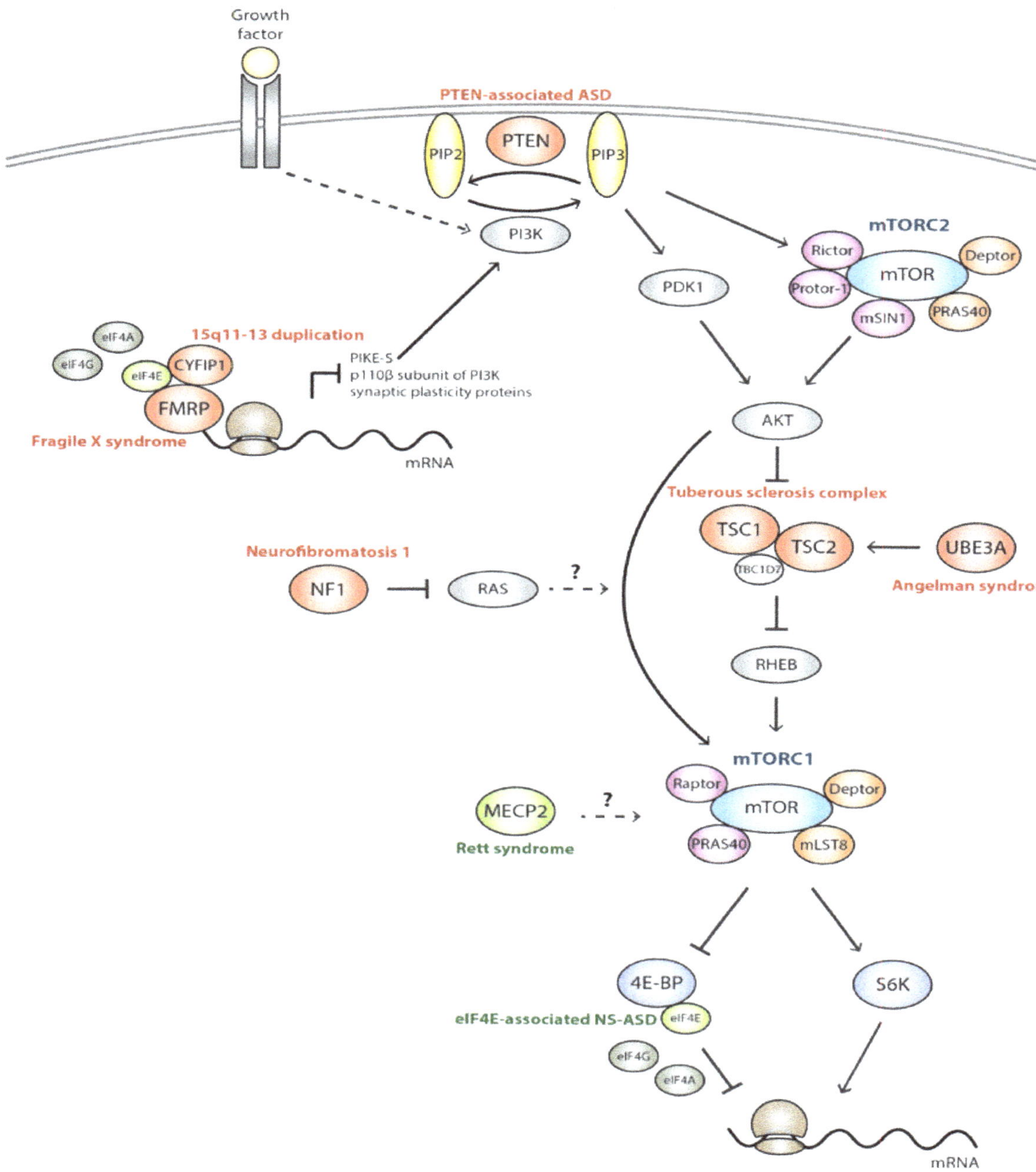

Figure 1. The mechanistic target of rapamycin complex 1 (mTORC1) signaling pathway. mTORC1 signaling components and proteins encoded by genes that inhibit (in red) or enhance (in green) mTORC1 pathway and cause autism spectrum disorder (ASD)-related syndromes and nonsyndromic ASD. Please see Box 1 for further details on mTORC1 signaling pathway. 4E-BP = eIF4E-binding protein; CYFIP1 = cytoplasmic FMR1 interacting protein 1; Deptor = DEP domain-containing mTOR-interacting protein; eIF = eukaryotic initiation factor; FMRP = fragile X mental retardation protein; MECP2 = methyl-CpG binding protein 2; mLST8 = mammalian lethal with SEC13 protein 8; mSIN1 = mammalian stress-activated protein kinase interacting protein 1; NF1 = neurofibromatosis 1; PDK1 = 3-phosphoinositide-dependent protein kinase 1; PI3K = phosphoinositide 3-kinase; PIKE = phosphoinositide 3-kinase enhancer; PIP = phosphatidylinositol; PRAS40 = proline-rich AKT substrate of 40 kDa; Protor-1 = protein observed with Rictor-1; PTEN = phosphatase and tensin homolog; Raptor = regulatory-associated protein of mTOR; RHEB = Ras homolog enriched in brain; Rictor = rapamycin-insensitive companion of mTOR; S6K = S6 kinase; TSC = tuberous sclerosis complex; UBE3A = ubiquitin-protein ligase E3A.

2.2. *Phosphatase and Tensin Homolog-Associated ASD (PTEN-ASD)*

Germline loss-of-function mutations in *PTEN* have been identified in patients with hamartoma tumor syndromes (PHTS) and in patients with ASD who also display macrocephaly with and without additional developmental features of PHTS (MIM#605309) [11,94,95]. Due to this reason and to the fact that higher lifetime risks for multiple cancers exist in patients with *PTEN* mutations, PTEN-ASD was included herein in the category of monogenic ASD-related syndromes. It has been estimated that the prevalence of *PTEN* mutations in patients with ASD and macrocephaly range from 7% to 27% [95–97]. *PTEN* encodes a lipid and protein phosphatase critical for modulating cellular growth, proliferation and survival [98]. PTEN counteracts the function of phosphoinositide 3-kinase (PI3K) and, similarly to TSC1/2, negatively regulates the mTORC1 pathway [99] (Figure 1). Therefore, *PTEN* deficiency is associated with constitutive activation of downstream AKT/mTORC1 pathways [41,100]. Except for macrocephaly, reports of brain pathological findings in patients are scarce and describe some structural abnormalities [101,102] and seizures in a few patients [103,104]. On the other hand, several heterozygous mice with constitutive *Pten* haploinsufficiency and conditional KO or knockdown mice with *Pten*-deficiency in different subsets of neuronal and glial cells have provided critical insights into the role of PTEN in the central nervous system (CNS), suggesting that it functions largely cell autonomously. Brain pathological features in these animals include seizures, macrocephaly, hypertrophy of both neurons and astrocytes throughout the brain [100,105–110]; enhanced glial cell number [105]; altered neuronal and glial migration [105,111,112]; severe abnormalities in myelination [107]; increased calibers, length and arborization of dendritic and axonal projections; increased dendritic spines density and length [100,106–110] (Table 1); and enhanced excitatory connectivity [108,109]. Importantly, treatment of *Pten*-deficient mice with rapamycin or pharmacological inhibition of S6 kinase 1 (S6K1) during early postnatal life prevented seizures, macrocephaly, aberrant neuronal migration, somatic, dendritic and axonal hypertrophy, increased neurite arborization and spine density (Table 1), enhanced excitatory connectivity, as well as reversed ASD-relevant symptoms [100,110,112], providing a causal link between elevated mTORC1 signaling and these neurobehavioral abnormalities in mouse models of *Pten* deficiency in the CNS (Table 1). Although alterations in glial cell growth, proliferation and migration, as well as in myelin production might be related to disease pathogenesis, further studies are needed to determine whether these abnormalities are linked to mTORC1 overactivation and affect ASD-relevant behaviors. Whereas increased/decreased number of immature-shaped spines [107,109] and reduced/increased LTP [107,113], decreased hippocampal mGluR-LTD [113] and cortical protein synthesis [110] are all neuropathological features also found in PTEN-ASD mouse models (Table 1), which might be in part linked to enhanced mTORC1 signaling activity as observed in TSC, a clear mechanistic link is still lacking and deserves deeper studies.

2.3. *Neurofibromatosis Type I (NF1)*

NF1 (MIM#162200) is a tumor predisposition syndrome which may also exhibit cognitive impairments and ASD-like symptoms [114]. The prevalence of ASD in NF1 patients has been estimated to be ~18% [63]. NF1 is caused by loss-of-function mutations in the *NF1* gene, which encodes the RAS GTPase-activating protein termed neurofibromin. Consequently, *NF1* defect triggers RAS signaling activation [115,116], a key driver of cancer. The first studies suggesting mTORC1 involvement in NF1 showed that RAS can induce PI3K activation and subsequent TSC2 inhibition by AKT, increasing mTORC1 activity in *Nf1*-null mouse embryonic fibroblasts and astrocytes, as well as in cells derived from NF1 patient tumors [117,118]. Thereafter, however, it was shown that NF1 regulates glial cell proliferation and tumor growth in an AKT/mTORC1 dependent but TSC/RHEB independent manner [119] (Figure 1). Although only less than 10% of NF1 patients report seizures [120–122], several brain pathological features were frequently described in patients, such as macrocephaly [123,124] and reduced myelination [125,126], as well as in mouse models of the disorder, including larger brains [127], structural malformations [128–130], abnormal cerebellar neuronal migration [131,132], increased proliferation and protein synthesis in astrocytes [118,119,133], decreased neurite length [134,135], reduced dendritic spine density [136,137] and impaired LTP [138,139] (Table 1). Among those phenotypic alterations, it has been shown that rapamycin inhibited proliferation and protein synthesis in astrocytes [118,119] (Table 1), indicating that mTORC1 overactivation regulates astrocyte function in NF1 and is probably linked to glioma formation, such that pharmacological inhibition of mTORC1 suppresses tumor growth both in NF1 patients [140,141] and in mouse models [142,143]. Interestingly, not only *Nf1* loss of function in astrocytes may promote astrogliosis [118,119,133], but also neuron-specific *Nf1* deletion induces an increase in astrocyte number via a non-cell autonomous mechanism [144]. Nevertheless, further studies are required to unravel whether a defective glial proliferation affects social and other ASD-associated behaviors. Most of the other neuropathological features found in NF1 has not yet been associated with disrupted mTORC1 activity, and might also be due to mTORC1-independent functions of NF1. In fact, impaired cerebellar neuronal migration and LTP were shown to be dependent on extracellular signal-regulated kinase (ERK) signaling [131,132,139], whereas reduced neurite length is caused by defective cyclic AMP (cAMP) generation independently of RAS signaling [134,135].

2.4. Fragile X Syndrome (FXS)

FXS (MIM#300624) is considered the most commonly inherited cause of intellectual disability and a large percentage of individuals with FXS (~30%) are codiagnosed with ASD [63,145]. FXS is caused by transcriptional silence of the X-linked gene *FMR1* and loss of the protein product, fragile X mental retardation protein (FMRP) [146,147]. FMRP is an RNA-binding protein that negatively regulates the translation, stability and transport of several mRNAs, many of which encode proteins that are essential to synapse maturation, stabilization and elimination and that are well-studied ASD risk genes, such as *SH3 and multiple ankyrin repeat domains 3* (*SHANK3*), *PTEN*, *TSC2*, *NF1*, *CYFIP1*, *Neuroligin 3* (*NLGN3*) and *Neurexin 1* (*NRXN1*) [147–149]. In addition to high incidence of epilepsy [150,151] and increased head circumference that may be present in FXS patients [152,153], consistent neuronal pathology includes increased dendritic spine density and overabundance of immature-shaped spines on neurons in various brain regions [154,155], which are thought to affect synaptic plasticity and network function (Table 1). In addition, it was shown that in vitro neurons derived from human FXS pluripotent stem cell lines show reduced cell size and neurite length [156–158] (Table 1). Accordingly, *Fmr1*KO mice, a model for human FXS, also exhibit a seizure phenotype [159,160], neurons with shorter neurite length [161] and with the atypical immature feature of FXS spines [160,162–166]. Additionally, it was shown that *Fmr1*KO mice exhibit altered neuronal migration and cortical circuitry [167], cerebellar astrogliosis [168], reduced cerebellar myelination [169], exaggerated hippocampal mGluR-LTD and protein synthesis [160,166,170–172], as well as overall brain hyperexcitability [173,174] (Table 1). Among these latter brain abnormalities, increased mGluR-LTD and protein synthesis were proved to play an important role in the neurological manifestations of FXS. In addition, less consistent results exist regarding decreased/normal neurite arborization in neurons derived from human FXS pluripotent stem cell lines [157,158], as well as normal/increased neuron size [175,176], increased/decreased/normal dendritic spine density [160,162–164,175,177] or length [165,175,178] and decreased/increased LTP [179–181] in *Fmr1*KO mice (Table 1). These discrepancies have been suggested to be due to differences in experimental conditions, brain regions examined, age and genetic background of the animals. It has been well documented that *Fmr1*KO mice exhibit upregulated mTORC1 signaling and elevated translation initiation complex formation in the brain [160,166,172], due at least in part to increased translation of the mRNAs encoding the p110β subunit of PI3K and its upstream activator PI3K enhancer (PIKE)-S, positive regulators of the mTORC1 pathway [172] (Figure 1). These findings suggest that in addition to its RNA-binding activity, FMRP also plays a role in the regulation of PI3K/mTORC1-mediated translation initiation. It is also noteworthy that although it has been suggested that mTORC1 signaling phosphorylates FMRP and inhibits its translation repressor activity [182], this finding was not confirmed in another study [183]. Importantly, pharmacological inhibition of either PI3K or mTORC1 rescues excessive synaptic protein synthesis in neurons from

*Fmr1*KO mice [177]. In addition, genetic deletion of *S6K1* and pharmacological or genetic ablation of eukaryotic translation initiation factor (eIF) 4E phosphorylation, downstream targets of both ERK and mTORC1 pathways (Box 1; Figure 1), in *Fmr1*KO mice prevented dendritic spine morphology defects, synaptic plasticity alterations, exaggerated protein synthesis (Table 1) and ASD-associated behavioral phenotypes [160,166], providing a direct evidence that upregulated mTORC1 signaling and cap-dependent translation play a role in FXS pathophysiology.

2.5. Angelman Syndrome (AS)

Most cases of AS (MIM#105830) are caused by loss of function of the maternally-inherited *ubiquitin protein ligase E3A (UBE3A)* allele in neuronal cells [184,185], which encodes a protein that targets other proteins for degradation. This gene is localized on a cluster of imprinted genes on chromosomal region 15q11-13 such that *UBE3A* is paternally imprinted and silenced by a non-coding antisense transcript [186]. A substantial portion of AS patients meets criteria for ASD [187], and the prevalence of ASD in AS has been estimated to be ~34% [63]. Brain pathological features already described in AS patients include epilepsy [188,189], microcephaly [190] and reduced myelination [191,192]. These abnormalities have been also observed in mice with a maternal null mutation in *Ube3a* (AS mice) [193–195], which additionally exhibit abnormal spine morphology, reduced dendritic spine density and length [44,45,196], suggesting that deficient synaptic development may underlie the neurological aspects of AS. Moreover, an overall excitatory network, due to a more severe decrease in inhibitory than excitatory inputs [197], possibly contributes to the increased seizure susceptibility observed in AS patients. In vitro studies using *Ube3a* knockdown or *Ube3a*KO neurons from mice have also shown that *Ube3a* loss of function decreased dendrite arborization, disrupted dendrite polarity and reduced apical dendrite length [198,199]. In addition, disrupted synaptic plasticity in the form of impaired LTP in different brain areas [45,193,200] and enhanced hippocampal mGluR-LTD [201] were also observed in AS mice (Table 1). This is believed to be mainly caused by increased levels of Arc due to its reduced ubiquitination by the UBE3A proteins and, consequently, reduced degradation [202]. Importantly, recent studies have also observed that the increased levels of Arc may also be the result of increased mTORC1 signaling and its downstream target S6K1 activation in the cerebellum and hippocampus of AS mice, triggered by increased inhibitory phosphorylation of TSC2 in the absence of UBE3A [44,45], although the precise mechanism is unknown. In addition to increasing Arc levels and improving LTP deficits, rapamycin or an S6K1 inhibitor also ameliorated dendritic spine density and morphology in Purkinje and pyramidal cells (Table 1), and consequently, motor dysfunction and learning deficits in AS mice [44,45], suggesting that mTORC1 activity may also be affecting synaptic plasticity and function in AS patients. Given the fact that the association between mTORC1 and UBE3A deficiency has been only recently demonstrated, further studies are necessary to test whether the other brain abnormalities found in AS are dependent on mTORC1 overactivation and would benefit from mTORC1-targeted therapies.

2.6. Rett Syndrome (RTT)

RTT (MIM#312750) is a severe progressive neurodevelopmental disorder that manifests mostly in girls during early childhood after a typical perinatal development. Although RTT is no longer considered an ASD in Diagnostic and Statistical Manual of Mental Disorders, fifth edition (DMS-5) [2], children afflicted with RTT often exhibit ASD-like behaviors, and the prevalence of ASD symptoms in RTT has been estimated to be ~61% in female patients [63]. RTT is mainly caused by loss-of-function mutations in the X-linked gene *MECP2* [203,204], which encodes a methyl-CpG binding protein that controls gene expression and chromatin remodeling [205]. In addition to epilepsy [206,207] and reduced brain size [208,209], brain pathology in human patients that are thought to contribute to the neurocognitive deficits in RTT includes reduced neuronal size but increased neuronal cell density in several brain regions [210,211], evidence of cortical astrogliosis [212], decreased dendritic arborization and length [213,214], as well as decreased spine density and maturation in the cortex and hippocampus [215–217] (Table 1). These neuronal abnormalities have been consistently reproduced by several studies using genetically distinct rodent models of RTT [218–225], which additionally exhibit abnormal activity-dependent synaptic plasticity in the form of attenuated LTP and LTD [226,227], and reduced number of excitatory synapses in hippocampal neurons [228] (Table 1). Notably, studies in RTT mouse models have suggested that cell autonomous and non-cell autonomous mechanisms drive neuronal morphology and function [229–231]. In addition, recent in vitro models of RTT using *MECP2*-deficient neurons derived from human pluripotent stem cells have recapitulated many neurological features of RTT [232–236], and have also shown neuronal migration defects [236] (Table 1). Interestingly, in contrast to the majority of the ASD-associated mTORopathies, neurons from *Mecp2*$^{-/-}$ and *Mecp2*$^{+/-}$ mice [43], as well as from *MECP2*-deficient human pluripotent stem cells [233], show decreased mTORC1 signaling activity, transcription and protein synthesis rate. These findings suggest that mTORC1 signaling deviations in either direction can adversely affect neuronal connectivity, cognition and social behavior. Although the mechanism by which MECP2 enhances mTORC1 signaling is still unknown (Figure 1), the levels of brain-derived neurotrophic factor (BDNF) are lower in RTT mouse models, possibly resulting in lower activation of PI3K/mTORC1 pathways [43]. Treatment of neurons derived from *MECP2*-deficient human pluripotent stem cells with exogenous growth factors (insulin-like growth factor 1 [IGF-1] or BNDF) or genetically ablation of *PTEN*, promoted protein synthesis via enhancing PI3K/mTORC1 signaling activity and rescued the soma size and neurite complexity deficits [233] (Table 1). These findings suggest that defects in the global control of transcription and PI3K/mTORC1-mediated translation might be the underlying pathomechanisms by which MECP2 dysfunction leads to RTT, although additional mechanistic exploration are needed.

3. mTORC1 Signaling Pathway in Nonsyndromic/Idiopathic Autism Spectrum Disorder

3.1. 15q11-13 Duplication (Dup15q)

Maternally inherited duplications at 15q11-13 (#MIN608636) is one of the most frequent and penetrant copy number variation in ASD, found in ~1%–2% of patients [237,238], suggesting that one or several genes from this region, when duplicated, can lead to ASD. Deletions at this same region give rise to Prader–Willi syndrome (PWS) or AS depending on whether the deletions are paternally or maternally inherited, respectively [239] and, as discussed above, ASD symptoms are usually reported in AS patients. Instability of this region is mediated by the presence of five low copy repeats, termed breakpoint (BP)1 through BP5. The PWS/AS critical region lies on the imprinted region between BP2 and BP3, and evidence from mouse models suggests that increased dosage of the *Ube3a* gene located in this region impairs excitatory synapse transmission and might underlie ASD-relevant behaviors [240]. It is noteworthy that, although duplications of paternal origin show low penetrance, a mouse model with a paternally inherited duplication of the BP2–BP3 interval (patDp/+ mice) displays behaviors associated with ASD [241], increased spine turnover [242] and impairment in cerebellar LTP [243] (Table 1). In addition, there is evidence suggesting that the more proximal non-imprinted region between BP1 and BP2 (15q11.2) is also a hot spot for ASD and that genes located in this region impact neurological and behavioral functions [244–246]. Among the four genes located between BP1 and BP2, *CYFIP1* became a prime candidate for a causal role in ASD [52,245]: it directly interacts with FMRP and with eIF4E and mediates the translational repression activity of FMRP in the brain [247], and also regulates actin polymerization and cytoskeleton remodeling through its interaction with the small GTPase Rac1 [248,249]. It was shown that CYFIP1 levels are increased in lymphoblastoid cells [52,250] and *postmortem* brain tissues (temporal cortex) [52] from ASD subjects with Dup15q, and its overexpression in cultured human and mouse neuronal cells leads to increased neuronal cell size, neurite arborization, as well as increased/decreased neurite length [52,251]. Similar abnormalities in neuronal cell size, neurite outgrowth and branching were also observed in transgenic mice overexpressing *Cyfip1*, which additionally exhibit increased spine density and number of mature spines in cortical neurons [52] (Table 1), defects previously shown to contribute to synaptopathology that drives ASD-related symptoms. However, further research should evaluate whether *Cyfip1* transgenic mice exhibits autistic traits. Importantly, evidence for increased mTORC1 signaling was observed in *postmortem* brains of ASD-Dup15q carriers ($n = 3$), as well as in embryonic *Cyfip1* transgenic mice and cultured mouse neuronal cells overexpressing *Cyfip1*. Pharmacological treatment of these cultured cells with rapamycin rescued the observed abnormalities in cell size, neurite length and branching [52]. Finally, evidence for hyperfunctional mTORC1 signaling was also observed in cultured stem cells from human exfoliated deciduous teeth (SHED) derived from one ASD patient with Dup15q [53]. Taken together these findings suggest that CYFIP1-mediated mTORC1 signaling overactivation may contribute to disease pathogenesis in ASD-Dup15 patients.

3.2. eIF4E-Associated NS-ASD (eIF4E-NS-ASD)

mTORC1 signaling phosphorylates eIF4E-binding proteins (4E-BPs) and releases them from eIF4E, allowing eIF4E to interact with eIF4G and eIF4A to form the eIF4F complex, a critical step in cap-dependent translation (Box 1; Figure 1). Interestingly, rare mutations in the promoter region of the *eIF4E* gene, which were suspected to enhance promoter activity, were found in few unrelated NS-ASD patients [48]. Later on, it was shown that transgenic mice overexpressing *eif4e* and mice lacking *4e-bp2* display increased dendritic spine density, altered synaptic plasticity, including augmented excitation, enhanced late-phase LTP and mGluR-LTD in the prefrontal cortex and hippocampus, as well as exaggerated brain cap-dependent translation [49,50] (Table 1). Treatment of *eif4e*-transgenic and *4e-bp2*KO mice with 4EGI-1, an inhibitor of eIF4E-eIF4G interaction, rescued protein synthesis and synaptic plasticity abnormalities (Table 1), as well as ASD-relevant behaviors [49,50]. These findings provided a causal link between NS-ASD and excessive cap-dependent translation, and suggest that this is one of the targets by which mTORC1 inhibitors reverse synaptic plasticity deficits and ASD symptoms.

3.3. Idiopathic Autism Spectrum Disorder

Paralleling neuropathological observations from ASD-related syndromes, children with ASD of unknown etiology also frequently display increased risk for developing epilepsy [252,253], macrocephaly in early childhood [254,255], increased neuronal density in several brain regions but reduced number of Purkinje cells [255,256], normal/decreased neuronal size [255,257], altered neuronal migration [258,259], astrogliosis and microglial activation [260], altered myelination [261,262], increased dendritic spine densities on cortical neurons [51,263] and impaired LTP [264]. In addition, increased number of inhibitory synaptic connections was described in cultured neurons derived from patient-induced pluripotent stem cells (iPSCs) [265], and increased spine turnover was found in the BTBR inbred mouse strain that displays the core behavioral deficits of ASD [242]. Although these abnormalities are most probably caused by different etiological origins, recent studies have shown that there is a subgroup of idiopathic ASD with defects in mTORC1 signaling activity. Hyperactivation of mTORC1 pathway was observed in *postmortem* brains from adolescent patients with idiopathic ASD ($n = 5$) and was shown to impair autophagy and spine pruning during childhood and adolescence, leading to increased basal dendritic spine density and, therefore, enhanced excitatory connectivity [51] (Table 1). As discussed above, similar findings were also observed in TSC mouse models in the same study, suggesting that downregulation of mTORC1 signaling is required for postnatal spine pruning [51]. In addition, mTORC1 pathway upregulation was also observed in non-neuronal cells derived from idiopathic ASD patients, such as in cultured stem cells from SHED derived from 2 out of 12 patients [53], and in lymphoblastoid cell lines (LCLs) derived from 4 out of 58 patients (7% of the patient sample) [55]. Interestingly, in LCLs from one of these patients with elevated mTORC1 pathway activity, it was also observed increased expression of the p110δ subunit of PI3K and enhanced protein synthesis rates, which were corrected by a p110δ-specific inhibitor [55] (Table 1). Curiously, contrary to these findings, a study reported evidence for decreased mTORC1 signaling in *postmortem* brains from patients with idiopathic ASD ($n = 11$; aged 5–56 years, mean 20.1 years) [54] (Table 1). The high etiological heterogeneity in this group of patients may account for these observed discrepancies in the direction of mTORC1 signaling activation, and additional investigations are needed to provide further mechanistic understanding of the causal link between mTORC1 pathway dysfunction and ASD in this group.

4. Discussion

Research on both ASD-related syndromes and NS-ASD and their corresponding mouse models has shown that abnormalities in brain size and structure, neuronal size, migration and myelination, astrocyte proliferation, neurite and dendritic spine morphology, synapse plasticity, imbalanced synaptic excitation/inhibition, as well as dysregulated brain protein synthesis are all common features of ASD across different etiologies. Although aberrant mTORC1 pathway activation has been suggested as a convergent molecular mechanism in ASD etiopathology, the evidence supporting a causal relationship between abnormal mTORC1 signaling and these brain anatomical and physiological deficits, as well as behavioral alterations found in patients and/or animal models, varies greatly depending on the ASD form involved. Herein, we will discuss only the neurobehavioral abnormalities that were experimentally linked to mTORC1, which include those phenotypes that were rescued or prevented by modulating mTORC1 cascade activity at different levels.

Seizures, enlarged brain and neuron size, neuronal migration abnormalities and increased neurite arborization were mechanistically linked to enhanced mTORC1 signaling in mouse models of ASD-related syndromes caused by mutations in upstream negative regulators of the pathway, such as TSC [69,70,72,75,76,78] and PTEN-ASD [100,112]. Interestingly, overactivation of mTORC1 was also associated with increased neuronal size and neurite arborization in cultured neuronal cells overexpressing *Cyfip1*, located in the 15q11.2 ASD risk locus [52]. On the other hand, diminished mTORC1 pathway seems to be associated with decreased neuronal size and neurite arborization in RTT models [233]. These results suggest that an optimal level of mTORC1 signaling activation is required to maintain proper brain and neuron size, as well as neurite branching patterns, such that abnormalities in these morphological features of neurons may contribute to ASD pathogenesis.

Atypical number and/or length and/or morphology of dendritic spines were mechanistically linked to disinhibited mTORC1 signaling in different mouse models of ASD-related syndromes, including TSC [75,76,86], PTEN-ASD [100], FXS [160,166] and AS [44,45], as well as in NS-ASD models, such as *Cyfip1* transgenic mice [52], eIF4E-NS-ASD mice [49,50] and idiopathic ASD patients [51]. Importantly, a recent study reported that disruption of mTORC1-dependent macroautophagy reduces spine pruning and consequently increases spine density in neurons of individuals with TSC or idiopathic ASD [51]. It would be important to address whether defects in mTORC1-mediated autophagy also play a role in impaired developmental pruning of neuronal connections in other ASD models. Together these findings suggest that mTORC1-mediated abnormalities in dendritic spine number and structure are central in ASD pathogenesis across multiple underlying causes.

Abnormal mTORC1-mediated brain protein synthesis was shown to play a role in the synaptic pathophysiology of TSC [84,86], FXS [160,166,177] and eIF4E-NS-ASD [49,50] mouse models. In addition, different responses for overactivated mTORC1 signaling in synaptic plasticity was observed depending on the ASD mouse model, i.e., mTORC1 may reduce mGluR-LTD in TSC [84] but enhance it in FXS [160,166] and eIF4E-NS-ASD [49,50], as well as decrease LTP in AS [44,45] and increase it in eIF4E-NS-ASD [49,50]. Interestingly, there is a tendency for those ASD forms with heightened mTORC1-dependent translation of synaptic proteins, such as FXS and eIF4E-NS-ASD, to display enhanced mGluR-LTD, whereas TSC, which show decreased mTORC1-dependent translation of synaptic proteins, exhibit impaired mGluR-LTD, suggesting that altered (either enhanced or reduced) mTORC1-mediated protein abundance of synaptic proteins, such as Arc, may influence mGluR-LTD and may be implicated in the synaptic defects and cognitive impairments associated with ASD pathogenesis across different genetic causes. Although PI3K/mTORC1-associated protein synthesis defects have also been observed in *Nf1*-deficient astrocytes [118], in *MECP2*-deficient human pluripotent stem cells (model of RTT) [233] and in lymphoblastoid cell lines from an idiopathic ASD patient [55], further investigation is required in order to unravel a potential link with synaptic plasticity abnormalities and ASD-like symptoms in these different ASD models.

Finally, and perhaps most importantly, a direct role for overactivated mTORC1 signaling in ASD core symptoms is supported by multiple evidence in mouse models of TSC [77,87,88], PTEN-ASD [100], FXS [160,166] and eIF4E-NS-ASD [49,50], showing that pharmacological or genetic inhibition of mTORC1 cascade both upstream and downstream of its kinase activity rescues or attenuates ASD-relevant behaviors, highlighting the potential therapeutic value of drugs targeting this pathway for patients. Indeed, based on evidence for the benefit of rapamycin and similar drugs on neurobehavioral deficits in TSC mouse models, clinical trials aimed to evaluate the effect of mTORC1 inhibitors on neurocognition in TSC patients are currently underway [266].

Therapeutic approaches based on mTORC1 inhibition might benefit NS-ASD patients as well. There are evidences that individuals with Dup15q, which accounts for 1%–2% of all ASD cases, display aberrant mTORC1 pathway activation [52] and, thus, it would be interesting to develop preclinical and clinical studies to evaluate the ability of drugs acting on mTORC1 cascade to ameliorate neurobehavioral function in Dup15q. Lastly, some studies have described mTORC1 signaling defects in a sub-cohort of patients with idiopathic ASD [51,53–55], although further functional studies are required to provide additional and mechanistic proof of a causal link between mTORC1 abnormalities and ASD development in this group of patients. While it is currently difficult to estimate the proportion of patients with ASD of unknown etiology that show aberrant mTORC1 pathway, pilot studies using patient-derived non-neuronal cells [53,55] have opened up the exciting possibility of large-scale screens for mTORC1 signaling defects using more easily accessible patient biological material, which might be used to select those patients who could possibly benefit from treatments targeting mTORC1 pathway. It is noteworthy that mTORC1 signaling abnormalities may be caused by a variety of factors in this group, including genetic, epigenetic and environmental risk factors, which may further complicate clinical studies; however, in spite of these challenges, identifying a subgroup of patients that will benefit from mTORC1-targeted therapies will be of paramount importance.

5. Conclusions and Future Directions

A causal relationship has been established between disturbed activation of mTORC1 signaling pathway and several neurological abnormalities observed in different well-characterized monogenic syndromes with high prevalence of ASD (TSC, PTEN-ASD, FXS, AS and RTT), and preclinical studies have shown that modulation of mTORC1 signaling may provide promising avenues for the treatment of ASD-relevant symptoms. The emerging evidence for aberrant mTORC1 signaling activation in a subgroup of patients with nonsyndromic/idiopathic ASD also provides an exciting possibility for the treatment of behavioral and cognitive deficits in these patients as well. The findings that defective mTORC1 activity can also be detected in non-neuronal more easily accessible cells suggest that mTORC1 cascade components may potentially be used as biomarkers to identify those patients most likely to benefit from mTORC1-targeted therapies. However, given the etiological complexity of ASD in this group, additional studies are required to further explore the mechanistic relevance of mTORC1 pathway alterations to the disease.

Box 1. mTOR signaling biology.

mTOR is a large (predicted molecular weight 280 kD) serine/threonine kinase that can combine with protein binding partners to form one of two functionally distinct mTOR complexes: mTORC1 and mTORC2. In addition to mTOR, mTORC1 consists of regulatory-associated protein of mTOR (Raptor) and mammalian lethal with SEC13 protein 8 (mLST8), which are essential for mTORC1 function, as well as proline-rich AKT substrate of 40 kDa (PRAS40) and DEP domain-containing mTOR-interacting protein (Deptor), inhibitors of mTORC1 activity (Figure 1). Although most of mTORC1 actions are sensitive to rapamycin, mTORC2 is mostly insensitive to rapamycin and contains the core components mTOR, mLST8, Deptor, mammalian stress-activated protein kinase interacting protein 1 (mSIN1), rapamycin-insensitive companion of mTOR (Rictor) and protein observed with Rictor-1 (Protor-1) (Figure 1). Although much less is known about mTORC2 than is known for mTORC1, a growing amount of literature demonstrates a role for mTORC2 in cytoskeletal integrity and neuronal morphology [267,268]. To date, the majority of neurological disorders associated with mTOR signaling have been linked to mTORC1 [39,269]. In the presence of growth factors, such as insulin, the PI3K is activated and stimulates phosphatidylinositol (3,4,5)-trisphosphate (PIP3) production. PIP3 accumulation in the plasma membrane promotes AKT recruitment, phosphorylation and activation by 3-phosphoinositide-dependent protein kinase 1 (PDK1) and mTORC2. When active, AKT phosphorylates and inhibits TSC2 that, together with TSC1 and TBC1D7 [58], is part of the tuberous sclerosis complex (TSC) [270]. TSC functions as a GTPase-activating protein (GAP) toward RAS homolog enriched in brain (RHEB), stimulating the conversion of RHEB-GTP to RHEB-GDP and inactivating this protein. Therefore, the inhibition of TSC by AKT promotes RHEB activation, which then activates mTORC1 in the presence of amino acids [271,272]. Among several processes, mTORC1 inhibits autophagy and stimulates mRNA translation, which is dependent on the phosphorylation and activation of S6 kinase (S6K) and inhibition of eukaryotic translation initiation factor 4E (eIF4E)-binding proteins (4E-BPs), releasing it from eIF4E and enabling interaction with eIF4G and eIF4A to form the eIF4F translation initiation complex, a critical step in cap-dependent translation (Figure 1). In addition to insulin and amino acids, other signals modulate mTORC1 activity, such as levels of ATP, glucose and oxygen. Therefore, mTORC1 is considered a sensor of internal and external cues that maintains cellular homeostasis through modulation of anabolic and catabolic processes [273].

Author Contributions: Juliana Magdalon and Andrea L. Sertie reviewed the literature and wrote the manuscript; Sandra M.S. Sánchez analyzed critically the literature review; Karina Griesi-Oliveira critically revised the manuscript; and Andrea L. Sertie conceived the manuscript. All the authors approved the final version of the manuscript.

References

1. Christensen, D.L.; Baio, J.; van Naarden Braun, K.; Bilder, D.; Charles, J.; Constantino, J.; Daniels, J.; Durkin, M.; Fitzgerald, R.T.; Kurzius-Spencer, M.; et al. Prevalence and Characteristics of Autism Spectrum Disorder among Children Aged 8 Years—Autism and Developmental Disabilities Monitoring Network, 11 Sites, United States, 2012. *MMWR Surveill. Summ.* **2016**, *65*, 1–23. [CrossRef] [PubMed]
2. American Psychiatric Association. *Diagnostic and Statistical Manual of Mental Disorders (5th ed.; DSM–5)*; American Psychiatric Publishing: Arlington, VA, USA, 2013.
3. Newschaffer, C.; Croen, L.A.; Daniels, J.; Giarelli, E.; Grether, J.K.; Levy, S.E.; Mandell, D.S.; Miller, L.A.; Pinto-Martin, J.; Reaven, J.; et al. The Epidemiology of Autism Spectrum Disorders. *Annu. Rev. Public Health* **2007**, *28*, 235–258. [CrossRef] [PubMed]
4. Fombonne, E. Epidemiology of pervasive developmental disorders. *Pediatr. Res.* **2009**, *65*, 591–598. [CrossRef] [PubMed]
5. Jeste, S.S.; Sahin, M.; Bolton, P. Characterization of Autism in Young Children with Tuberous Sclerosis Complex. *J. Child Neurol.* **2008**, *23*, 520–525. [CrossRef] [PubMed]
6. Budimirovic, D.B.; Kaufmann, W.E. What Can We Learn about Autism from Studying Fragile X Syndrome? *Dev. Neurosci.* **2011**, *33*, 379–394. [CrossRef] [PubMed]
7. Chahrour, M.; Zoghbi, H.Y. The Story of Rett Syndrome: From Clinic to Neurobiology. *Neuron* **2007**, *56*, 422–437. [CrossRef] [PubMed]
8. Neul, J.L. The relationship of Rett syndrome and MECP2 disorders to autism. *Dialogues Clin. Neurosci.* **2012**, *14*, 253–262. [PubMed]

9. Williams, C.A.; Beaudet, A.L.; Clayton-Smith, J.; Knoll, J.H.; Kyllerman, M.; Laan, L.A.; Magenis, R.E.; Moncla, A.; Schinzel, A.A.; Summers, J.A.; et al. Angelman Syndrome 2005: Updated Consensus for Diagnostic Criteria. *Am. J. Med. Genet.* **2006**, *140*, 413–418. [CrossRef] [PubMed]
10. Buiting, K. Prader-Willi syndrome and Angelman syndrome. *Am. J. Med. Genet. Part C Semin. Med. Genet.* **2010**, *154*, 365–376. [CrossRef] [PubMed]
11. Butler, M.G.; Dasouki, M.J.; Zhou, X.; Talebizadeh, Z.; Brown, M.; Takahashi, T.N.; Miles, J.H.; Wang, C.H.; Stratton, R.; Pilarski, R.; et al. Subset of individuals with autism spectrum disorders and extreme macrocephaly associated with germline PTEN tumour suppressor gene mutations. *J. Med. Genet.* **2005**, *42*, 318–321. [CrossRef] [PubMed]
12. Ratner, N.; Miller, S.J. A RASopathy gene commonly mutated in cancer: The neurofibromatosis type 1 tumour suppressor. *Nat. Rev. Cancer* **2015**, *15*, 290–301. [CrossRef] [PubMed]
13. Splawski, I.; Timothy, K.W.; Sharpe, L.M.; Decher, N.; Kumar, P.; Bloise, R.; Napolitano, C.; Schwartz, P.J.; Joseph, R.M.; Condouris, K.; et al. CaV1.2 Calcium Channel Dysfunction Causes a Multisystem Disorder Including Arrhythmia and Autism. *Cell* **2004**, *119*, 19–31. [CrossRef] [PubMed]
14. Phelan, K.; McDermid, H.E. The 22q13.3 deletion syndrome (Phelan-McDermid syndrome). *Mol. Syndromol.* **2011**, *2*, 186–201. [CrossRef] [PubMed]
15. Kelleher, R.J.; Bear, M.F. The Autistic Neuron: Troubled Translation? *Cell* **2008**, *135*, 401–406. [CrossRef] [PubMed]
16. Ebrahimi-Fakhari, D.; Sahin, M. Autism and the synapse: Emerging mechanisms and mechanism-based therapies. *Curr. Opin. Neurol.* **2015**, *28*, 91–102. [CrossRef] [PubMed]
17. Sztainberg, Y.; Zoghbi, H.Y. Lessons learned from studying syndromic autism spectrum disorders. *Nat. Neurosci.* **2016**, *19*, 1408–1418. [CrossRef] [PubMed]
18. Ronald, A.; Hoekstra, R.A. Autism spectrum disorders and autistic traits: A decade of new twin studies. *Am. J. Med. Genet. Part B Neuropsychiatr. Genet.* **2011**, *156*, 255–274. [CrossRef] [PubMed]
19. Sandin, S.; Lichtenstein, P.; Larsson, H.; Cm, H.; Reichenberg, A. The familial risk of autism. *JAMA* **2014**, *311*, 1770–1777. [CrossRef] [PubMed]
20. Gaugler, T.; Klei, L.; Sanders, S.J.; Bodea, C.A.; Goldberg, A.P.; Lee, A.B.; Mahajan, M.; Manaa, D.; Pawitan, Y.; Reichert, J.; et al. Most genetic risk for autism resides with common variation. *Nat. Genet.* **2014**, *46*, 881–885. [CrossRef] [PubMed]
21. State, M.W.; Levitt, P. The conundrums of understanding genetic risks for autism spectrum disorders. *Nat. Neurosci.* **2011**, *14*, 1499–1506. [CrossRef] [PubMed]
22. Devlin, B.; Scherer, S.W. Genetic architecture in autism spectrum disorder. *Curr. Opin. Genet. Dev.* **2012**, *22*, 229–237. [CrossRef] [PubMed]
23. Klei, L.; Sanders, S.J.; Murtha, M.T.; Hus, V.; Lowe, J.K.; Willsey, A.J.; Moreno-De-Luca, D.; Yu, T.W.; Fombonne, E.; Geschwind, D.; et al. Common genetic variants, acting additively, are a major source of risk for autism. *Mol. Autism* **2012**, *3*, 9. [CrossRef] [PubMed]
24. Sebat, J.; Lakshmi, B.; Malhotra, D.; Troge, J.; Lese-martin, C.; Walsh, T.; Yamrom, B.; Yoon, S.; Krasnitz, A.; Kendall, J.; et al. Strong Association of De Novo Copy Number Mutations with Autism. *Science* **2007**, *316*, 445–449. [CrossRef] [PubMed]
25. Glessner, J.; Wang, K.; Cai, G.; Korvatska, O. Autism genome-wide copy number variation reveals ubiquitin and neuronal genes. *Nature* **2009**, *459*, 569–573. [CrossRef] [PubMed]
26. Pinto, D.; Pagnamenta, A.T.; Klei, L.; Anney, R.; Merico, D.; Regan, R.; Conroy, J.; Magalhaes, T.R.; Correia, C.; Brett, S.; et al. Functional Impact of Global Rare Copy Number Variation in Autism Spectrum Disorder. *Nature* **2010**, *466*, 368–372. [CrossRef] [PubMed]
27. Betancur, C. Etiological heterogeneity in autism spectrum disorders: More than 100 genetic and genomic disorders and still counting. *Brain Res.* **2011**, *1380*, 42–77. [CrossRef] [PubMed]
28. Iossifov, I.; Ronemus, M.; Levy, D.; Wang, Z.; Hakker, I.; Yamrom, B.; Lee, Y.; Narzisi, G.; Leotta, A.; Grabowska, E.; et al. De novo Gene Disruptions in children on the Autistic Spectrum. *Neuron* **2012**, *74*, 285–299. [CrossRef] [PubMed]
29. Neale, B.; Kou, Y.; Liu, L.; Ma'ayan, A. Patterns and rates of exonic de novo mutations in autism spectrum disorders. *Nature* **2013**, *485*, 242–245. [CrossRef] [PubMed]

30. O'Roak, B.J.; Vives, L.; Girirajan, S.; Karakoc, E.; Krumm, N.; Coe, B.P.; Levy, R.; Ko, A.; Lee, C.; Smith, J.D.; et al. Sporadic autism exomes reveal a highly interconnected protein network of de novo mutations. *Nature* **2012**, *485*, 246–250. [CrossRef] [PubMed]
31. Sanders, S.J.; Murtha, M.T.; Gupta, A.R.; Murdoch, J.D.; Raubeson, M.J.; Willsey, A.J.; Ercan-Sencicek, A.G.; DiLullo, N.M.; Parikshak, N.N.; Stein, J.L.; et al. De novo mutations revealed by whole-exome sequencing are strongly associated with autism. *Nature* **2012**, *485*, 237–241. [CrossRef] [PubMed]
32. De Rubeis, S.; He, X.; Goldberg, A.P.; Poultney, C.S.; Samocha, K.; Ercument Cicek, A.; Kou, Y.; Liu, L.; Fromer, M.; Walker, S.; et al. Synaptic, transcriptional and chromatin genes disrupted in autism. *Nature* **2014**, *515*, 209–215. [CrossRef] [PubMed]
33. Ronemus, M.; Iossifov, I.; Levy, D.; Wigler, M. The role of de novo mutations in the genetics of autism spectrum disorders. *Nat. Rev. Genet.* **2014**, *15*, 133–141. [CrossRef] [PubMed]
34. Simons Foundation Autism Research Initiative (SFARI). Available online: https://gene.sfari.org (accessed on 16 March 2017).
35. Bourgeron, T. From the genetic architecture to synaptic plasticity in autism spectrum disorder. *Nat. Rev. Neurosci.* **2015**, *16*, 551–563. [CrossRef] [PubMed]
36. Gilman, S.R.; Iossifov, I.; Levy, D.; Ronemus, M.; Wigler, M.; Vitkup, D. Rare De Novo Variants Associated with Autism Implicate a Large Functional Network of Genes Involved in Formation and Function of Synapses. *Neuron* **2011**, *70*, 898–907. [CrossRef]
37. Baudouin, S.J.; Gaudias, J.; Gerharz, S.; Hatstatt, L.; Zhou, K.; Punnakkal, P.; Tanaka, K.F.; Spooren, W.; Hen, R.; De Zeeuw, C.I.; et al. Shared Synaptic Pathophysiology in Syndromic and Nonsyndromic Rodent Models of Autism. *Science* **2012**, *338*, 128–132. [CrossRef] [PubMed]
38. Pinto, D.; Delaby, E.; Merico, D.; Barbosa, M.; Merikangas, A.; Klei, L.; Thiruvahindrapuram, B.; Xu, X.; Ziman, R.; Wang, Z.; et al. Convergence of Genes and Cellular Pathways Dysregulated in Autism Spectrum Disorders. *Am. J. Hum. Genet.* **2014**, *94*, 677–694. [CrossRef] [PubMed]
39. Costa-Mattioli, M.; Monteggia, L.M. mTOR complexes in neurodevelopmental and neuropsychiatric disorders. *Nat. Neurosci* **2013**, *16*, 1537–1543. [CrossRef] [PubMed]
40. Lipton, J.O.; Sahin, M. The Neurology of mTOR. *Neuron* **2014**, *84*, 275–291. [CrossRef] [PubMed]
41. Ehninger, D.; Silva, A.J. Rapamycin for treating Tuberous sclerosis and Autism spectrum disorders. *Trends Mol. Med.* **2011**, *17*, 78–87. [CrossRef] [PubMed]
42. Huber, K.M.; Klann, E.; Costa-Mattioli, M.; Zukin, R.S. Dysregulation of Mammalian Target of Rapamycin Signaling in Mouse Models of Autism. *J. Neurosci.* **2015**, *35*, 13836–13842. [CrossRef] [PubMed]
43. Ricciardi, S.; Boggio, E.M.; Grosso, S.; Lonetti, G.; Forlani, G.; Stefanelli, G.; Calcagno, E.; Morello, N.; Landsberger, N.; Biffo, S.; et al. Reduced AKT/mTOR signaling and protein synthesis dysregulation in a Rett syndrome animal model. *Hum. Mol. Genet.* **2011**, *20*, 1182–1196. [CrossRef] [PubMed]
44. Sun, J.; Liu, Y.; Moreno, S.; Baudry, M.; Bi, X. Imbalanced Mechanistic Target of Rapamycin C1 and C2 Activity in the Cerebellum of Angelman Syndrome Mice Impairs Motor Function. *J. Neurosci.* **2015**, *35*, 4706–4718. [CrossRef] [PubMed]
45. Sun, J.; Liu, Y.; Tran, J.; O'Neal, P.; Baudry, M.; Bi, X. mTORC1-S6K1 inhibition or mTORC2 activation improves hippocampal synaptic plasticity and learning in Angelman syndrome mice. *Cell. Mol. Life Sci.* **2016**, *73*, 4303–4314. [CrossRef] [PubMed]
46. Jiang, M.; Ash, R.T.; Baker, S.A.; Suter, B.; Ferguson, A.; Park, J.; Rudy, J.; Torsky, S.P.; Chao, H.-T.; Zoghbi, H.Y.; et al. Dendritic arborization and spine dynamics are abnormal in the mouse model of MECP2 duplication syndrome. *J. Neurosci.* **2013**, *33*, 19518–19533. [CrossRef] [PubMed]
47. Della Sala, G.; Putignano, E.; Chelini, G.; Melani, R.; Calcagno, E.; Michele Ratto, G.; Amendola, E.; Gross, C.T.; Giustetto, M.; Pizzorusso, T. Dendritic Spine Instability in a Mouse Model of CDKL5 Disorder Is Rescued by Insulin-like Growth Factor 1. *Biol. Psychiatry* **2016**, *80*, 302–311. [CrossRef] [PubMed]
48. Neves-Pereira, M.; Müller, B.; Massie, D.; Williams, J.H.G.; O'Brien, P.C.M.; Hughes, A.; Shen, S.-B.; Clair, D.S.; Miedzybrodzka, Z. Deregulation of EIF4E: A novel mechanism for autism. *J. Med. Genet.* **2009**, *46*, 759–765. [CrossRef] [PubMed]
49. Gkogkas, C.G.; Khoutorsky, A.; Ran, I.; Rampakakis, E.; Nevarko, T.; Weatherill, D.B.; Vasuta, C.; Yee, S.; Truitt, M.; Dallaire, P.; et al. Autism-related deficits via dysregulated eIF4E-dependent translational control. *Nature* **2013**, *493*, 371–377. [CrossRef] [PubMed]

50. Santini, E.; Huynh, T.N.; Macaskill, A.F.; Carter, A.G.; Pierre, P.; Ruggero, D.; Kaphzan, H.; Klann, E. Exaggerated Translation Causes Synaptic and Behavioural Aberrations Associated with Autism. *Nature* **2013**, *493*, 411–415. [CrossRef] [PubMed]
51. Tang, G.; Gudsnuk, K.; Kuo, S.H.; Cotrina, M.L.; Rosoklija, G.; Sosunov, A.; Sonders, M.S.; Kanter, E.; Castagna, C.; Yamamoto, A.; et al. Loss of mTOR-Dependent Macroautophagy Causes Autistic-like Synaptic Pruning Deficits. *Neuron* **2014**, *83*, 1131–1143. [CrossRef] [PubMed]
52. Oguro-Ando, A.; Rosensweig, C.; Herman, E.; Nishimura, Y.; Werling, D.; Bill, B.R.; Berg, J.M.; Gao, F.; Coppola, G.; Abrahams, B.S.; et al. Increased CYFIP1 dosage alters cellular and dendritic morphology and dysregulates mTOR. *Mol. Psychiatry* **2015**, *20*, 1069–1078. [CrossRef] [PubMed]
53. Suzuki, A.M.; Griesi-Oliveira, K.; de Oliveira Freitas Machado, C.; Vadasz, E.; Zachi, E.C.; Passos-Bueno, M.R.; Sertie, A.L. Altered mTORC1 signaling in multipotent stem cells from nearly 25% of patients with nonsyndromic autism spectrum disorders. *Mol. Psychiatry* **2015**, *20*, 551–552. [CrossRef] [PubMed]
54. Nicolini, C.; Ahn, Y.; Michalski, B.; Rho, J.M.; Fahnestock, M. Decreased mTOR signaling pathway in human idiopathic autism and in rats exposed to valproic acid. *Acta Neuropathol. Commun.* **2015**, *3*, 3. [CrossRef] [PubMed]
55. Poopal, A.C.; Schroeder, L.M.; Horn, P.S.; Bassell, G.J.; Gross, C. Increased expression of the PI3K catalytic subunit p110δ underlies elevated S6 phosphorylation and protein synthesis in an individual with autism from a multiplex family. *Mol. Autism* **2016**, *7*, 3. [CrossRef] [PubMed]
56. The European Chromosome 16 Tuberous Sclerosis Consortium. Identification and Characterization of the Tuberous Sclerosis Gene on Chromosome 16. *Cell* **1993**, *75*, 1305–1315.
57. Slegtenhorst, V.; de Hoogt, R.; Hermans, C.; Nellist, M.; Janssen, B.; Verhoef, S.; Lindhout, D.; van den Ouweland, AH.D.; Young, J.; Burley, M.; et al. Identification of the Tuberous Sclerosis Gene TSC1 on Chromosome 9q34. *Science* **1997**, *277*, 805–808. [CrossRef] [PubMed]
58. Dibble, C.C.; Elis, W.; Menon, S.; Qin, W.; Klekota, J.; Asara, J.M.; Finan, P.M.; Kwiatkowski, D.J.; Murphy, L.O.; Manning, B.D. TBC1D7 Is a Third Subunit of the TSC1-TSC2 Complex Upstream of mTORC1. *Mol. Cell* **2012**, *47*, 535–546. [CrossRef] [PubMed]
59. Garami, A.; Zwartkruis, F.J.T.; Nobukuni, T.; Joaquin, M.; Roccio, M.; Stocker, H.; Kozma, S.C.; Hafen, E.; Bos, J.L.; Thomas, G. Insulin Activation of Rheb, a Mediator of mTOR/S6K/4E-BP Signaling, Is Inhibited by TSC1 and 2. *Mol. Cell* **2003**, *11*, 1457–1466. [CrossRef]
60. Tee, A.R.; Manning, B.D.; Roux, P.P.; Cantley, L.C.; Blenis1, J. Tuberous Sclerosis Complex Gene Products, Tuberin and Hamartin, Control mTOR Signaling by Acting as a GTPase-Activating Protein Complex toward Rheb. *Curr. Biol.* **2003**, *13*, 1259–1268. [CrossRef]
61. Curatolo, P.; Bombardieri, R.; Jozwiak, S. Tuberous sclerosis. *Lancet* **2008**, *372*, 657–668. [CrossRef]
62. Curatolo, P.; Moavero, R. mTOR Inhibitors in Tuberous Sclerosis Complex. *Curr. Neuropharmacol.* **2012**, *10*, 404–415. [CrossRef] [PubMed]
63. Richards, C.; Jones, C.; Groves, L.; Moss, J.; Oliver, C. Prevalence of autism spectrum disorder phenomenology in genetic disorders: A systematic review and meta-analysis. *Lancet Psychiatry* **2015**, *2*, 909–916. [CrossRef]
64. Chu-Shore, C.J.; Major, P.; Camposano, S.; Muzykewicz, D.; Thiele, E.A. The natural history of epilepsy in tuberous sclerosis complex. *Epilepsia* **2010**, *51*, 1236–1241. [CrossRef] [PubMed]
65. Wang, Y.; Greenwood, J.S.F.; Calcagnotto, M.E.; Kirsch, H.E.; Barbaro, N.M.; Baraban, S.C. Neocortical Hyperexcitability in a Human Case of Tuberous Sclerosis Complex and Mice Lacking Neuronal Expression of TSC1. *Ann. Neurol.* **2007**, *61*, 139–152. [CrossRef] [PubMed]
66. Talos, D.M.; Kwiatkowski, D.J.; Cordero, K.; Black, P.M.; Jensen, F.E. Cell-Specific Alterations of Glutamate Receptor Expression in Tuberous Sclerosis Complex Cortical Tubers. *Ann. Neurol.* **2008**, *63*, 454–465. [CrossRef] [PubMed]
67. Ruppe, V.; Dilsiz, P.; Reiss, C.S.; Carlson, C.; Devinsky, O.; Zagzag, D.; Weiner, H.L.; Talos, D.M. Developmental brain abnormalities in tuberous sclerosis complex: A comparative tissue analysis of cortical tubers and perituberal cortex. *Epilepsia* **2014**, *55*, 539–550. [CrossRef] [PubMed]
68. Uhlmann, E.J.; Wong, M.; Baldwin, R.L.; Bajenaru, M.L.; Onda, H.; Kwiatkowski, D.J.; Yamada, K.; Gutmann, D.H. Astrocyte-Specific TSC1 Conditional Knockout Mice Exhibit Abnormal Neuronal Organization and Seizures. *Ann. Neurol.* **2002**, *52*, 285–296. [CrossRef] [PubMed]
69. Zeng, L.H.; Xu, L.; Gutmann, D.H.; Wong, M. Rapamycin prevents epilepsy in a mouse model of tuberous sclerosis complex. *Ann. Neurol.* **2008**, *63*, 444–453. [CrossRef] [PubMed]

70. Zeng, L.H.; Rensing, N.R.; Zhang, B.; Gutmann, D.H.; Gambello, M.J.; Wong, M. Tsc2 gene inactivation causes a more severe epilepsy phenotype than Tsc1 inactivation in a mouse model of Tuberous Sclerosis Complex. *Hum. Mol. Genet.* **2011**, *20*, 445–454. [CrossRef] [PubMed]
71. Fu, C.; Ess, K.C. Conditional and domain-specific inactivation of the Tsc2 gene in neural progenitor cells. *Genesis* **2013**, *51*, 284–292. [CrossRef] [PubMed]
72. Magri, L.; Cambiaghi, M.; Cominelli, M.; Alfaro-Cervello, C.; Cursi, M.; Pala, M.; Bulfone, A.; Garca-Verdugo, J.M.; Leocani, L.; Minicucci, F.; et al. Sustained Activation of mTOR Pathway in Embryonic Neural Stem Cells Leads to Development of Tuberous Sclerosis Complex-Associated Lesions. *Cell Stem Cell* **2011**, *9*, 447–462. [CrossRef] [PubMed]
73. Crowell, B.; Hwa Lee, G.; Nikolaeva, I.; Dal Pozzo, V.; D'Arcangelo, G. Complex Neurological Phenotype in Mutant Mice Lacking Tsc2 in Excitatory Neurons of the Developing Forebrain. *eNeuro* **2015**, *2*. [CrossRef] [PubMed]
74. Moon, U.Y.; Park, J.Y.; Park, R.; Cho, J.Y.; Hughes, L.J.; McKenna, J.; Goetzl, L.; Cho, S.-H.; Crino, P.B.; Gambello, M.J.; et al. Impaired Reelin-Dab1 Signaling Contributes to Neuronal Migration Deficits of Tuberous Sclerosis Complex. *Cell Rep.* **2015**, *12*, 965–978. [CrossRef] [PubMed]
75. Tavazoie, S.F.; Alvarez, V.A.; Ridenour, D.A.; Kwiatkowski, D.J.; Sabatini, B.L. Regulation of neuronal morphology and function by the tumor suppressors Tsc1 and Tsc2. *Nat. Neurosci.* **2005**, *8*, 1727–1734. [CrossRef] [PubMed]
76. Meikle, L.; Pollizzi, K.; Egnor, A.; Kramvis, I.; Lane, H.; Sahin, M.; Kwiatkowski, D.J. Response of a Neuronal Model of Tuberous Sclerosis to Mammalian Target of Rapamycin (mTOR) Inhibitors: Effects on mTORC1 and Akt Signaling Lead to Improved Survival and Function. *J. Neurosci.* **2008**, *28*, 5422–5432. [CrossRef] [PubMed]
77. Tsai, P.T.; Hull, C.; Chu, Y.; Greene-Colozzi, E.; Sadowski, A.R.; Leech, J.M.; Steinberg, J.; Crawley, J.N.; Regehr, W.G.; Sahin, M. Autistic-like behaviour and cerebellar dysfunction in Purkinje cell Tsc1 mutant mice. *Nature* **2012**, *488*, 647–651. [CrossRef] [PubMed]
78. Choi, Y.; Di Nardo, A.; Kramvis, I.; Meikle, L.; Kwiatkowski, D.J.; Sahin, M.; He, X. Tuberous sclerosis complex proteins control axon formation. *Genes Dev.* **2008**, *22*, 2485–2495. [CrossRef] [PubMed]
79. Ebrahimi-fakhari, D.; Saffari, A.; Wahlster, L.; Di Nardo, A.; Turner, D.; Lewis, T.L., Jr.; Conrad, C.; Rothberg, J.M.; Jonathan, O.; Kölker, S.; et al. Impaired Mitochondrial Dynamics and Mitophagy in Neuronal Models of Tuberous Sclerosis Complex. *Cell Rep.* **2016**, *17*, 1053–1070. [CrossRef] [PubMed]
80. Bateup, H.S.; Takasaki, K.T.; Saulnier, J.L.; Denefrio, C.L.; Sabatini, B.L. Loss of Tsc1 In Vivo Impairs Hippocampal mGluR-LTD and Increases Excitatory Synaptic Function. *J. Neurosci.* **2011**, *31*, 8862–8869. [CrossRef] [PubMed]
81. Bateup, H.S.; Johnson, C.A.; Denefrio, C.L.; Saulnier, J.L.; Kornacker, K.; Sabatini, B.L. Excitatory/Inhibitory Synaptic Imbalance Leads to Hippocampal Hyperexcitability in Mouse Models of Tuberous Sclerosis. *Neuron* **2013**, *78*, 510–522. [CrossRef] [PubMed]
82. Von Der Brelie, C.; Waltereit, R.; Zhang, L.; Beck, H.; Kirschstein, T. Impaired synaptic plasticity in a rat model of tuberous sclerosis. *Eur. J. Neurosci.* **2006**, *23*, 686–692. [CrossRef] [PubMed]
83. Zeng, L.H.; Ouyang, Y.; Gazit, V.; Cirrito, J.R.; Jansen, L.A.; Ess, K.C.; Yamada, K.A.; Wozniak, D.F.; Holtzman, D.M.; Gutmann, D.H.; et al. Abnormal glutamate homeostasis and impaired synaptic plasticity and learning in a mouse model of tuberous sclerosis complex. *Neurobiol. Dis.* **2007**, *28*, 184–196. [CrossRef] [PubMed]
84. Auerbach, B.D.; Osterweil, E.K.; Bear, M.F. Mutations causing syndromic autism define an axis of synaptic pathophysiology. *Nature* **2011**, *480*, 63–68. [CrossRef] [PubMed]
85. Yasuda, S.; Sugiura, H.; Katsurabayashi, S.; Shimada, T.; Tanaka, H.; Takasaki, K.; Iwasaki, K.; Kobayashi, T.; Hino, O.; Yamagata, K. Activation of Rheb, but not of mTORC1, impairs spine synapse morphogenesis in tuberous sclerosis complex. *Sci. Rep.* **2014**, *4*, 5155. [CrossRef] [PubMed]
86. Nie, D.; Chen, Z.; Ebrahimi-Fakhari, D.; Di Nardo, A.; Julich, K.; Robson, V.K.; Cheng, Y.-C.; Woolf, C.J.; Heiman, M.; Sahin, M. The Stress-Induced Atf3-Gelsolin Cascade Underlies Dendritic Spine Deficits in Neuronal Models of Tuberous Sclerosis Complex. *J. Neurosci.* **2015**, *35*, 10762–10772. [CrossRef] [PubMed]
87. Ehninger, D.; Han, S.; Shilyansky, C.; Zhou, Y.; Li, W.; David, J. Reversal of learning deficits in a Tsc2+/− mouse model of tuberous sclerosis. *Nat. Med.* **2008**, *14*, 843–848. [CrossRef] [PubMed]

88. Sato, A.; Kasai, S.; Kobayashi, T.; Takamatsu, Y.; Hino, O.; Ikeda, K.; Mizuguchi, M. Rapamycin reverses impaired social interaction in mouse models of tuberous sclerosis complex. *Nat. Commun.* **2012**, *3*, 1292. [CrossRef] [PubMed]
89. Ercan, E.; Han, J.M.; Di Nardo, A.; Winden, K.; Han, M.-J.; Hoyo, L.; Saffari, A.; Leask, A.; Geschwind, D.H.; Sahin, M. Neuronal CTGF/CCN2 negatively regulates myelination in a mouse model of tuberous sclerosis complex. *J. Exp. Med.* **2017**, *214*, 681–697. [CrossRef] [PubMed]
90. Verstreken, P.; Ly, C.V.; Venken, K.J. T.; Koh, T.W.; Zhou, Y.; Bellen, H.J. Synaptic mitochondria are critical for mobilization of reserve pool vesicles at Drosophila neuromuscular junctions. *Neuron* **2005**, *47*, 365–378. [CrossRef] [PubMed]
91. Ma, H.; Cai, Q.; Lu, W.; Sheng, Z.-H.; Mochida, S. KIF5B Motor Adaptor Syntabulin Maintains Synaptic Transmission in Sympathetic Neurons. *J. Neurosci.* **2009**, *29*, 13019–13029. [CrossRef] [PubMed]
92. Di Nardo, A.; Wertz, M.H.; Kwiatkowski, E.; Tsai, P.T.; Leech, J.D.; Greene-Colozzi, E.; Goto, J.; Dilsiz, P.; Talos, D.M.; Clish, C.B.; et al. Neuronal Tsc1/2 complex controls autophagy through AMPK-dependent regulation of ULK1. *Hum. Mol. Genet.* **2014**, *23*, 3865–3874. [CrossRef] [PubMed]
93. Rossignol, D.A.; Frye, R.E. Evidence linking oxidative stress, mitochondrial dysfunction, and inflammation in the brain of individuals with autism. *Front. Physiol.* **2014**, *5*, 150. [CrossRef] [PubMed]
94. Buxbaum, J.D.; Cai, G.; Chaste, P.; Nygren, G.; Goldsmith, J.; Reichert, J.; Anckarsäter, H.; Rastam, M.; Smith, C.J.; Silverman, J.M.; et al. Mutation Screening of the PTEN Gene in Patients With Autism Spectrum Disorders and Macrocephaly. *Am. J. Med. Genet. Part B Neuropsychiatr. Genet.* **2007**, *144*, 484–491. [CrossRef] [PubMed]
95. McBride, K.L.; Varga, E.A.; Pastore, M.T.; Prior, T.W.; Manickam, K.; Atkin, J.F.; Herman, G.E. Confirmation study of PTEN mutations among individuals with autism or developmental delays/mental retardation and macrocephaly. *Autism Res.* **2010**, *3*, 137–141. [CrossRef] [PubMed]
96. Varga, E.A.; Pastore, M.; Prior, T.; Herman, G.E.; McBride, K.L. The prevalence of PTEN mutations in a clinical pediatric cohort with autism spectrum disorders, developmental delay, and macrocephaly. *Genet. Med.* **2009**, *11*, 111–117. [CrossRef] [PubMed]
97. Hobert, J.A.; Embacher, R.; Mester, J.L.; Frazier, T.W.; Eng, C. Biochemical screening and PTEN mutation analysis in individuals with autism spectrum disorders and macrocephaly. *Eur. J. Hum. Genet.* **2014**, *22*, 273–276. [CrossRef] [PubMed]
98. Song, M.S.; Salmena, L.; Pandolfi, P.P. The functions and regulation of the PTEN tumour suppressor. *Nat. Rev. Mol. Cell. Biol.* **2012**, *13*, 283–296. [CrossRef] [PubMed]
99. Maehama, A.J.; Dixon, J.E. The Tumor Suppressor PTEN/MMAC1, Dephosphorylates the Lipid Second Messenger, Phosphatidylinositol 3,4,5-Trisphosphate. *J. Biol. Chem.* **1998**, *273*, 13375–13379. [CrossRef] [PubMed]
100. Zhou, J.; Blundell, J.; Ogawa, S.; Kwon, C.-H.; Zhang, W.; Sinton, C.; Powell, C.M.; Parada, L.F. Pharmacological inhibition of mTORC1 suppresses anatomical, cellular, and behavioral abnormalities in neural-specific Pten knock-out mice. *J. Neurosci.* **2009**, *29*, 1773–1783. [CrossRef] [PubMed]
101. Vanderver, A.; Tonduti, D.; Kahn, I.; Schmidt, J.; Medne, L.; Vento, J.; Chapman, K.A.; Lanpher, B.; Pearl, P.; Gropman, A.; et al. Characteristic brain magnetic resonance imaging pattern in patients with macrocephaly and PTEN mutations. *Am. J. Med. Genet. Part A* **2014**, *164*, 627–633. [CrossRef] [PubMed]
102. Jansen, L.A.; Mirzaa, G.M.; Ishak, G.E.; O'Roak, B.J.; Hiatt, J.B.; Roden, W.H.; Gunter, S.A.; Christian, S.L.; Collins, S.; Adams, C.; et al. PI3K/AKT pathway mutations cause a spectrum of brain malformations from megalencephaly to focal cortical dysplasia. *Brain* **2015**, *138*, 1613–1628. [CrossRef] [PubMed]
103. Conti, S.; Condo, M.; Posar, A.; Mari, F.; Resta, N.; Renieri, A.; Neri, I.; Patrizi, A.; Parmeggiani, A. Phosphatase and Tensin Homolog (PTEN) Gene Mutations and Autism: Literature Review and a Case Report of a Patient With Cowden Syndrome, Autistic Disorder, and Epilepsy. *J. Child Neurol.* **2012**, *27*, 392–397. [CrossRef] [PubMed]
104. Marchese, M.; Conti, V.; Valvo, G.; Moro, F.; Muratori, F.; Tancredi, R.; Santorelli, F.M.; Guerrini, R.; Sicca, F. Autism-epilepsy phenotype with macrocephaly suggests PTEN, but not GLIALCAM, genetic screening. *BMC Med. Genet.* **2014**, *15*, 26. [CrossRef] [PubMed]
105. Fraser, M.M.; Zhu, X.; Kwon, C.H.; Uhlmann, E.J.; Gutmann, D.H.; Baker, S.J. Pten loss causes hypertrophy and increased proliferation of astrocytes in vivo. *Cancer Res.* **2004**, *64*, 7773–7779. [CrossRef] [PubMed]

106. Kwon, C.H.; Luikart, B.W.; Powell, C.M.; Zhou, J.; Matheny, S.A.; Zhang, W.; Li, Y.; Baker, S.J.; Parada, L.F. Pten Regulates Neuronal Arborization and Social Interaction in Mice. *Neuron* **2006**, *50*, 377–388. [CrossRef] [PubMed]
107. Fraser, M.M.; Bayazitov, I.T.; Zakharenko, S.S.; Baker, S.J. Phosphatase and tensin homolog, deleted on chromosome 10 deficiency in brain causes defects in synaptic structure, transmission and plasticity, and myelination abnormalities. *Neuroscience* **2008**, *151*, 476–488. [CrossRef] [PubMed]
108. Luikart, B.W.; Schnell, E.; Washburn, E.K.; Bensen, A.L.; Tovar, K.R.; Westbrook, G.L. Pten Knockdown In Vivo Increases Excitatory Drive onto Dentate Granule Cells. *J. Neurosci.* **2011**, *31*, 4345–4354. [CrossRef] [PubMed]
109. Williams, M.R.; DeSpenza, T.; Li, M.; Gulledge, A.T.; Luikart, B.W. Hyperactivity of Newborn Pten Knock-out Neurons Results from Increased Excitatory Synaptic Drive. *J. Neurosci.* **2015**, *35*, 943–959. [CrossRef] [PubMed]
110. Huang, W.-C.; Chen, Y.; Page, D.T. Hyperconnectivity of prefrontal cortex to amygdala projections in a mouse model of macrocephaly/autism syndrome. *Nat. Commun.* **2016**, *7*, 13421. [CrossRef] [PubMed]
111. Marino, S.; Krimpenfort, P.; Leung, C.; van der Korput, H.A.G.M.; Trapman, J.; Camenisch, I.; Berns, A.; Brandner, S. PTEN is essential for cell migration but not for fate determination and tumourigenesis in the cerebellum. *Development* **2002**, *129*, 3513–3522. [PubMed]
112. Getz, S.A.; DeSpenza, T.; Li, M.; Luikart, B.W. Rapamycin prevents, but does not reverse, aberrant migration in Pten knockout neurons. *Neurobiol. Dis.* **2016**, *93*, 12–20. [CrossRef] [PubMed]
113. Takeuchi, K.; Gertner, M.J.; Zhou, J.; Parada, L.F.; Bennett, M.V.L.; Zukin, R.S. Dysregulation of synaptic plasticity precedes appearance of morphological defects in a Pten conditional knockout mouse model of autism. *Proc. Natl. Acad. Sci. USA* **2013**, *110*, 4738–4743. [CrossRef] [PubMed]
114. Garg, S.; Green, J.; Leadbitter, K.; Emsley, R.; Lehtonen, A.; Evans, G.; Huson, S.M. Neurofibromatosis type 1 and autism spectrum disorder. *Pediatrics* **2013**, *132*, e1642–e1648. [CrossRef] [PubMed]
115. Xu, G.; Lin, B.; Tanaka, K.; Dunn, D.; Wood, D.; Gesteland, R.; White, R.; Weiss, R.; Tamanoi, F. The catalytic domain of the neurofibromatosis type 1 gene product stimulates ras GTPase and complements ira mutants of *S. cerevisiae*. *Cell* **1990**, *63*, 835–841. [CrossRef]
116. Cawthon, R.M.; Weiss, R.; Xu, G.; Viskochil, D.; Culver, M.; Stevens, J.; Robertson, M.; Dunn, D.; Gesteland, R.; O'Connell, P.; et al. A major segment of the neurofibromatosis type 1 gene: cDNA sequence, genomic structure, and point mutations. *Cell* **1990**, *62*, 193–201. [CrossRef]
117. Johannessen, C.M.; Reczek, E.E.; James, M.F.; Brems, H.; Legius, E.; Cichowski, K. The NF1 tumor suppressor critically regulates TSC2 and mTOR. *Proc. Natl. Acad. Sci. USA* **2005**, *102*, 8573–8578. [CrossRef] [PubMed]
118. Dasgupta, B.; Yi, Y.; Chen, D.Y.; Weber, J.D.; Gutmann, D.H. Proteomic Analysis Reveals Hyperactivation of the Mammalian Target of Rapamycin Pathway in Neurofibromatosis 1—Associated Human and Mouse Brain Tumors. *Cancer Res.* **2005**, *65*, 2755–2760. [CrossRef] [PubMed]
119. Banerjee, S.; Crouse, N.R.; Emnett, R.J.; Gianino, S.M.; Gutmann, D.H. Neurofibromatosis-1 regulates mTOR-mediated astrocyte growth and glioma formation in a TSC/Rheb-independent manner. *Proc. Natl. Acad. Sci. USA* **2011**, *108*, 15996–16001. [CrossRef] [PubMed]
120. Kulkantrakorn, K.; Geller, T.J. Seizures in neurofibromatosis 1. *Pediatr. Neurol.* **1998**, *19*, 347–350. [CrossRef]
121. Vivarelli, R.; Grosso, S.; Calabrese, F.; Farnetani, M.; Di, B.R.; Morgese, G.; Balestri, P. Epilepsy in neurofibromatosis 1. *J. Child Neurol.* **2003**, *18*, 338–342. [CrossRef] [PubMed]
122. Ostendorf, A.P.; Gutmann, D.H.; Weisenberg, J.L.Z. Epilepsy in individuals with neurofibromatosis type 1. *Epilepsia* **2013**, *54*, 1810–1814. [CrossRef] [PubMed]
123. Moore, B.D.; Slopis, J.M.; Jackson, E.F.; De Winter, A.E.; Leeds, N.E. Brain volume in children with neurofibromatosis type 1. *Neurology* **2000**, *54*, 914–920. [CrossRef] [PubMed]
124. Cutting, L.E.; Koth, C.W.; Burnette, C.P.; Abrams, M.T.; Kaufmann, W.E.; Denckla, M.B. Relationship of Cognitive Functioning, Whole Brain Volumes, and T2-Weighted Hyperintensities in Neurofibromatosis-1. *J. Child Neurol.* **2000**, *15*, 157–160. [CrossRef] [PubMed]
125. Margariti, P.N.; Blekas, K.; Katzioti, F.G.; Zikou, A.K.; Tzoufi, M.; Argyropoulou, M.I. Magnetization transfer ratio and volumetric analysis of the brain in macrocephalic patients with neurofibromatosis type 1. *Eur. Radiol.* **2007**, *17*, 433–438. [CrossRef] [PubMed]
126. Karlsgodt, K.H.; Rosser, T.; Lutkenhoff, E.S.; Cannon, T.D.; Silva, A.; Bearden, C.E. Alterations in White Matter Microstructure in Neurofibromatosis-1. *PLoS ONE* **2012**, *7*, e47854. [CrossRef] [PubMed]

127. Petrella, L.I.; Cai, Y.; Sereno, J.V.; Gon??alves, S.I.; Silva, A.J.; Castelo-Branco, M. Brain and behaviour phenotyping of a mouse model of neurofibromatosis type-1: An MRI/DTI study on social cognition. *Genes Brain Behav.* **2016**, *15*, 637–646. [CrossRef] [PubMed]
128. Korf, B.R.; Schneider, G.; Poussaint, T.Y. Structural anomalies revealed by neuroimaging studies in the brains of patients with neurofibromatosis type 1 and large deletions. *Genet. Med.* **1999**, *1*, 136–140. [CrossRef] [PubMed]
129. Balestri, P.; Vivarelli, R.; Grosso, S.; Santori, L.; Farnetani, M.A.; Galluzzi, P.; Vatti, G.P.; Calabrese, F.; Morgese, G. Malformations of cortical development in neurofibromatosis type 1. *Neurology* **2003**, *61*, 1799–1801. [CrossRef] [PubMed]
130. Huijbregts, S.C.; Loitfelder, M.; Rombouts, S.A.; Swaab, H.; Verbist, B.M.; Arkink, E.B.; van Buchem, M.A.; Veer, I.M. Cerebral volumetric abnormalities in Neurofibromatosis type 1: Associations with parent ratings of social and attention problems, executive dysfunction, and autistic mannerisms. *J. Neurodev. Disord.* **2015**, *7*, 32. [CrossRef] [PubMed]
131. Kim, E.; Wang, Y.; Kim, S.-J.; Bornhorst, M.; Jecrois, E.S.; Anthony, T.E.; Wang, C.; Li, Y.E.; Guan, J.-L.; Murphy, G.G.; et al. Transient inhibition of the ERK pathway prevents cerebellar developmental defects and improves long-term motor functions in murine models of neurofibromatosis type 1. *Elife* **2014**, *3*, e05151. [CrossRef] [PubMed]
132. Sanchez-Ortiz, E.; Cho, W.; Nazarenko, I.; Mo, W.; Chen, J.; Parada, L.F. NF1 regulation of RAS/ERK signaling is required for appropriate granule neuron progenitor expansion and migration in cerebellar development. *Genes Dev.* **2014**, *28*, 2407–2420. [CrossRef] [PubMed]
133. Bajenaru, M.L.; Zhu, Y.; Hedrick, N.M.; Donahoe, J.; Parada, L.F.; Gutmann, D.H. Astrocyte-specific inactivation of the neurofibromatosis 1 gene (NF1) is insufficient for astrocytoma formation. *Mol. Cell. Biol.* **2002**, *22*, 5100–5113. [CrossRef] [PubMed]
134. Hegedus, B.; Dasgupta, B.; Shin, J.E.; Emnett, R.J.; Hart-Mahon, E.K.; Elghazi, L.; Bernal-Mizrachi, E.; Gutmann, D.H. Neurofibromatosis-1 Regulates Neuronal and Glial Cell Differentiation from Neuroglial Progenitors In Vivo by Both cAMP- and Ras-Dependent Mechanisms. *Cell Stem Cell* **2007**, *1*, 443–457. [CrossRef] [PubMed]
135. Brown, J.A.; Gianino, S.M.; Gutmann, D.H. Defective cAMP generation underlies the sensitivity of CNS neurons to neurofibromatosis-1 heterozygosity. *J. Neurosci.* **2010**, *30*, 5579–5589. [CrossRef] [PubMed]
136. Lin, Y.L.; Lei, Y.T.; Hong, C.J.; Hsueh, Y.P. Syndecan-2 induces filopodia and dendritic spine formation via the neurofibromin-PKA-Ena/VASP pathway. *J. Cell Biol.* **2007**, *177*, 829–841. [CrossRef] [PubMed]
137. Wang, H.F.; Shih, Y.T.; Chen, C.Y.; Chao, H.W.; Lee, M.J.; Hsueh, Y.P. Valosin-containing protein and neurofibromin interact to regulate dendritic spine density. *J. Clin. Investig.* **2011**, *121*, 4820–4837. [CrossRef] [PubMed]
138. Costa, R.M.; Federov, N.B.; Kogan, J.H.; Murphy, G.G.; Stern, J.; Ohno, M.; Kucherlapati, R.; Jacks, T.; Silva, A.J. Mechanism for the learning deficits in a mouse model of neurofibromatosis type 1. *Nature* **2002**, *415*, 526–530. [CrossRef] [PubMed]
139. Guilding, C.; McNair, K.; Stone, T.W.; Morris, B.J. Restored plasticity in a mouse model of neurofibromatosis type 1 via inhibition of hyperactive ERK and CREB. *Eur. J. Neurosci.* **2007**, *25*, 99–105. [CrossRef] [PubMed]
140. Weiss, B.; Widemann, B.C.; Wolters, P.; Dombi, E.; Vinks, A.; Cantor, A.; Perentesis, J.; Schorry, E.; Ullrich, N.; Gutmann, D.H.; et al. Sirolimus for progressive neurofibromatosis type 1-associated plexiform neurofibromas: A neurofibromatosis clinical trials consortium phase II study. *Neurol. Oncol.* **2015**, *17*, 596–603. [CrossRef] [PubMed]
141. Hua, C.; Zehou, O.; Ducassou, S.; Minard-Colin, V.; Hamel-Teillac, D.; Wolkenstein, P.; Valeyrie-Allanore, L. Sirolimus Improves Pain in NF1 Patients with Severe Plexiform Neurofibromas. *Pediatrics* **2014**, *133*, e1792–e1797. [CrossRef] [PubMed]
142. Johannessen, C.M.; Johnson, B.W.; Williams, S.M.G.; Chan, A.W.; Reczek, E.E.; Lynch, R.C.; Rioth, M.J.; McClatchey, A.; Ryeom, S.; Cichowski, K. TORC1 Is Essential for NF1-Associated Malignancies. *Curr. Biol.* **2008**, *18*, 56–62. [CrossRef] [PubMed]
143. Bhola, P.; Banerjee, S.; Mukherjee, J.; Balasubramanium, A.; Arun, V.; Karim, Z.; Burrell, K.; Croul, S.; Gutmann, D.H.; Guha, A. Preclinical in vivo evaluation of rapamycin in human malignant peripheral nerve sheath explant xenograft. *Int. J. Cancer* **2010**, *126*, 563–571. [CrossRef] [PubMed]

144. Zhu, Y.; Romero, M.I.; Ghosh, P.; Ye, Z.; Charnay, P.; Rushing, E.J.; Marth, J.D.; Parada, L.F. Ablation of NF1 function in neurons induces abnormal development of cerebral cortex and reactive gliosis in the brain. *Genes Dev.* **2001**, *15*, 859–876. [CrossRef] [PubMed]
145. Hagerman, R.; Hoem, G.; Hagerman, P. Fragile X and autism: Intertwined at the molecular level leading to targeted treatments. *Mol. Autism* **2010**, *1*, 12. [CrossRef] [PubMed]
146. Verkerk, A.J.M.H.; Pieretti, M.; Sutcliffe, J.S.; Fu, Y.H.; Kuhl, D.P.A.; Pizzuti, A.; Reiner, O.; Richards, S.; Victoria, M.F.; Zhang, F.; et al. Identification of a gene (FMR-1) containing a CGG repeat coincident with a breakpoint cluster region exhibiting length variation in fragile X syndrome. *Cell* **1991**, *65*, 905–914. [CrossRef]
147. Bagni, C.; Greenough, W.T. From mRNP trafficking to spine dysmorphogenesis: The roots of fragile X syndrome. *Nat. Rev. Neurosci.* **2005**, *6*, 376–387. [CrossRef] [PubMed]
148. Darnell, J.C.; van Driesche, S.J.; Zhang, C.; Hung, K.Y.S.; Mele, A.; Fraser, C.E.; Stone, E.F.; Chen, C.; Fak, J.J.; Chi, S.W.; et al. FMRP stalls ribosomal translocation on mRNAs linked to synaptic function and autism. *Cell* **2011**, *146*, 247–261. [CrossRef] [PubMed]
149. Darnell, J.C.; Klann, E. The translation of translational control by FMRP: Therapeutic targets for FXS. *Nat. Neurosci.* **2013**, *16*, 1530–1536. [CrossRef] [PubMed]
150. Incorpora, G.; Sorge, G.; Sorge, A.; Pavone, L. Epilepsy in fragile X syndrome. *Brain Dev.* **2002**, *24*, 766–769. [CrossRef]
151. Hagerman, P.J.; Stafstrom, C.E. Origins of Epilepsy in Fragile X Syndrome. *Epilepsy Curr.* **2009**, *9*, 108–112. [CrossRef] [PubMed]
152. Butler, M.G.; Brunschwig, A.; Miller, L.K.; Hagerman, R.J. Standards for Selected Anthropometric Measurements in Males With the Fragile X Syndrome. *Pediatrics* **1992**, *89*, 1059–1062. [PubMed]
153. Chiu, S.; Wegelin, J.A.; Blank, J.; Jenkins, M.; Day, J.; Hessl, D.; Tassone, F.; Hagerman, R. Early acceleration of head circumference in children with fragile x syndrome and autism. *J. Dev. Behav. Pediatr.* **2007**, *28*, 31–35. [CrossRef] [PubMed]
154. Hinton, V.J.; Brown, W.T.; Wisniewski, K.; Rudelli, R.D. Analysis of neocortex in three males with the fragile X syndrome. *Am. J. Med. Genet.* **1991**, *41*, 289–294. [CrossRef] [PubMed]
155. Irwin, S.A.; Patel, B.; Idupulapati, M.; Harris, J.B.; Crisostomo, R.A.; Larsen, B.P.; Kooy, F.; Willems, P.J.; Cras, P.; Kozlowski, P.B.; et al. Abnormal Dendritic Spine Characteristics in the Temporal and Visual Cortices of Patients With Fragile-X Syndrome: A Quantitative Examination. *Am. J. Med. Genet.* **2001**, *98*, 161–167. [CrossRef]
156. Sheridan, S.D.; Theriault, K.M.; Reis, S.A.; Zhou, F.; Madison, J.M.; Daheron, L.; Loring, J.F.; Haggarty, S.J. Epigenetic Characterization of the FMR1 Gene and Aberrant Neurodevelopment in Human Induced Pluripotent Stem Cell Models of Fragile X Syndrome. *PLoS ONE* **2011**, *6*, e26203. [CrossRef] [PubMed]
157. Doers, M.E.; Musser, M.T.; Nichol, R.; Berndt, E.R.; Baker, M.; Gomez, T.M.; Zhang, S.-C.; Abbeduto, L.; Bhattacharyya, A. iPSC-Derived Forebrain Neurons from FXS Individuals Show Defects in Initial Neurite Outgrowth. *Stem Cells Dev.* **2014**, *23*, 1777–1787. [CrossRef] [PubMed]
158. Telias, M.; Kuznitsov-Yanovsky, L.; Segal, M.; Ben-Yosef, D. Functional Deficiencies in Fragile X Neurons Derived from Human Embryonic Stem Cells. *J. Neurosci.* **2015**, *35*, 15295–15306. [CrossRef] [PubMed]
159. Musumeci, S.A.; Calabrese, G.; Bonaccorso, C.M.; D'Antoni, S.; Brouwer, J.R.; Bakker, C.E.; Elia, M.; Ferri, R.; Nelson, D.L.; Oostra, B.A.; et al. Audiogenic seizure susceptibility is reduced in fragile X knockout mice after introduction of FMR1 transgenes. *Exp. Neurol.* **2007**, *203*, 233–240. [CrossRef] [PubMed]
160. Bhattacharya, A.; Kaphzan, H.; Alvarez-Dieppa, A.C.; Murphy, J.P.; Pierre, P.; Klann, E. Genetic Removal of p70 S6 Kinase 1 Corrects Molecular, Synaptic, and Behavioral Phenotypes in Fragile X Syndrome Mice. *Neuron* **2012**, *76*, 325–337. [CrossRef] [PubMed]
161. Uutela, M.; Lindholm, J.; Louhivuori, V.; Wei, H.; Louhivuori, L.M.; Pertovaara, A.; Åkerman, K.; Castrén, E.; Castrén, M.L. Reduction of BDNF expression in Fmr1 knockout mice worsens cognitive deficits but improves hyperactivity and sensorimotor deficits. *Genes Brain Behav.* **2012**, *11*, 513–523. [CrossRef] [PubMed]
162. Comery, T.A.; Harris, J.B.; Willems, P.J.; Oostra, B.A.; Irwin, S.A.; Weiler, I.J.; Greenough, W.T. Abnormal dendritic spines in fragile X knockout mice: Maturation and pruning deficits. *Proc. Natl. Acad. Sci. USA* **1997**, *94*, 5401–5404. [CrossRef] [PubMed]
163. Galvez, R.; Greenough, W.T. Sequence of abnormal dendritic spine development in primary somatosensory cortex of a mouse model of the fragile X mental retardation syndrome. *Am. J. Med. Genet.* **2005**, *135A*, 155–160. [CrossRef] [PubMed]

164. Grossman, A.W.; Elisseou, N.M.; McKinney, B.C.; Greenough, W.T. Hippocampal pyramidal cells in adult Fmr1 knockout mice exhibit an immature-appearing profile of dendritic spines. *Brain Res.* **2006**, *1084*, 158–164. [CrossRef] [PubMed]
165. Liu, Z.-H.; Chuang, D.-M.; Smith, C.B. Lithium ameliorates phenotypic deficits in a mouse model of fragile X syndrome. *Int. J. Neuropsychopharmacol.* **2011**, *14*, 618–630. [CrossRef] [PubMed]
166. Gkogkas, C.G.; Khoutorsky, A.; Cao, R.; Jafarnejad, S.M.; Prager-Khoutorsky, M.; Giannakas, N.; Kaminari, A.; Fragkouli, A.; Nader, K.; Price, T.J.; et al. Pharmacogenetic Inhibition of eIF4E-Dependent Mmp9 mRNA Translation Reverses Fragile X Syndrome-like Phenotypes. *Cell Rep.* **2014**, *9*, 1742–1755. [CrossRef] [PubMed]
167. La Fata, G.; Gärtner, A.; Domínguez-Iturza, N.; Dresselaers, T.; Dawitz, J.; Poorthuis, R.B.; Averna, M.; Himmelreich, U.; Meredith, R.M.; Achsel, T.; et al. FMRP regulates multipolar to bipolar transition affecting neuronal migration and cortical circuitry. *Nat. Neurosci.* **2014**, *17*, 1693–1700. [CrossRef] [PubMed]
168. Pacey, L.K.K.; Guan, S.; Tharmalingam, S.; Thomsen, C.; Hampson, D.R. Persistent astrocyte activation in the fragile X mouse cerebellum. *Brain Behav.* **2015**, *5*, e00400. [CrossRef] [PubMed]
169. Pacey, L.K.K.; Xuan, I.C.Y.; Guan, S.; Sussman, D.; Henkelman, R.M.; Chen, Y.; Thomsen, C.; Hampson, D.R. Delayed myelination in a mouse model of fragile X syndrome. *Hum. Mol. Genet.* **2013**, *22*, 3920–3930. [CrossRef] [PubMed]
170. Huber, K.M.; Gallagher, S.M.; Warren, S.T.; Bear, M.F. Altered synaptic plasticity in a mouse model of fragile X mental retardation. *Proc. Natl. Acad. Sci. USA* **2002**, *99*, 7746–7750. [CrossRef] [PubMed]
171. Nosyreva, E.D.; Huber, K.M.; Elena, D.; Metabotropic, K.M. H. Metabotropic Receptor-Dependent Long-Term Depression Persists in the Absence of Protein Synthesis in the Mouse Model of Fragile X Syndrome. *J. Neurophysiol.* **2006**, *95*, 3291–3295. [CrossRef] [PubMed]
172. Sharma, A.; Hoeffer, C.A.; Takayasu, Y.; Miyawaki, T.; McBride, S.M.; Klann, E.; Zukin, R.S. Dysregulation of mTOR signaling in fragile X syndrome. *J. Neurosci.* **2010**, *30*, 694–702. [CrossRef] [PubMed]
173. Gonçalves, J.T.; Anstey, J.E.; Golshani, P.; Portera-Cailliau, C. Circuit level defects in the developing neocortex of Fragile X mice. *Nat. Neurosci.* **2013**, *16*, 903–909. [CrossRef] [PubMed]
174. Deng, P.Y.; Rotman, Z.; Blundon, J.A.; Cho, Y.; Cui, J.; Cavalli, V.; Zakharenko, S.S.; Klyachko, V.A. FMRP Regulates Neurotransmitter Release and Synaptic Information Transmission by Modulating Action Potential Duration via BK Channels. *Neuron* **2013**, *77*, 696–711. [CrossRef] [PubMed]
175. Braun, K.; Segal, M. FMRP involvement in formation of synapses among cultured hippocampal neurons. *Cereb. Cortex* **2000**, *10*, 1045–1052. [CrossRef] [PubMed]
176. Selby, L.; Zhang, C.; Sun, Q. Major Defects in Neocortical GABAergic Inhibitory Circuits in Mice Lacking the Fragile X Mental Retardation Protein. *Neurosci. Lett.* **2007**, *412*, 227–232. [CrossRef] [PubMed]
177. Gross, C.; Nakamoto, M.; Yao, X.; Chan, C.; Yim, S.Y.; Warren, S.T.; Bassell, G.J. Excess PI3K subunit synthesis and activity as a novel therapeutic target in Fragile X Syndrome. *Neuroscience* **2010**, *30*, 10624–10638. [PubMed]
178. Hayashi, M.L.; Rao, B.S.S.; Seo, J.-S.; Choi, H.-S.; Dolan, B.M.; Choi, S.-Y.; Chattarji, S.; Tonegawa, S. Inhibition of p21-activated kinase rescues symptoms of fragile X syndrome in mice. *Proc. Natl. Acad. Sci. USA* **2007**, *104*, 11489–11494. [CrossRef] [PubMed]
179. Zhao, M.-G.; Toyoda, H.; Ko, S.W.; Ding, H.-K.; Wu, L.-J.; Zhou, M. Deficits in Trace Fear Memory and Long-Term Potentiation in a Mouse Model for Fragile X Syndrome. *J. Neurosci.* **2005**, *25*, 7385–7392. [CrossRef] [PubMed]
180. Pilpel, Y.; Kolleker, A.; Berberich, S.; Ginger, M.; Frick, A.; Mientjes, E.; Oostra, B.A.; Seeburg, P.H. Synaptic ionotropic glutamate receptors and plasticity are developmentally altered in the CA1 field of Fmr1 knockout mice. *J. Physiol.* **2009**, *587*, 787–804. [CrossRef] [PubMed]
181. Seese, R.R.; Babayan, A.H.; Katz, A.M.; Cox, C.D.; Lauterborn, J.C.; Lynch, G.; Gall, C.M. LTP induction translocates cortactin at distant synapses in wild-type but not Fmr1 knock-out mice. *J. Neurosci.* **2012**, *32*, 7403–7413. [CrossRef] [PubMed]
182. Narayanan, U.; Nalavadi, V.; Nakamoto, M.; Thomas, G.; Ceman, S.; Bassell, G.J.; Warren, S.T. S6K1 phosphorylates and regulates fragile X mental retardation protein (FMRP) with the neuronal protein synthesis-dependent mammalian target of rapamycin (mTOR) signaling cascade. *J. Biol. Chem.* **2008**, *283*, 18478–18482. [CrossRef] [PubMed]
183. Bartley, C.M.; O'Keefe, R.A.; Bordey, A. FMRP S499 is phosphorylated independent of mTORC1-S6K1 activity. *PLoS ONE* **2014**, *9*, e96956.

184. Vu, T.H.; Hoffman, A.R. Imprinting of the Angelman syndrome gene, UBE3A, is restricted to brain. *Nat. Genet.* **1997**, *17*, 12–13. [CrossRef] [PubMed]
185. Grier, M.D.; Carson, R.P.; Lagrange, A.H. Toward a broader view of Ube3a in a mouse model of Angelman Syndrome: Expression in brain, spinal cord, sciatic nerve, glial cells. *PLoS ONE* **2015**, *10*, 1–14. [CrossRef] [PubMed]
186. Buiting, K.; Williams, C.; Horsthemke, B. Angelman syndrome—Insights into a rare neurogenetic disorder. *Nat. Rev. Neurol.* **2016**, *12*, 584–593. [CrossRef] [PubMed]
187. Bonati, M.T.; Russo, S.; Finelli, P.; Valsecchi, M.R.; Cogliati, F.; Cavalleri, F.; Roberts, W.; Elia, M.; Larizza, L. Evaluation of autism traits in Angelman syndrome: A resource to unfold autism genes. *Neurogenetics* **2007**, *8*, 169–178. [CrossRef] [PubMed]
188. Matsumoto, A.; Kumagai, T.; Miura, K.; Miyazaki, S.; Hayakawa, C.; Yamanaka, T. Epilepsy in Angelman Syndrome Associated with Chromosome 15q Deletion. *Epilepsia* **1992**, *33*, 1083–1090. [CrossRef] [PubMed]
189. Clayton-Smith, J. Clinical research on Angelman syndrome in the United Kingdom: Observations on 82 affected individuals. *Am. J. Med. Genet.* **1993**, *46*, 12–15. [CrossRef] [PubMed]
190. Tan, W.H.; Bacino, C.A.; Skinner, S.A.; Anselm, I.; Barbieri-Welge, R.; Bauer-Carlin, A.; Beaudet, A.L.; Bichell, T.J.; Gentile, J.K.; Glaze, D.G.; et al. Angelman syndrome: Mutations influence features in early childhood. *Am. J. Med. Genet. Part A* **2011**, *155*, 81–90. [CrossRef] [PubMed]
191. Harting, I.; Seitz, A.; Rating, D.; Sartor, K.; Zschocke, J.; Janssen, B.; Ebinger, F.; Wolf, N.I. Abnormal myelination in Angelman syndrome. *Eur. J. Paediatr. Neurol.* **2009**, *13*, 271–276. [CrossRef] [PubMed]
192. Castro-Gago, M.; Gómez-Lado, C.; Eirís-Puñal, J. Abnormal myelination in Angelman syndrome. *Eur. J. Paediatr. Neurol.* **2010**, *14*, 292. [CrossRef] [PubMed]
193. Jiang, Y.-H.; Armstrong, D.; Albrecht, U.; Atkins, C.M.; Noebels, J.L.; Eichele, G.; Sweatt, J.D.; Beaudet, A.L. Mutation of the Angelman ubiquitin ligase in mice causes increased cytoplasmic p53 and deficits of contextual learning and long-term potentiation. *Neuron* **1998**, *21*, 799–811. [CrossRef]
194. Miura, K.; Kishino, T.; Li, E.; Webber, H.; Dikkes, P.; Holmes, G.L.; Wagstaff, J. Neurobehavioral and electroencephalographic abnormalities in Ube3a maternal-deficient mice. *Neurobiol. Dis.* **2002**, *9*, 149–159. [CrossRef] [PubMed]
195. Grier, M.D.; Carson, R.P.; Lagrange, A.H. Of mothers and myelin: Aberrant myelination phenotypes in mouse model of Angelman syndrome are dependent on maternal and dietary influences. *Behav. Brain Res.* **2015**, *291*, 260–267. [CrossRef] [PubMed]
196. Dindot, S.V.; Antalffy, B.A.; Bhattacharjee, M.B.; Beaudet, A.L. The Angelman syndrome ubiquitin ligase localizes to the synapse and nucleus, and maternal deficiency results in abnormal dendritic spine morphology. *Hum. Mol. Genet.* **2008**, *17*, 111–118. [CrossRef] [PubMed]
197. Wallace, M.L.; Burette, A.C.; Weinberg, R.J.; Philpot, B.D. Maternal Loss of Ube3a Produces an Excitatory/Inhibitory Imbalance through Neuron Type-Specific Synaptic Defects. *Neuron* **2012**, *74*, 793–800. [CrossRef] [PubMed]
198. Miao, S.; Chen, R.; Ye, J.; Tan, G.-H.; Li, S.; Zhang, J.; Jiang, Y.-H.; Xiong, Z.-Q. The Angelman Syndrome Protein Ube3a Is Required for Polarized Dendrite Morphogenesis in Pyramidal Neurons. *J. Neurosci.* **2013**, *33*, 327–333. [CrossRef] [PubMed]
199. Tonazzini, I.; Meucci, S.; van Woerden, G.M.; Elgersma, Y.; Cecchini, M. Impaired Neurite Contact Guidance in Ubiquitin Ligase E3a (Ube3a)-Deficient Hippocampal Neurons on Nanostructured Substrates. *Adv. Healthc. Mater.* **2016**, *5*, 850–862. [CrossRef] [PubMed]
200. Yashiro, K.; Riday, T.T.; Condon, K.H.; Roberts, A.C.; Bernardo, D.R.; Prakash, R.; Weinberg, R.J.; Ehlers, M.D.; Philpot, B.D. Ube3a is required for experience-dependent maturation of the neocortex. *Nat. Neurosci.* **2009**, *12*, 777–783. [CrossRef]
201. Pignatelli, M.; Piccinin, S.; Molinaro, G.; Di Menna, L.; Riozzi, B.; Cannella, M.; Motolese, M.; Vetere, G.; Catania, M.V.; Battaglia, G.; et al. Changes in mGlu5 receptor-dependent synaptic plasticity and coupling to homer proteins in the hippocampus of Ube3A hemizygous mice modeling angelman syndrome. *J. Neurosci.* **2014**, *34*, 4558–4566. [CrossRef] [PubMed]
202. Greer, P.L.; Hanayama, R.; Bloodgood, B.L.; Mardinly, A.R.; Lipton, D.M.; Flavell, S.W.; Kim, T.K.; Griffith, E.C.; Waldon, Z.; Maehr, R.; et al. The Angelman Syndrome Protein Ube3A Regulates Synapse Development by Ubiquitinating Arc. *Cell* **2010**, *140*, 704–716. [CrossRef] [PubMed]

203. Amir, R.E.; van den Veyver, I.B.; Wan, M.; Tran, C.Q.; Francke, U.; Zoghbi, H.Y. Rett syndrome is caused by mutations in X-linked MECP2, encoding methyl-CpG-binding protein 2. *Nat. Genet.* **1999**, *23*, 185–188. [PubMed]
204. Bienvenu, T.; Chelly, J. Molecular genetics of Rett syndrome: When DNA methylation goes unrecognized. *Nat. Rev. Genet.* **2006**, *7*, 415–426. [CrossRef] [PubMed]
205. Chahrour, M.; Jung, S.Y.; Shaw, C.; Zhou, X.; Wong, S.T.C.; Qin, J.; Zoghbi, H.Y. MeCP2, a key contributor to neurological disease, activates and represses transcription. *Science* **2008**, *320*, 1224–1229. [CrossRef] [PubMed]
206. Cardoza, B.; Clarke, A.; Wilcox, J.; Gibbon, F.; Smith, P.E.M.; Archer, H.; Hryniewiecka-Jaworska, A.; Kerr, M. Epilepsy in Rett syndrome: Association between phenotype and genotype, and implications for practice. *Seizure* **2011**, *20*, 646–649. [CrossRef] [PubMed]
207. Dolce, A.; Ben-Zeev, B.; Naidu, S.; Kossoff, E.H. Rett syndrome and epilepsy: An update for child neurologists. *Pediatr. Neurol.* **2013**, *48*, 337–345. [CrossRef] [PubMed]
208. Jellinger, K.; Armstrong, D.; Zoghbi, H.Y.; Percy, A.K.; Boltzmann, L.; Wien, A. Neuropathology of Rett syndrome. *Acta Neuropathol.* **1988**, *76*, 142–158. [CrossRef] [PubMed]
209. Hagberg, G.; Stenbom, Y.; Witt Engerström, I. Head growth in Rett syndrome. *Brain Dev.* **2001**, *23*, 227–229. [CrossRef]
210. Bauman, M.L.; Kemper, T.L.; Arin, D.M. Microscopic observations of the brain in Rett syndrome. *Neuropediatrics* **1995**, *26*, 105–108. [CrossRef] [PubMed]
211. Bauman, M.L.; Kemper, T.L.; Arin, D.M. Pervasive neuroanatomic abnormalities of the brain in three cases of Rett's syndrome. *Neurology* **1995**, *45*, 1581–1586. [CrossRef] [PubMed]
212. Lipani, J.D.; Bhattacharjee, M.B.; Corey, D.M.; Lee, D.A. Reduced nerve growth factor in Rett syndrome postmortem brain tissue. *J. Neuropathol. Exp. Neurol.* **2000**, *59*, 889–895. [CrossRef] [PubMed]
213. Armstrong, D.; Dunn, J.K.; Antalffy, B.T.R. Selective dendritic alterations in the cortex of Rett syndrome. *J. Neuropathol. Exp. Neurol.* **1995**, *54*, 195–201. [CrossRef] [PubMed]
214. Armstrong, D.D. Neuropathology of Rett syndrome. *J. Child Neurol.* **2005**, *20*, 747–753. [CrossRef] [PubMed]
215. Belichenko, P.V.; Oldfors, A.; Hagberg, B.; Dahlström, A. Rett syndrome: 3-D confocal microscopy of cortical pyramidal dendrites and afferents. *Neuroreport* **1994**, *5*, 1509–1513. [CrossRef] [PubMed]
216. Kaufmann, W.E.; Taylor, C.; Hohmann, C.; Sanwal, I.; Naidu, S. Abnormalities in neuronal maturation in Rett syndrome neocortex: Preliminary molecular correlates. *Eur. Child Adolesc. Psychiatry* **1997**, *6*, 75–77.
217. Chapleau, C.A.; Larimore, J.L.; Theibert, A.; Pozzo-Miller, L. Modulation of dendritic spine development and plasticity by BDNF and vesicular trafficking: Fundamental roles in neurodevelopmental disorders associated with mental retardation and autism. *J. Neurodev. Disord.* **2009**, *1*, 185–196. [CrossRef] [PubMed]
218. Chen, R.Z.; Akbarian, S.; Tudor, M.; Jaenisch, R. Deficiency of methyl-CpG binding protein-2 in CNS neurons results in a Rett-like phenotype in mice. *Nat. Genet.* **2001**, *27*, 327–331. [CrossRef] [PubMed]
219. Shahbazian, M.D.; Young, J.I.; Yuva-Paylor, L.A.; Spencer, C.M.; Antalffy, B.A.; Noebels, J.L.; Armstrong, D.L.; Paylor, R.; Zoghbi, H.Y. Mice with truncated MeCP2 recapitulate many Rett syndrome features and display hyperacetylation of histone H3. *Neuron* **2002**, *35*, 243–254. [CrossRef]
220. Kishi, N.; Macklis, J.D. MECP2 is progressively expressed in post-migratory neurons and is involved in neuronal maturation rather than cell fate decisions. *Mol. Cell. Neurosci.* **2004**, *27*, 306–321. [CrossRef] [PubMed]
221. Fukuda, T.; Yamashita, Y.; Nagamitsu, S.; Miyamoto, K.; Jin, J.J.; Ohmori, I.; Ohtsuka, Y.; Kuwajima, K.; Endo, S.; Iwai, T.; et al. Methyl-CpG binding protein 2 gene (MECP2) variations in Japanese patients with Rett syndrome: Pathological mutations and polymorphisms. *Brain Dev.* **2005**, *27*, 211–217. [CrossRef] [PubMed]
222. Tropea, D.; Giacometti, E.; Wilson, N.R.; Beard, C.; McCurry, C.; Fu, D.D.; Flannery, R.; Jaenisch, R.; Sur, M. Partial reversal of Rett Syndrome-like symptoms in MeCP2 mutant mice. *Proc. Natl. Acad. Sci. USA* **2009**, *106*, 2029–2034. [CrossRef] [PubMed]
223. Nguyen, M.V.C.; Du, F.; Felice, C.A.; Shan, X.; Nigam, A.; Mandel, G.; Robinson, J.K.; Ballas, N. MeCP2 is critical for maintainng mature neuronal networks and global brain anatomy during late stages of postnatal brain development and in the mature adult brain. *J. Neurosci.* **2012**, *32*, 10021–10034. [CrossRef] [PubMed]

224. Castro, J.; Garcia, R.I.; Kwok, S.; Banerjee, A.; Petravicz, J.; Woodson, J.; Mellios, N.; Tropea, D.; Sur, M. Functional recovery with recombinant human IGF1 treatment in a mouse model of Rett Syndrome. *Proc. Natl. Acad. Sci. USA* **2014**, *111*, 9941–9946. [CrossRef] [PubMed]
225. Baj, G.; Patrizio, A.; Montalbano, A.; Sciancalepore, M.; Tongiorgi, E. Developmental and maintenance defects in Rett syndrome neurons identified by a new mouse staging system in vitro. *Front. Cell. Neurosci.* **2014**, *8*, 18. [CrossRef] [PubMed]
226. Asaka, Y.; Jugloff, D.G.M.; Zhang, L.; Eubanks, J.H.; Fitzsimonds, R.M. Hippocampal synaptic plasticity is impaired in the Mecp2-null mouse model of Rett syndrome. *Neurobiol. Dis.* **2006**, *21*, 217–227. [CrossRef] [PubMed]
227. Moretti, P. Learning and Memory and Synaptic Plasticity Are Impaired in a Mouse Model of Rett Syndrome. *J. Neurosci.* **2006**, *26*, 319–327. [CrossRef] [PubMed]
228. Chao, H.T.; Zoghbi, H.Y.; Rosenmund, C. MeCP2 Controls Excitatory Synaptic Strength by Regulating Glutamatergic Synapse Number. *Neuron* **2007**, *56*, 58–65. [CrossRef] [PubMed]
229. Ballas, N.; Lioy, D.T.; Grunseich, C.; Mandel, G. Non-cell autonomous influence of MeCP2-deficient glia on neuronal dendritic morphology. *Nat. Neurosci.* **2009**, *12*, 311–317. [CrossRef] [PubMed]
230. Maezawa, I.; Swanberg, S.; Harvey, D.; LaSalle, J.M.; Jin, L.-W. Rett Syndrome Astrocytes Are Abnormal and Spread MeCP2 Deficiency through Gap Junctions. *J. Neurosci.* **2009**, *29*, 5051–5061. [CrossRef] [PubMed]
231. Kishi, N.; Macklis, J.D. MeCP2 functions largely cell-autonomously, but also non-cell-autonomously, in neuronal maturation and dendritic arborization of cortical pyramidal neurons. *Exp. Neurol.* **2010**, *222*, 51–58. [CrossRef] [PubMed]
232. Marchetto, M.C.N.; Carromeu, C.; Acab, A.; Yu, D.; Yeo, G.W.; Mu, Y.; Chen, G.; Gage, F.H.; Muotri, A.R. A model for neural development and treatment of rett syndrome using human induced pluripotent stem cells. *Cell* **2010**, *143*, 527–539. [CrossRef] [PubMed]
233. Li, Y.; Wang, H.; Muffat, J.; Cheng, A.W.; Orlando, D.A.; Lovén, J.; Kwok, S.M.; Feldman, D.A.; Bateup, H.S.; Gao, Q.; et al. Global transcriptional and translational repression in human-embryonic- stem-cell-derived rett syndrome neurons. *Cell Stem Cell* **2013**, *13*, 446–458. [CrossRef] [PubMed]
234. Williams, E.C.; Zhong, X.; Mohamed, A.; Li, R.; Liu, Y.; Dong, Q.; Ananiev, G.E.; Choongmok, J.C.; Lin, B.R.; Lu, J.; et al. Mutant astrocytes differentiated from Rett syndrome patients-specific iPSCs have adverse effects on wildtype neurons. *Hum. Mol. Genet.* **2014**, *23*, 2968–2980. [CrossRef] [PubMed]
235. Djuric, U.; Cheung, A.Y.L.; Zhang, W.; Mok, R.S.; Lai, W.; Piekna, A.; Hendry, J.A.; Ross, P.J.; Pasceri, P.; Kim, D.S.; et al. MECP2e1 isoform mutation affects the form and function of neurons derived from Rett syndrome patient iPS cells. *Neurobiol. Dis.* **2015**, *76*, 37–45. [CrossRef] [PubMed]
236. Zhang, Z.-N.; Freitas, B.C.; Qian, H.; Lux, J.; Acab, A.; Trujillo, C.A.; Herai, R.H.; Nguyen Huu, V.A.; Wen, J.H.; Joshi-Barr, S.; et al. Layered hydrogels accelerate iPSC-derived neuronal maturation and reveal migration defects caused by MeCP2 dysfunction. *Proc. Natl. Acad. Sci. USA* **2016**, *113*, 3185–3190. [CrossRef] [PubMed]
237. Cook, E.H.; Lindgren, V.; Leventhal, B.L.; Courchesne, R.; Lincoln, A.; Shulman, C.; Lord, C.; Courchesne, E. Autism or Atypical Autism in Maternally but Not Paternally Derived Proximal 15q Duplication. *Am. J. Hum. Genet.* **1997**, *60*, 928–934. [PubMed]
238. Cook, E.H.; Scherer, S.W. Copy-number variations associated with neuropsychiatric conditions. *Nature* **2008**, *455*, 919–923. [CrossRef] [PubMed]
239. Driscoll, D.; Waters, M.; Williams, C.; Zori, R.; Glenn, C.; Avidano, K.; Nicholls, R. A DNA methylation imprint, determined by the sex of the parent, distinguishes the Angelman and Prader-Willi syndromes. *Genomics* **1992**, *13*, 917–924. [CrossRef]
240. Smith, S.E. P.; Zhou, Y.-D.; Zhang, G.; Jin, Z.; Stoppel, D.C.; Anderson, M.P. Increased gene dosage of Ube3a results in autism traits and decreased glutamate synaptic transmission in mice. *Sci. Transl. Med.* **2011**, *3*, 103ra97. [CrossRef] [PubMed]
241. Nakatani, J.; Tamada, K.; Hatanaka, F.; Ise, S.; Ohta, H.; Inoue, K.; Tomonaga, S.; Watanabe, Y.; Chung, Y.J.; Banerjee, R.; et al. Abnormal Behavior in a Chromosome- Engineered Mouse Model for Human 15q11-13 Duplication Seen in Autism. *Cell* **2009**, *137*, 1235–1246. [CrossRef] [PubMed]
242. Isshiki, M.; Tanaka, S.; Kuriu, T.; Tabuchi, K.; Takumi, T.; Okabe, S. Enhanced synapse remodelling as a common phenotype in mouse models of autism. *Nat. Commun.* **2014**, *5*, 4742. [CrossRef] [PubMed]

243. Piochon, C.; Kloth, A.D.; Grasselli, G.; Titley, H.K.; Nakayama, H.; Hashimoto, K.; Wan, V.; Simmons, D.H.; Eissa, T.; Nakatani, J.; et al. Masanobu Kano8, Samuel S-H Wang2, 3, and C.H. Cerebellar Plasticity and Motor Learning Deficits in a Copy Number Variation Mouse Model of Autism. *Nat. Commun.* **2014**, *5*, 5586. [CrossRef] [PubMed]
244. Doornbos, M.; Sikkema-Raddatz, B.; Ruijvenkamp, C.A.L.; Dijkhuizen, T.; Bijlsma, E.K.; Gijsbers, A.C.J.; Hilhorst-Hofstee, Y.; Hordijk, R.; Verbruggen, K.T.; Kerstjens-Frederikse, W.S.; et al. Nine patients with a microdeletion 15q11.2 between breakpoints 1 and 2 of the Prader-Willi critical region, possibly associated with behavioural disturbances. *Eur. J. Med. Genet.* **2009**, *52*, 108–115. [CrossRef] [PubMed]
245. Van Der Zwaag, B.; Staal, W.G.; Hochstenbach, R.; Poot, M.; Spierenburg, H.; De Jonge, M.V.; Verbeek, N.E.; van 't Slot, R.; van Es, M.A.; Staal, F.J.; et al. A co-segregating microduplication of chromosome 15q11.2 pinpoints two risk genes for autism spectrum disorder. *Am. J. Med. Genet. Part B Neuropsychiatr. Genet.* **2009**, *153*, 960–966. [CrossRef] [PubMed]
246. Burnside, R.D.; Pasion, R.; Mikhail, F.M.; Carroll, A.J.; Robin, N.H.; Youngs, E.L.; Gadi, I.K.; Keitges, E.; Jaswaney, V.L.; Papenhausen, P.R.; et al. Microdeletion/microduplication of proximal 15q11.2 between BP1 and BP2: A susceptibility region for neurological dysfunction including developmental and language delay. *Hum. Genet.* **2011**, *130*, 517–528. [CrossRef] [PubMed]
247. Napoli, I.; Mercaldo, V.; Boyl, P.P.; Eleuteri, B.; Zalfa, F.; De Rubeis, S.; Di Marino, D.; Mohr, E.; Massimi, M.; Falconi, M.; et al. The Fragile X Syndrome Protein Represses Activity-Dependent Translation through CYFIP1, a New 4E-BP. *Cell* **2008**, *134*, 1042–1054. [CrossRef] [PubMed]
248. Kobayashi, K.; Kuroda, S.; Fukata, M.; Nakamura, T.; Nagase, T.; Nomura, N.; Matsuura, Y.; Yoshida-Kubomura, N.; Iwamatsu, A.; Kaibuchi, K. p140Sra-1 (specifically Rac1-associated protein) is a novel specific target for Rac1 small GTPase. *J. Biol. Chem.* **1998**, *273*, 291–295. [CrossRef] [PubMed]
249. DeRubeis, S.; Pasciuto, E.; Li, K.W.; Fernández, E.; DiMarino, D.; Buzzi, A.; Ostroff, L.E.; Klann, E.; Zwartkruis, F.J.T.; Komiyama, N.H.; Grant, S.G.N.; et al. CYFIP1 coordinates mRNA translation and cytoskeleton remodeling to ensure proper dendritic Spine formation. *Neuron* **2013**, *79*, 1169–1182. [CrossRef] [PubMed]
250. Nishimura, Y.; Martin, C.L.; Vazquez-Lopez, A.; Spence, S.J.; Alvarez-Retuerto, A.I.; Sigman, M.; Steindler, C.; Pellegrini, S.; Schanen, N.C.; Warren, S.T.; et al. Genome-wide expression profiling of lymphoblastoid cell lines distinguishes different forms of autism and reveals shared pathways. *Hum. Mol. Genet.* **2007**, *16*, 1682–1698. [CrossRef] [PubMed]
251. Pathania, M.; Davenport, E.C.; Muir, J.; Sheehan, D.F.; López-Doménech, G.; Kittler, J.T. The autism and schizophrenia associated gene CYFIP1 is critical for the maintenance of dendritic complexity and the stabilization of mature spines. *Transl. Psychiatry* **2014**, *4*, e374. [CrossRef] [PubMed]
252. Spence, S.J.; Schneider, M.T. The role of epilepsy and epileptiform EEGs in autism spectrum disorders. *Pediatr. Res.* **2009**, *65*, 599–606. [CrossRef] [PubMed]
253. Tuchman, R.; Alessandri, M.; Cuccaro, M. Autism spectrum disorders and epilepsy: Moving towards a comprehensive approach to treatment. *Brain Dev.* **2010**, *32*, 719–730. [CrossRef] [PubMed]
254. Courchesne, E.; Pierce, K.; Schumann, C.M.; Redcay, E.; Buckwalter, J.A.; Kennedy, D.P.; Morgan, J.T. Mapping early brain development in autism. *Neuron* **2007**, *56*, 399–413. [CrossRef] [PubMed]
255. Courchesne, E.; Campbell, K.; Solso, S. Brain growth across the life span in autism: Age-specific changes in anatomical pathology. *Brain Res.* **2011**, *1380*, 138–145. [CrossRef] [PubMed]
256. Casanova, M.F.; Pickett, J. The Neuropathology of Autism. In *Imaging the Brain in Autism*; Casanova, M., El-Baz, A., Suri, J., Eds.; Springer: New York, NY, USA, 2013; pp. 27–41.
257. Bauman, M.L.; Kemper, T.L. Neuroanatomic observations of the brain in autism: A review and future directions. *Int. J. Dev. Neurosci.* **2005**, *23*, 183–187. [CrossRef] [PubMed]
258. Wegiel, J.; Kuchna, I.; Nowicki, K.; Imaki, H.; Wegiel, J.; Marchi, E.; Ma, S.Y.; Chauhan, A.; Chauhan, V.; Bobrowicz, T.W.; et al. The neuropathology of autism: Defects of neurogenesis and neuronal migration, and dysplastic changes. *Acta Neuropathol.* **2010**, *119*, 755–770. [CrossRef] [PubMed]
259. Stoner, R.; Chow, M.L.; Boyle, M.P.; Sunkin, S.M.; Mouton, P.R.; Roy, S.; Wynshaw-Boris, A.; Colamarino, S.A.; Lein, E.S.; Courchesne, E. Patches of disorganization in the neocortex of children with autism. *N. Engl. J. Med.* **2014**, *370*, 1209–1219. [CrossRef] [PubMed]
260. Laurence, J.A.; Fatemi, S.H. Glial fibrillary acidic protein is elevated in superior frontal, parietal and cerebellar cortices of autistic subjects. *Cerebellum* **2005**, *4*, 206–210. [CrossRef] [PubMed]

261. Gozzi, M.; Nielson, D.M.; Lenroot, R.K.; Ostuni, J.L.; Luckenbaugh, D.A.; Thurm, A.E.; Giedd, J.N.; Swedo, S.E. A magnetization transfer imaging study of corpus callosum myelination in young children with autism. *Biol. Psychiatry* **2012**, *72*, 215–220. [CrossRef] [PubMed]
262. Deoni, S.C. L.; Dean, D.C.; Remer, J.; Dirks, H.; O'Muircheartaigh, J. Cortical maturation and myelination in healthy toddlers and young children. *Neuroimage* **2015**, *115*, 147–161. [CrossRef] [PubMed]
263. Hutsler, J.J.; Zhang, H. Increased dendritic spine densities on cortical projection neurons in autism spectrum disorders. *Brain Res.* **2010**, *1309*, 83–94. [CrossRef] [PubMed]
264. Jung, N.H.; Janzarik, W.G.; Delvendahl, I.; Münchau, A.; Biscaldi, M.; Mainberger, F.; Bäumer, T.; Rauh, R.; Mall, V. Impaired induction of long-term potentiation-like plasticity in patients with high-functioning autism and Asperger syndrome. *Dev. Med. Child Neurol.* **2012**, *55*, 83–89. [CrossRef] [PubMed]
265. Mariani, J.; Coppola, G.; Zhang, P.; Abyzov, A.; Provini, L.; Tomasini, L.; Amenduni, M.; Szekely, A.; Palejev, D.; Wilson, M.; et al. FOXG1-Dependent Dysregulation of GABA/Glutamate Neuron Differentiation in Autism Spectrum Disorders. *Cell* **2015**, *162*, 375–390. [CrossRef] [PubMed]
266. Capal, J.K.; Franz, D.N. Profile of everolimus in the treatment of tuberous sclerosis complex: An evidence-based review of its place in therapy. *Neuropsychiatr. Dis. Treat.* **2016**, *12*, 2165–2172. [PubMed]
267. Angliker, N.; Rüegg, M. In vivo evidence for mTORC2-mediated actin cytoskeleton rearrangement in Neurons. *Bioarchitecture* **2013**, *3*, 113–118. [CrossRef] [PubMed]
268. Thomanetz, V.; Angliker, N.; Cloëtta, D.; Lustenberger, R.M.; Schweighauser, M.; Oliveri, F.; Suzuki, N.; Rüegg, M.A. Ablation of the mTORC2 component rictor in brain or Purkinje cells affects size and neuron morphology. *J. Cell Biol.* **2013**, *201*, 293–308. [CrossRef] [PubMed]
269. Crino, P.B. The mTOR signalling cascade: Paving new roads to cure neurological disease. *Nat. Rev. Neurol.* **2016**, *12*, 379–392. [CrossRef] [PubMed]
270. Sengupta, S.; Peterson, T.R.; Sabatini, D.M. Regulation of the mTOR Complex 1 Pathway by Nutrients, Growth Factors, and Stress. *Mol. Cell* **2010**, *40*, 310–322. [CrossRef] [PubMed]
271. Inoki, K.; Li, Y.; Xu, T.; Guan, K. Rheb GTPase is a direct target of TSC2 GAP activity and regulates mTOR signaling. *Genes Dev.* **2003**, *17*, 1829–1834. [CrossRef] [PubMed]
272. Menon, S.; Dibble, C.C.; Talbott, G.; Hoxhaj, G.; Valvezan, A.J.; Takahashi, H.; Cantley, L.C.; Manning, B.D. Spatial Control of the TSC Complex Integrates Insulin and Nutrient Regulation of mTORC1 at the Lysosome. *Cell* **2014**, *156*, 771–785. [CrossRef] [PubMed]
273. Laplante, M.; Sabatini, D.M. mTOR Signaling in Growth Control and Disease. *Cell* **2012**, *149*, 274–293. [CrossRef] [PubMed]

12

Genome, Environment, Microbiome and Metabolome in Autism (GEMMA) Study Design: Biomarkers Identification for Precision Treatment and Primary Prevention of Autism Spectrum Disorders by an Integrated Multi-Omics Systems Biology Approach

Jacopo Troisi [1,*], Reija Autio [2], Thanos Beopoulos [3], Carmela Bravaccio [4], Federica Carraturo [5], Giulio Corrivetti [6], Stephen Cunningham [7], Samantha Devane [8], Daniele Fallin [9], Serguei Fetissov [10], Manuel Gea [3], Antonio Giorgi [11], François Iris [3], Lokesh Joshi [7], Sarah Kadzielski [8], Aletta Kraneveld [12], Himanshu Kumar [13], Christine Ladd-Acosta [9], Geraldine Leader [7], Arlene Mannion [7], Elise Maximin [14], Alessandra Mezzelani [15], Luciano Milanesi [15], Laurent Naudon [14], Lucia N. Peralta Marzal [12], Paula Perez Pardo [12], Naika Z. Prince [12], Sylvie Rabot [14], Guus Roeselers [13], Christophe Roos [16], Lea Roussin [14], Giovanni Scala [1], Francesco Paolo Tuccinardi [5] and Alessio Fasano [17]

1. Theoreo srl spin off company of the University of Salerno, Via degli Ulivi, 3, 84090 Montecorvino Pugliano (SA), Italy; scala@theoreosrl.com
2. Faculty of Social Sciences, Health Sciences Unit, Tampere University, Arvo Ylpön Katu 34, 33014 Tampere, Finland; reija.autio@tuni.fi
3. Bio-Modeling System, 3, Rue De L'arrivee. 75015 Paris, France; thanos.beopoulos@bmsystems.org (T.B.); manuel.gea@bmsystems.org (M.G.); francois.iris@bmsystems.org (F.I.)
4. Department of science medicine translational, University of Naples Federico II, Via Pansini 5, 80131 Naples, Italy; carmela.bravaccio@unina.it
5. Promete srl, Piazzale Tecchio 45, 80125 Napoli, Italy; federica.carraturo@unina.it (F.C.); tuccinardi@promete.it (F.P.T.)
6. Azienda Sanitaria Locale (ASL) Salerno, Via Nizza, 146, 84125 Salerno (SA), Italy; corrivetti@gmail.com
7. National University of Ireland Galaway, University Road, Galaway, Ireland; stephen.cunningham@nuigalway.ie (S.C.); lokesh.joshi@nuigalway.ie (L.J.); geraldine.leader@nuigalway.ie (G.L.); arlene.mannion@nuigalway.ie (A.M.)
8. Massachusetts General Hospital, Fruit Street, 55, Boston, MA 02114, USA; SDEVANE@mgh.harvard.edu (S.D.); smkadzielski@mgh.harvard.edu (S.K.)
9. John Hopkins School of Public Health and the Wendy Klag Center for Autism and Developmental Disabilities, 615 N. Wolfe St, Baltimore, MD 21205, USA; dfallin@jhu.edu (D.F.); claddac1@jhu.edu (C.L.-A.)
10. Laboratory of Neuronal and Neuroendocrine Differentiation and Communication, Inserm UMR 1239, Rouen University of Normandy, 25 rue Tesnière, 76130 Mont-Saint-Aignan, France; Serguei.Fetissov@univ-rouen.fr
11. Medinok Spa, Via Palazziello, 80040 Volla (NA), Italy; a.giorgi@perfexia.it
12. Division of Pharmacology, Utrecht Institute for Pharmaceutical Sciences, Faculty of Science, Utrecht University, Universiteitsweg 99, 3508 TB Utrecht, The Netherlands; a.d.kraneveld@uu.nl (A.K.); l.n.peraltamarzal@uu.nl (L.N.P.M.); p.perezpardo@uu.nl (P.P.P.); n.z.prince@uu.nl (N.Z.P.)
13. Danone Nutricia Research, Uppsalalaan, 12, 3584 CT Utrecht, The Netherlands; Himanshu.KUMAR@nutricia.com (H.K.); Guus.ROESELERS@danone.com (R.G.)
14. Institut National de Recherche Pour L'agriculture, L'alimentation et L'environnement (INRAE), AgroParisTech, Micalis Institute, Université Paris-Saclay, 78350 Jouy-en-Josas, France; Elise.Maximin@inrae.fr (E.M.); laurent.naudon@inrae.fr (L.N.); sylvie.rabot@inrae.fr (S.R.); lea.roussin@inrae.fr (L.R.)
15. Consiglio Nazionale delle Ricerche (CNR), Piazzale Aldo Moro, 7, 00185 Roma, Italy; alessandra.mezzelani@itb.cnr.it (A.M.); luciano.milanesi@itb.cnr.it (L.M.)
16. Euformatics, Tekniikantie, 02150 Espoo, Finland; christophe.roos@euformatics.com
17. European Biomedical Research Institute of Salerno (EBRIS), Via S. de Renzi, 3, 84125 Salerno (SA), Italy; afasano@mgh.harvard.edu

* Correspondence: troisi@theoreosrl.com

Abstract: Autism Spectrum Disorder (ASD) affects approximately 1 child in 54, with a 35-fold increase since 1960. Selected studies suggest that part of the recent increase in prevalence is likely attributable to an improved awareness and recognition, and changes in clinical practice or service availability. However, this is not sufficient to explain this epidemiological phenomenon. Research points to a possible link between ASD and intestinal microbiota because many children with ASD display gastro-intestinal problems. Current large-scale datasets of ASD are limited in their ability to provide mechanistic insight into ASD because they are predominantly cross-sectional studies that do not allow evaluation of perspective associations between early life microbiota composition/function and later ASD diagnoses. Here we describe GEMMA (Genome, Environment, Microbiome and Metabolome in Autism), a prospective study supported by the European Commission, that follows at-risk infants from birth to identify potential biomarker predictors of ASD development followed by validation on large multi-omics datasets. The project includes clinical (observational and interventional trials) and pre-clinical studies in humanized murine models (fecal transfer from ASD probands) and in vitro colon models. This will support the progress of a microbiome-wide association study (of human participants) to identify prognostic microbiome signatures and metabolic pathways underlying mechanisms for ASD progression and severity and potential treatment response.

Keywords: microbiome; metabolomics; autism; study design; biomarker discovery; precise medicine

---

1. Introduction

Autism Spectrum Disorder (ASD) is a lifelong neurodevelopmental disorder characterized by deficits in social communication and social interaction, in addition to restricted, repetitive patterns of behavior, interests, or activities [1]. As a spectrum disorder, its symptoms may range from mild to severe. Some children may have strong language and intellectual abilities whereas others may not be verbal and may require lifelong care. Globally, ASD incidence has shown a 35-fold increase compared to the 1960s and 1970s, when the first epidemiological studies were conducted [2–6]. As documented by the Centers for Disease Control and Prevention, ASD affects 1 in 54 children in USA [7] and 1 in 89 in Europe [8].

Children born in a family with an affected sibling show a ten-fold higher risk of developing the condition [9]. These data, including a large-scale exome sequencing study [10], suggest a combination of non-Mendelian genetic and environmental factors in ASD pathogenesis [11,12]. One environmental factor that is emerging as important for ASD risk is the immune system [13–16]. Indeed, individuals with ASD show increased expression of genes encoding mediators of the innate immune response [15]. Low-grade systemic inflammatory events [17,18], combined with the hypofunction of protective, anti-inflammatory mechanisms [19], lead to mechanisms related to the biochemical and neuroanatomical characteristics associated with autism pathogenesis [20–22]. Immunoregulation, in addition to dysregulated immunoregulation, particularly during the first 1000 days of life [23], are guided by the gut microbiome. Low-grade systemic inflammatory responses can lead to psychiatric disorders, such as ASD and psychological stress, which leads to further inflammation through pathways involved in the intestinal microbiota homeostasis [24,25].

Many individuals with ASD have symptoms of associated comorbidities. These include medical comorbidities, such as gastrointestinal (GI) and immune system disorders (namely gut dysbiosis, susceptibility to infections, and increased prevalence of autoimmune disorders), sleep problems, feeding problems and epilepsy; comorbid psychopathology, including Attention-Deficit/Hyperactivity

Disorder (AD/HD), anxiety, mood problems, disruptive behavior; and developmental comorbidity, namely the presence of an intellectual disability.

A large number of individuals are living with ASD. Thus, ASD is a serious public health concern. The medical expenditure for ASD is higher than that for cancer, heart disease, and stroke combined [26,27]. Blumberg et al. [28] suggested that the recent increase in prevalence could be in part attributed to greater recognition and awareness, or changes in clinical practice or service availability. However, these changes are not sufficient to explain this phenomenon [6]. ASD is a multifactorial disorder; therefore, the contribution of environmental factors could explain its development in addition to why different therapeutic approaches, based on gene/environment interaction theory, have achieved conflicting results [29–31]. The GEMMA (Genome, Environment, Microbiome and Metabolome in Autism) team hypothesizes that many environmental factors can alter intestinal microbiota composition and activity, causing epigenetic modifications, changes in the metabolome profile, and increases in intestinal barrier permeability and macromolecule trafficking with the alteration of immune responses, thus contributing to the progression and development of ASD. Furthermore, it is hypothesized that the genome/metagenome interaction determines the switch from immune tolerance to immune response. Environmental stimuli, including dietary and microbial factors, can trigger an immune response, such as the neuroinflammation responsible for the behavioral changes that characterize ASD and intestinal inflammation causing its GI comorbidity.

The existence of a gut–brain axis was hypothesized by Bolte in the late 1990s [32]. This was one of the first reports of unhealthy changes in the intestinal tract's resident community (microbiome), driving both behavioral and GI problems in babies with ASD. Finegold et al. [33] showed that the increase in toxin-producing gut bacteria populations directly affects the brain via the vagus nerve. Currently, changes in gut microbiota of ASD patients with and without GI symptoms are well established [34–36], suggesting the potential beneficial effect of fecal transplantation [37,38].

Unfortunately, current large-scale studies of ASD are mainly of cross-sectional study design, which can provide information about associations between microbiome changes and ASD diagnoses but lack the information regarding the temporality of these changes. This limits inferences about causality or utility as an early life biomarker. Indeed, currently, there are no established biomarkers for ASD to enable its clinical diagnosis, which relies on behavioral evaluations. In addition, no medications are currently available to treat the core symptoms of ASD and results from intervention research are mixed [39].

2. Study Design

GEMMA is a multi-center, prospective, open-label, uncontrolled study with an observational and an interventional arm, comprised of collaborators in the European Union and the United States. It is coordinated by the European Biomedical Research Institute of Salerno (EBRIS), in Campania, Italy. GEMMA aims to study genomic, environmental, microbiome, and metabolomic factors that, via the immune system, may contribute to the development of ASD longitudinally. This study offers the potential to identify the mechanisms and/or biomarkers involved in either development or exacerbation of ASD signs and symptoms, which will potentially broaden the range of available therapeutic interventions (Figure 1).

The project includes clinical (observational and interventional trials) and pre-clinical studies. Several pre-clinical studies in humanized murine models (fecal transfer from ASD probands) and in vitro colon models will be performed simultaneously with clinical studies from the moment of recruitment of at-risk infants and their affected ASD sibling. This will support the progress of a microbiome-wide association study (of human participants) to identify prognostic microbiome signatures and metabolic pathways underlying mechanisms for ASD progression and severity and potential treatment response. The preclinical work will provide valuable information regarding validation of specific biomarkers mechanistically linked to the onset of ASD, which will be used to rationalize future patient stratification for primary intervention.

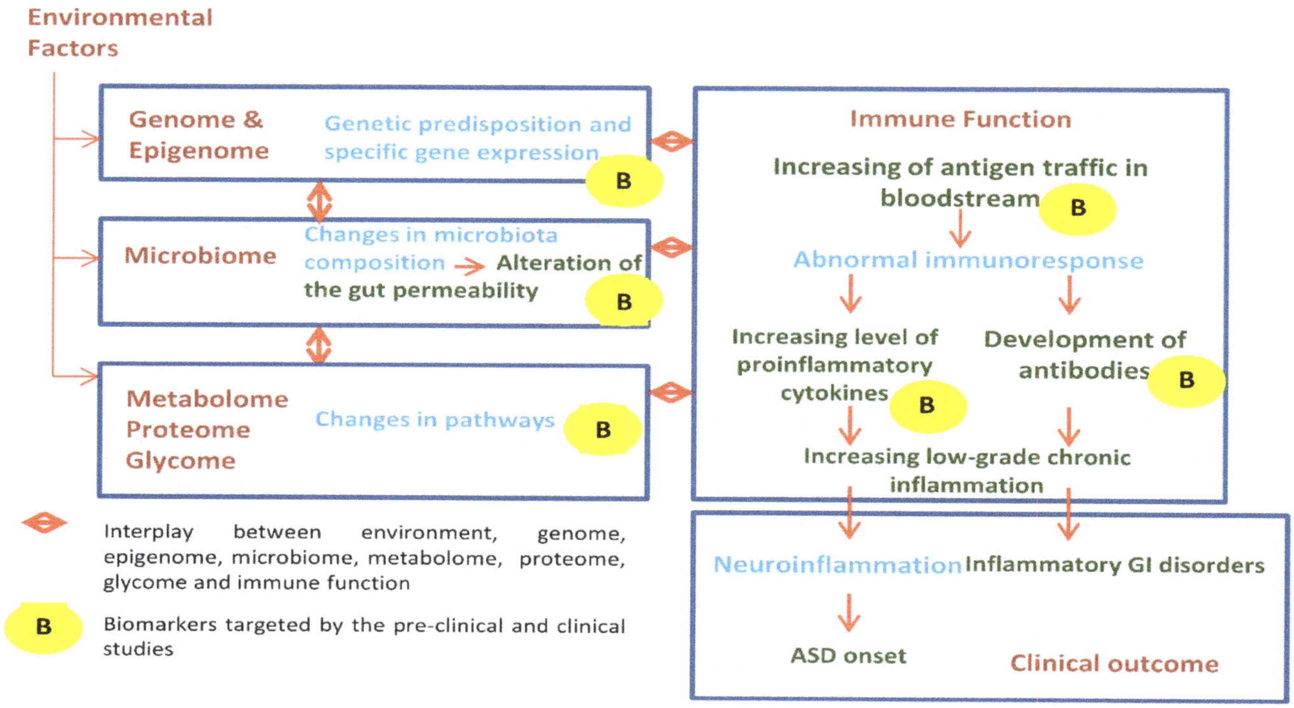

Figure 1. GEMMA (Genome, Environment, Microbiome and Metabolome in Autism) study design.

2.1. Pre-Clinical Studies

An in vitro micro-scale colon microbiota model or "colon microcosm" that mimics the microbiota of the human colon will be used to investigate effects of various combinations of prebiotic fiber types and probiotics on microbiota composition and functionality. The colon microcosms will be inoculated with fecal samples collected from children diagnosed with ASD with and without a history of GI problems, and from healthy siblings (controls) between the ages of 3 and 14. Samples will be excluded if the participants have used psychotropic medications in the previous 6 months and antibiotics and/or probiotics in the previous 2 months (Figure 2).

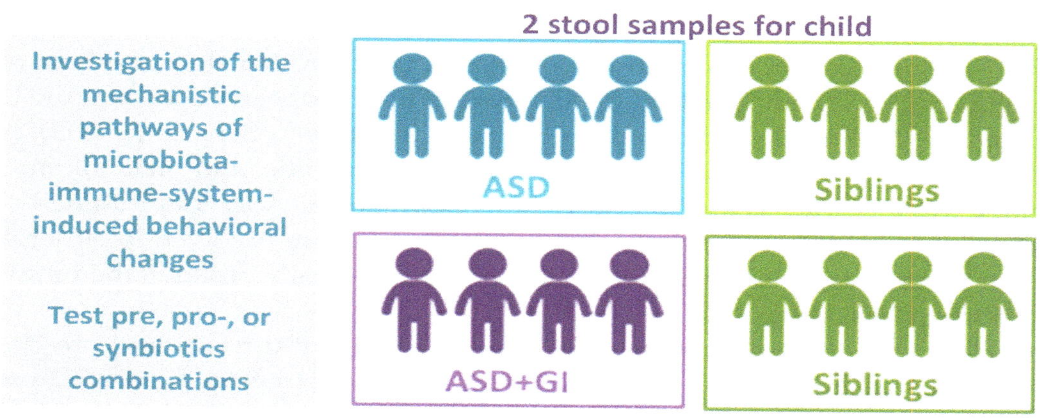

Figure 2. Preclinical studies—development of humanized mouse models by transplanting fecal samples from a well-characterized ASD diagnosed proband (and sibling controls). Four groups of children, each with 4 children, recruited in one center in Europe (Italy): autistic with no GI problems, autistic with GI problems, controls without or with GI problems. Ongoing.

The impact of pre- and probiotic combinations on microbiota composition and function will be measured by 16S rRNA gene sequencing, metagenomics, and targeted and untargeted metabolites analyses.

The preclinical studies in murine models will be carried out simultaneously with the other studies for two reasons: to provide further information on validation of specific biomarkers mechanistically linked to the onset of ASD and, consequently, to treat future patients primarily with a more precise intervention.

The preclinical studies in murine models include the development of humanized mouse models through transplanting fecal samples from a well-characterized ASD diagnosed proband (and sibling controls) in the families included in the clinical observational study. The fecal samples will be the same as those collected for the in vitro studies described above. In addition to wild type naïve mice, fecal transplantation will be conducted in genetically vulnerable (PCDH-KO), food allergic (CMA), and valproate-treated (VPA) male mice which have been previously demonstrated to show ASD-like behavior [40–43]. The natural gut microbiota of these mice will be depleted before transplantation with the human fecal samples. This will be achieved at the age of 3 weeks, with antibiotic treatment followed by a bowel cleansing according to procedures described by Le Roy and coworkers [44]. Fecal transplantation will also be conducted in germ-free male mice, which have abnormal development of the nervous system and show deficits in cognition, social behavior, and stress-related behaviors [45–51]. The microbial content of human donors will be orally administered to recipient microbiota-depleted or germ-free mice. Behavior, microbiota composition, gut permeability, metabolites, mucosal and systemic immune profiles (intestinal tract, mesenteric lymph nodes, blood, and spleen), neurotransmitters, and neuroinflammation in the brain will be evaluated to investigate the mechanistic evidence of the intestinal microbiota–brain axis in ASD. In addition, ASD-humanized VPA and CMA male mice will be suitable splenocyte donors for transferring their behavioral phenotype to naïve mice to reveal whether the ASD-like phenotype is microbiome-immune system-dependent. A second series of preclinical studies will establish whether correction of intestinal microbial dysbiosis by pre/pro/synbiotic intervention prevents and/or treats ASD-like behavior in ASD murine models. Selected ASD humanized murine models will be fed diets supplemented with selected pre/pro/synbiotics, which will be prescreened using microcosms systems as described above. Those that affect neurodevelopment, behavior, and the GI tract positively will be used in the clinical intervention trial.

2.2. Clinical Study

2.2.1. Participants

GEMMA aims to enroll 600 infants younger than 6 months/26 weeks of age, who have an older sibling with ASD for the observational trial. The recruitment will be carried out in three different centers: Irish Center for Autism and Neurodevelopmental Research (ICAN) at the National University of Ireland, Galway, Azienda Sanitaria Locale Salerno (ASL), and satellite centers in Italy, and Mass General Hospital for Children (MGHFC) Lurie Center for Autism in USA. The first study samples must be collected prior to the introduction of solid foods. Children who have started any other therapeutic intervention for ASD will also be excluded from the study. According to our previous experience with similar projects involving two cohorts of infants at-risk of celiac disease [52,53], enrollment will be performed by inviting parents' of the autistic patients who are followed by the recruitment clinics to participate in the study in the case of newborns, and advertising the study among ASD support and ASD patients' groups. Moreover, a traditional and social media diffusion plan was created to increase the project knowledge and support. No compensation will be provided to the participant.

Infants aged 18–36 months who were recruited, completed the observational study, developed clinical signs and symptoms of ASD, and whose parents permit the intervention of solely dietary and oral therapy in this study, will be invited to enroll for a follow-on dietary interventional trial.

2.2.2. Observational Trial

This study phase will evaluate infants at high risk of ASD. To achieve the sample size needed for clinical and biological comparisons, and ensure there is a reasonable representation across study sites, each site will target recruitment of 200 infants at high risk of developing ASD, over a 3 year period. All recruited children will undergo regular clinical and laboratory evaluations for 36 months, or more in the case of ASD development based on the annual intermediate clinical data check. Blood, urine, stools, and saliva samples will be collected every 6 months until 36 months of age.

Regarding GI symptoms, children will be evaluated for chronic irregular bowel movements (constipation, diarrhea), encopresis, recurrent abdominal pain, gastroesophageal reflux, and vomiting or food aversion. On these bases, the evaluable target study population (see Table 1 for inclusion/exclusion criteria) will be divided into four groups (depending on their clinical outcome: neuro competent at-risk infants with (NC-GI) and without GI symptoms (NC), ASD infants with GI symptoms (ASD-GI) and ASD infants without GI symptoms (ASD)). Maternal and paternal genomic samples will be taken from parents of infants at the time of enrollment and analyzed to examine inherited and de novo genetic traits.

Table 1. Inclusion and exclusion criteria for the observational trial.

Inclusion Criteria (All Must be Met)	Exclusion Criteria (Participant Will be Excluded from the Study if Any of the Criteria are Met)
1. Healthy newborns or infants 2. First-degree relatives of ASD participant (at least one sibling affected by ASD) 3. Younger than 6 months/26 weeks 4. Have never received solid food (elementary formula feeding permitted)	1. Newborns with significant health issues that require surgical treatments or continuous medical treatments and/or surgical treatments 2. Infants older than 6 months/26 weeks 3. Infants who have been introduced to solid food (including occasional use) 4. Severe GI problems requiring immediate treatment (life-threatening) 5. Severely underweight/malnourished children 6. Dietary restriction in the previous 3 months 7. Tube feeding 8. Drugs since birth which may affect the biomarkers being assessed, for example 9. Antibiotics within one month prior to enrollment; antibiotics used as a continuous course for ≥28 days prior to enrolment

Autism Diagnostic Observation Schedule (ADOS Toddler) evaluation [54] will be conducted every 6 months by a trained physician, starting at 12 months of age. For children younger than 24 months who test positive in the ADOS Toddler evaluation, the evaluation will be repeated one month later to confirm diagnosis to enroll the infant in an interventional study, and will be used to divide the participants into two groups: ASD children or non-ASD children (typically developing). Typically developing children will be followed until 36 months (see Figure 3) of age and their data will be selected at the end of the study to provide the information for the matched control comparisons.

Additional behavioral assessments include Early Screening for Autism and Communication Disorders and Repetitive Behavior Scale [55,56], Mullen Scales of Early Learning (MSEL) [57], and Vineland Adaptive Behavior Scales (VABS) [58]. These assessments will take place at 24 and 36 months of age.

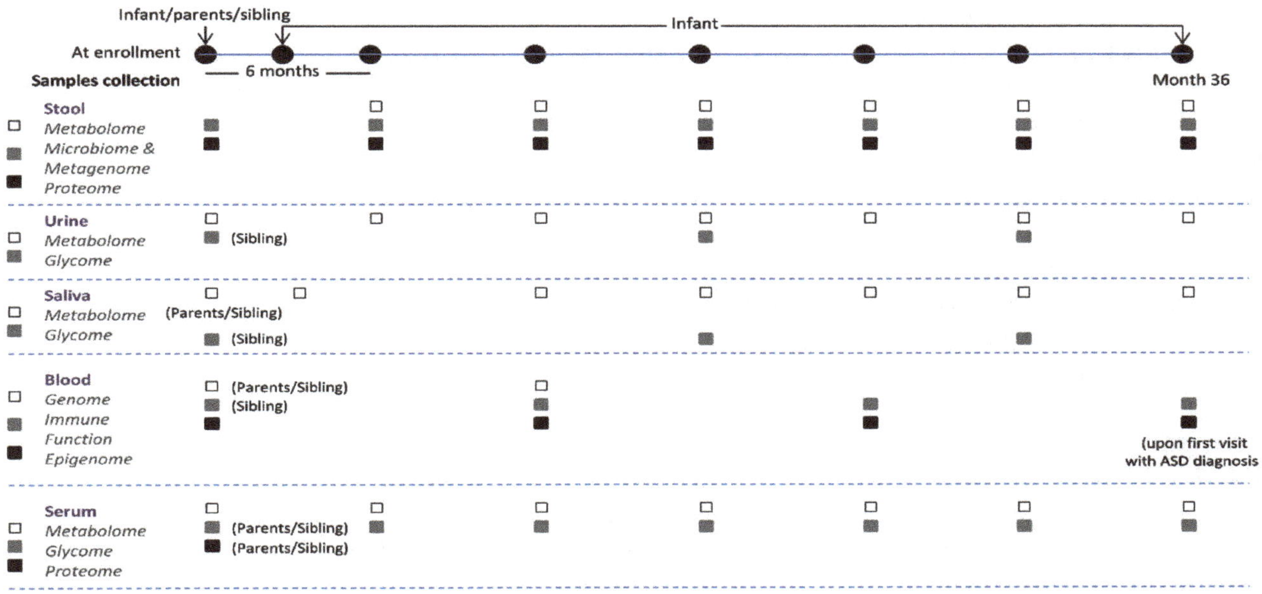

Figure 3. Clinical trials—prospective multi-center observational study evaluating infants at risk of ASD. 600 infants—newborns, less than 6 months of age—at risk, i.e., first-degree relatives of ASD individuals, recruited in US, Italy, and Ireland (200 infants at each site, over a 3-year period). Ongoing.

2.2.3. Interventional Trial

This prospective, multi-center, open-label, uncontrolled study (Figure 4) evaluates the effects of pre/pro/synbiotics supplementation started in infants between the ages of 18 and 36 months with a diagnosis of ASD.

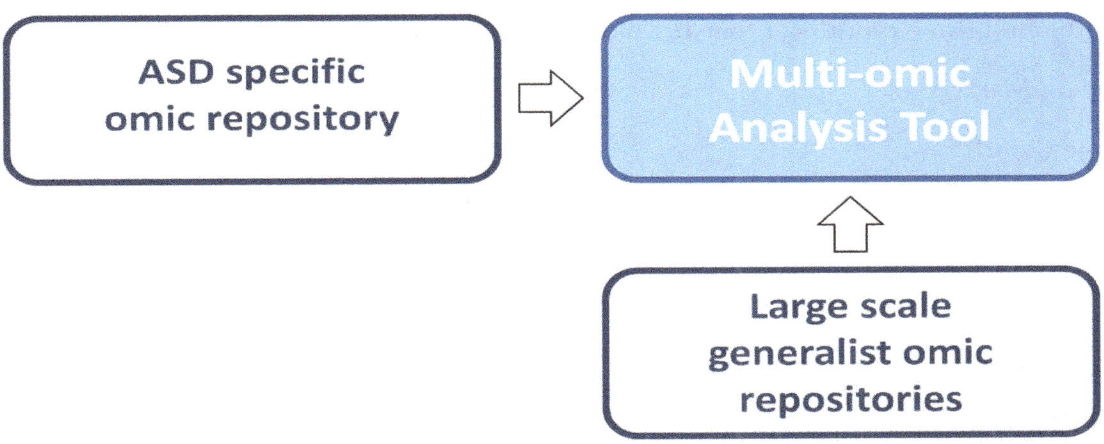

Figure 4. Interventional trial—prospective, multi-center, open-label, uncontrolled study to evaluate the effects of pre/pro/synbiotics supplementation in infants with a diagnosis of ASD. Forty children between the ages of 18 and 36 months diagnosed with ASD from the observational trial will be recruited (with parental consent).

A minimum of 40 children diagnosed with ASD from the observational trial will be recruited to the interventional trial, subject to parental consent. Each ASD infant will undergo a Positron Emission Tomography (PET) scan of their brain, at the beginning and end of the interventional study, to obtain information on the degree of neuro-inflammation and the potential effect of the intervention. The presence/absence of GI symptoms will also be evaluated.

Clinical and laboratory assessments will be made at the time of enrollment, monthly for 3 months, and then at the conclusion of the 6 month study.

The study was approved by the relevant ethics committee of each enrolling country. In particular: CE Campania Sud (IRB n.30/2019) for Italy; Partners Human Research (IRB ver.01/04/2019) for USA; and Clinical Research Ethics Committee of Galway University Hospital (IRB n. C.A. 2127/19) for Ireland. A written consent form will be signed by each participant or their legal representative. The clinical trial was registered with the access number: NCT04271774 (https://clinicaltrials.gov).

2.3. *Data Collection*

The timetables of data and sample collection are shown in Supplementary Tables S1–S3 and in Figure 3. Pre-screening may occur verbally via a telephone call or in person at a hospital clinic. Parents who wish to enroll their infant in the study will provide proof of ASD diagnosis for the child with the condition. Each clinical site will be responsible for its own data collection and management. Data will be monitored remotely for completeness and coherence by the project management team. All data will be collected through a secure, internet-based electronic capture system (REDCap) [59]. Participating institutions will be granted access to the electronic storage module with all appropriate forms and schedules pre-loaded. Each institution will only be able to view data for participants enrolled at their site. The coordinating center will be granted access to unidentified data from all sites through the electronic data capture system.

Parental and Child Questionnaires

An online questionnaire will be filled out by the family every month during the 6 months of intervention. Moreover, it will be filled out by the family at 9, 15, 21, 27, and 33 months of age and will include infant dietary data and the use of concomitant medication (vaccinations and antibiotics), demographics, infant clinical history including but not limited to infections, onset of food intolerance, and chronic stress. Parents will also be requested to complete the Aberrant Behavior Checklist (ABC) at all visits and at 9 months. Assessment scales for infant development (Rome 3 Criteria GSRS, ADOS-Toddler, Mullen scale, CGI-S, CGI-I) will be assessed, during the interventional trial, every month for the first three months of the study, and three months later at the final 6-month study visit.

2.4. *Serological Markers*

2.4.1. Whole Blood

Blood sampling will take place at enrollment, 0–6 months post birth, and at 12, 18, 24, 30, and 36 months of age. Blood for hematology, biochemistry evaluation, biomarker identification, and genetic assays will be collected from infants fasting for at least 3 h. The blood collection procedure is as follows: via umbilical cord for infants enrolled during gestation, or by heel sampling at enrollment (at 0–6 months of at-risk infant age), 1 mL every 6 months from 12 months of age, and finally at development of ASD or at the 36-month (observational study termination visit). The assays that will be performed on blood include whole genome sequencing on infants that develop ASD. Furthermore, DNA methylation (DNAm) will be measured among infants that develop ASD using samples obtained at three time points: (1) enrollment, (2) the time of ASD diagnosis, and (3) the completion of the interventional trial. In preparation for future testing, a biorepository will be established. A blood sample will be taken after 12 months for peripheral blood mononuclear cell (PBMC) isolation and immune profiling analysis.

Moreover, serum testing will take place at enrollment of the clinical study, 0–6 months post birth, and at 12, 18, 24, 30, and 36 months of age. A quantity of 500 uL of serum will be taken from the infant fasting for 3 h to evaluate serum zonulin (20 μL); serum IgA and IgG anti-gliadin and anti-casein antibody determination (40 μL) by the ELISA method; serum pro-inflammatory cytokines, including cIL-1, TNF-α, IFN-, IL-10, IL-12, IL-6, IL15, and IL-8 by Bioplex assay (75 μL) [60]; and cytokine gene expression by RT-PCR.

If ASD is developed, whole genome sequencing of the infant and of both parents will be performed.

2.4.2. Stool, Urine, and Saliva Samples

Every 3 months after enrollment, urine and stool samples will be collected at home and shipped to the laboratory for biomarker assay. Because patient samples are divided according to the presence and absence of a history of GI problems with an onset earlier than the initiation of toilet training, the aim is to select children with a biological rather than psychological etiology of GI discomfort. The control group includes fecal samples from age- and gender-matched control participants without previous diagnosis of a neurodevelopmental disorder and without a history of GI problems. Exclusion criteria for the use of patients and control samples include the use of psychotropic medication for the previous 6 months and antibiotics and/or probiotics for the previous 2 months.

Saliva samples will be taken for microbiome and glycome (the whole set of carbohydrates) analysis. Moreover, when possible subsequent analysis/correlation with blood biomarker levels either within this protocol or at a later timepoint will be performed. The saliva samples will be analyzed for pro-inflammatory markers and for six inflammatory markers selected from a previous study [61].

3. Factor of Interest

3.1. Environmental

Birthing delivery mode, method of infant feeding, and introduction of solid food and allergen to the infant diet could represent potential environmental factors causing ASD, so these will be recorded for each enrolled participant [53,62,63]. A diary of antibiotic usage will be completed by the parents monthly for the first year of life, and food diaries completed at the same time points will assess duration of breastfeeding (or other preferred feeding mode).

After the first year of life, detailed, although less frequent, records of antibiotic use will be obtained with each stool sample for the remaining duration of the study. Although the food diary will be discontinued at this time, pertinent dietary habits of both the mother and child will continue to be carefully recorded approximately every six months.

Moreover, details such as antibiotic exposure in early infancy, family living address, exposure to pets, and gastrointestinal sporadic symptoms will also be recorded.

3.2. Genetics

Currently, ASD heritability based on mono- and dizygotic twins is estimated to be about 79–80% [64,65]. Concordance is higher in monozygotic twins than dizygotic twins.

First-degree relatives of ASD probands show behavioral or cognitive features associated with autism intensification, such as language and social dysfunction, albeit in lesser forms [66], known as "broader phenotype" [67–70].

ASD-related social impairments are heritable [71] and increase in unaffected parents and children of autistic probands [72]. Several studies evaluating sub-threshold ASD traits in population cohorts suggested that different components, separately representing language, social function, and repetitive or stereotyped behaviors contribute to ASD [73–75]. Globally, these results suggest that ASD features represent a continuum of function that may be inherited in distinct patterns. This is consistent with the knowledge that specific genetic factors contribute to the development and function of specific brain structures, and that distinct brain circuits may underlie different components of autism [76].

Moreover, several genetic syndromes, including Fragile X, Tuberous Sclerosis, Joubert Syndrome and Smith Lemli Opitz, are known to cause, although with low penetrance, ASD-like symptoms [76,77]. This evidence further favors a genetic cause for ASD [78].

To assess the contribution of genetic risk factors, in combination with exposure and other omics data, we will perform whole genome sequencing in all participants with ASD, in addition to their parents. This will enable investigation of both common and rare variants that contribute to ASD risk.

3.3. *GI Microbiome and Metabolome*

The complete understanding of the host-GI microbiome genomics is necessary for the prediction of the activation of metabolic pathways linked with functional and clinical outcomes. Urine and stool samples will be collected and analyzed for a metabolomic phenotype of the GI microbiota and metabolomics profiles, including metabolites linked to bacterial activity in ASD. The metabolomic profiles, exploratory semi-quantitative assays, and targeted quantitative assays will be conducted throughout the study. Systems models of integrated metabolomic phenotypes will be created with the statistically linked data between the microbiota and immune function. By conjoining microbiota data and metabolomic data we will be able to understand the functions associated with GI comorbidity of children with ASD and the ASD patient-derived microbiota. Dietary interventions with pre/pro/synbiotics will be created based on the results found in the humanized mouse models undergoing fecal transplantation with ASD-specific microbiota.

3.4. *Immune Function*

The peripheral blood mononuclear cells (PBMCs) will be harvested and studied for immune functions. Standard flow cytometry will be used to measure monocyte and T-cell intracellular cytokine patterns. By looking at the T cell populations in children with ASD with and without GI symptoms we will be able to understand what cellular activation and functional alterations are present. Assays performed on serum samples collected at clinical visits include: serum zonulin determination; serum IgA and IgG anti-gliadin and anti-casein determination by the ELISA method; serum pro-inflammatory cytokines, including IL-1, TNF, IFN, IL-10, IL-12, IL-6, IL-15, and IL-8 by Bioplex assay; and cytokine gene expression by RT-PCR. Protein glycosylation is directly involved in nearly every biological process presenting altered glycosylation as potential biomarkers in many human conditions including inflammation, diabetes, rheumatism, cancer, and neurological disorders [79]. Serum immunoglobulin glyco-signaturing will be performed using lectin microarrays and anti-glycan ELISA profiling. Saliva samples will also be analyzed for proinflammatory cytokines and inflammatory markers selected from a previous study [61], and altered glycan and glycation products.

4. Statistical Approach

4.1. *Statistical Methods*

Categorical data will be described using frequency counts and percentages, and continuous data with mean, standard deviation, median, minimum, and maximum. Both parametric and non-parametric methods will be used to analyze the data. All omics data will be preprocessed with appropriate methods. The multi-omics analyses will be performed with statistical tests, regression models, and more advanced methods such as sparse canonical correlation analysis and random forest analysis. The false discovery rate (FDR) method will be used to adjust the p-values for multiple comparisons. Statistical significance will be set at $p < 0.05$.

4.2. *Power Analysis*

We estimated a conservative drop-off of 20% based on our previous experience with similar projects involving two cohorts of infants at-risk of celiac disease, one that has been followed for 10 years with a 20% drop-off [52] and a second that has been followed up to 7 years with a 12% drop-off [53]. The final cohort will comprise approximately 500 at-risk infants. Expected prevalence of ASD at 18–24 months in first-degree relatives is 14.7% [9], so in this study we estimate 73 ASD diagnoses. The expected prevalence of GI symptoms in an ASD population is 60% [80], so we anticipate 44 of the 73 ASD diagnosed infants to also present GI symptoms.

4.3. Developing an Integrative Multilevel Model to Predict ASD

Path a: A causal path between the genetics and the final effect on the onset of ASD, with the microbiome as the mediator (a1 × a2), so that the intestinal microbiome will be altered for the genetics to ultimately influence the development of the disorder (microbiome-mediated epigenetic pressure).

Path b: A causal path of the microbiome's effect on ASD mediated (b1 × b2) by the metabolic activity of intestinal bacteria, which, through the production of metabolites, affects the intestinal transcriptome and proteome. Including a bidirectional path between microbiome and metabolomics to capture how metabolism could alter the microbial metabolism and ultimately the risk for ASD.

Path c: A bidirectional path between the transcriptome and the microbiome because their causal relationship will depend on each other.

Path d: A direct relationship between lifestyle factors and the onset of the disorder mediated (d1 × d2) by alterations in the microbiome.

Path e: The environment affecting the onset of the disorder as a mediator and affecting the composition of the microbiome and resulting metabolome, in turn, influencing gene and protein expression.

Full Model: Time points will be clustered within individual characteristics; analyzing all of the paths listed above, individuals will be clustered within families, and families within regions.

5. Discussions and Conclusions

The implementation of primary prevention strategies for ASD via manipulation of the intestinal microbiota represents a complete paradigm shift of treatment and prevention of ASD. The identification of specific ASD metagenomics and metabolomics phenotypes can also help to define additional biomarker-based diagnostic tools and therapeutic interventions. Additionally, GEMMA's biorepository will encourage future epigenetic studies and validation of biomarkers. Our findings may also impact the prevention and treatment of other neuroinflammatory conditions.

Author Contributions: Conceptualization, A.F., A.K., C.L.-A., G.C., G.L., J.T., M.G., R.A. and S.R.; methodology, A.G., A.M. (Alessandra Mezzelani), A.M. (Arlene Mannion), C.B., C.R., D.F., E.M., F.I., G.R., H.K., L.J., L.M., L.N., N.Z.P., P.P.P., S.C., S.D., S.F., S.K. and T.B.; writing—original draft preparation, J.T.; writing—review and editing, A.F., A.K., C.L.-A., G.C., G.L., M.G., R.A., S.R., A.G., A.M. (Alessandra Mezzelani), A.M. (Arlene Mannion), C.B., C.R., D.F., E.M., F.C., F.I., F.P.T., G.R., G.S., H.K., L.J., L.M., L.N., L.N.P.M., L.R., N.Z.P., P.P.P., S.C., S.D., S.F., S.K. and T.B.; supervision, A.F.; project administration, F.C., F.P.T. All authors have read and agreed to the published version of the manuscript.

Acknowledgments: This work is conducted with support from the Advisory Board Members (California Institute of Technology, Winclove Probiotics, University of California Davis, Center for Autism and the Developing Brain, Ohio State University, the Autism Speaks Autism Treatment Network, Arizona State University, University College Cork), from the Consortium Partners: Fondazione EBRIS, in charge of project management and coordination and providing the gut permeability and immunological evaluation of the enrolled subjects; Nutricia Research Bv in charge of nutritional formulation development for interventional trial; Medinok Spa and Consiglio Nazionale Delle Ricerche (CNR) in charge of data analysis and multi-omics platform development; Bio Modeling Systems in charge of the mechanistic pathway hypothesis development; Euformatics in charge of analysis and the interpretation of the genomic variants of the patient material, and for the comparison of the variants from the different patient cohorts, Theoreo Srl and Imperial College Of Science in charge of metabolomics analysis and interpretation; National University of Ireland Galway, Azienda Sanitaria, Locale (ASL) Salerno and Massachusettse General Hospital for Children, in charge of enrollments for observation and interventional trials; Institut National de Recherche pour l'Agriculture, l'Alimentation et l'Environnement in charge of analyzing the genomic and transcriptomic profiles of the host microbiota; Institut National de la Santé et de la Recherche Médicale, in charge of proteomics analysis; Utrecht University, in charge of pre-clinical studies; Tampereen Yliopisto, in charge of experimental design; Johns Hopkins University in charge of epigenomic evaluation and interpretation. Financial contributions were made by European Union.

References

1. Evans, B. How autism became autism: The radical transformation of a central concept of child development in Britain. *Hist. Hum. Sci.* **2013**, *26*, 3–31. [CrossRef] [PubMed]

2. Elsabbagh, M.; Divan, G.; Koh, Y.-J.; Kim, Y.S.; Kauchali, S.; Marcín, C.; Montiel-Nava, C.; Patel, V.; Paula, C.S.; Wang, C.; et al. Global prevalence of autism and other pervasive developmental disorders. *Autism Res.* **2012**, *5*, 160–179. [CrossRef]
3. Newschaffer, C.J.; Croen, L.A.; Daniels, J.; Giarelli, E.; Grether, J.K.; Levy, S.E.; Mandell, D.S.; Miller, L.A.; Pinto-Martin, J.; Reaven, J.; et al. The epidemiology of autism spectrum disorders. *Annu. Rev. Public Health* **2007**, *28*, 235–258. [CrossRef] [PubMed]
4. Wing, L.; Potter, D. The epidemiology of autistic spectrum disorders: Is the prevalence rising? *Ment. Retard. Dev. Disabil. Res. Rev.* **2002**, *8*, 151–161. [CrossRef]
5. Fombonne, E. The prevalence of autism. *JAMA* **2003**, *289*, 87–89. [CrossRef] [PubMed]
6. Centers for Disease Control and Prevention. *(CDC) Prevalence of Autism Spectrum Disorders—Autism and Developmental Disabilities Monitoring Network, 14 Sites USA, 2008*; Centers for Disease Control and Prevention: Atlanta, GA, USA, 2012.
7. Maenner, M.J. Prevalence of Autism Spectrum Disorder Among Children Aged 8 Years—Autism and Developmental Disabilities Monitoring Network, 11 Sites, United States, 2016. *MMWR Surveill. Summ.* **2020**, *69*, 1–12. [CrossRef] [PubMed]
8. Autism Spectrum Disorders in the European Union (ASDEU). Consortium Autism Spectrum Disorders in the European Union (ASDEU): Final Report: Main Results of the ASDEU Project, ASDEU, Madrid: 28 August 2018. Available online: http://repositorio.insa.pt/handle/10400.18/6188 (accessed on 15 October 2020).
9. Ozonoff, S.; Young, G.S.; Carter, A.; Messinger, D.; Yirmiya, N.; Zwaigenbaum, L.; Bryson, S.; Carver, L.J.; Constantino, J.N.; Dobkins, K.; et al. Recurrence risk for autism spectrum disorders: A Baby Siblings Research Consortium study. *Pediatrics* **2011**, *128*, e488–e495. [CrossRef]
10. Satterstrom, F.K.; Kosmicki, J.A.; Wang, J.; Breen, M.S.; De Rubeis, S.; An, J.-Y.; Peng, M.; Collins, R.; Grove, J.; Klei, L.; et al. Large-Scale Exome Sequencing Study Implicates Both Developmental and Functional Changes in the Neurobiology of Autism. *Cell* **2020**, *180*, 568–584.e23. [CrossRef] [PubMed]
11. Bai, D.; Yip, B.H.K.; Windham, G.C.; Sourander, A.; Francis, R.; Yoffe, R.; Glasson, E.; Mahjani, B.; Suominen, A.; Leonard, H.; et al. Association of Genetic and Environmental Factors With Autism in a 5-Country Cohort. *JAMA Psychiatry* **2019**, *76*, 1035–1043. [CrossRef]
12. Sandin, S.; Lichtenstein, P.; Kuja-Halkola, R.; Larsson, H.; Hultman, C.M.; Reichenberg, A. The familial risk of autism. *JAMA* **2014**, *311*, 1770–1777. [CrossRef]
13. Brucato, M.; Ladd-Acosta, C.; Li, M.; Caruso, D.; Hong, X.; Kaczaniuk, J.; Stuart, E.A.; Fallin, M.D.; Wang, X. Prenatal exposure to fever is associated with autism spectrum disorder in the boston birth cohort. *Autism Res.* **2017**, *10*, 1878–1890. [CrossRef]
14. Croen, L.A.; Qian, Y.; Ashwood, P.; Zerbo, O.; Schendel, D.; Pinto-Martin, J.; Daniele Fallin, M.; Levy, S.; Schieve, L.A.; Yeargin-Allsopp, M.; et al. Infection and Fever in Pregnancy and Autism Spectrum Disorders: Findings from the Study to Explore Early Development. *Autism Res.* **2019**, *12*, 1551–1561. [CrossRef] [PubMed]
15. DiStasio, M.M.; Nagakura, I.; Nadler, M.J.; Anderson, M.P. T-lymphocytes and Cytotoxic Astrocyte Blebs Correlate Across Autism Brains. *Ann. Neurol.* **2019**, *86*, 885–898. [CrossRef] [PubMed]
16. Hornig, M.; Bresnahan, M.A.; Che, X.; Schultz, A.F.; Ukaigwe, J.E.; Eddy, M.L.; Hirtz, D.; Gunnes, N.; Lie, K.K.; Magnus, P.; et al. Prenatal fever and autism risk. *Mol. Psychiatry* **2018**, *23*, 759–766. [CrossRef] [PubMed]
17. Nankova, B.B.; Agarwal, R.; MacFabe, D.F.; La Gamma, E.F. Enteric bacterial metabolites propionic and butyric acid modulate gene expression, including CREB-dependent catecholaminergic neurotransmission, in PC12 cells–possible relevance to autism spectrum disorders. *PLoS ONE* **2014**, *9*, e103740. [CrossRef]
18. Macfabe, D. Autism: Metabolism, mitochondria, and the microbiome. *Glob. Adv. Health Med.* **2013**, *2*, 52–66. [CrossRef] [PubMed]
19. Scumpia, P.O.; Kelly-Scumpia, K.; Stevens, B.R. Alpha-lipoic acid effects on brain glial functions accompanying double-stranded RNA antiviral and inflammatory signaling. *Neurochem. Int.* **2014**, *64*, 55–63. [CrossRef]
20. Zielinski, B.A.; Prigge, M.B.D.; Nielsen, J.A.; Froehlich, A.L.; Abildskov, T.J.; Anderson, J.S.; Fletcher, P.T.; Zygmunt, K.M.; Travers, B.G.; Lange, N.; et al. Longitudinal changes in cortical thickness in autism and typical development. *Brain* **2014**, *137*, 1799–1812. [CrossRef]

21. Stoner, R.; Chow, M.L.; Boyle, M.P.; Sunkin, S.M.; Mouton, P.R.; Roy, S.; Wynshaw-Boris, A.; Colamarino, S.A.; Lein, E.S.; Courchesne, E. Patches of Disorganization in the Neocortex of Children with Autism. *N. Engl. J. Med.* **2014**, *370*, 1209–1219. [CrossRef]
22. Rossignol, D.A.; Frye, R.E. A review of research trends in physiological abnormalities in autism spectrum disorders: Immune dysregulation, inflammation, oxidative stress, mitochondrial dysfunction and environmental toxicant exposures. *Mol. Psychiatry* **2012**, *17*, 389–401. [CrossRef]
23. Kostic, A.D.; Gevers, D.; Siljander, H.; Vatanen, T.; Hyotylainen, T.; Hamalainen, A.-M.; Peet, A.; Tillmann, V.; Poho, P.; Mattila, I.; et al. The dynamics of the human infant gut microbiome in development and in progression toward type 1 diabetes. *Cell Host Microbe* **2015**, *17*, 260–273. [CrossRef] [PubMed]
24. Rook, G.A.; Raison, C.L.; Lowry, C.A. Microbiota, immunoregulatory old friends and psychiatric disorders. In *Microbial Endocrinology: The Microbiota-Gut-Brain Axis in Health and Disease*; Springer: Berlin/Heidelberg, Germany, 2014; pp. 319–356.
25. Borre, Y.E.; Moloney, R.D.; Clarke, G.; Dinan, T.G.; Cryan, J.F. The impact of microbiota on brain and behavior: Mechanisms & therapeutic potential. In *Microbial Endocrinology: The Microbiota-Gut-Brain Axis in Health and Disease*; Springer: Berlin/Heidelberg, Germany, 2014; pp. 373–403.
26. Shimabukuro, T.T.; Grosse, S.D.; Rice, C. Medical expenditures for children with an autism spectrum disorder in a privately insured population. *J. Autism Dev. Disord.* **2008**, *38*, 546–552. [CrossRef] [PubMed]
27. Peacock, G.; Amendah, D.; Ouyang, L.; Grosse, S.D. Autism spectrum disorders and health care expenditures: The effects of co-occurring conditions. *J. Dev. Behav. Pediatr.* **2012**, *33*, 2–8. [CrossRef]
28. Blumberg, S.J.; Bramlett, M.D.; Kogan, M.D.; Schieve, L.A.; Jones, J.R.; Lu, M.C. Changes in prevalence of parent-reported autism spectrum disorder in school-aged U.S. children: 2007 to 2011–2012. *Natl. Health Stat. Rep.* **2013**, *65*, 1–11.
29. Fletcher-Watson, S.; McConnell, F.; Manola, E.; McConachie, H. Interventions based on the Theory of Mind cognitive model for autism spectrum disorder (ASD). *Cochrane Database Syst. Rev.* **2014**, *3*, CD008785. [CrossRef]
30. Sukhodolsky, D.G.; Bloch, M.H.; Panza, K.E.; Reichow, B. Cognitive-behavioral therapy for anxiety in children with high-functioning autism: A meta-analysis. *Pediatrics* **2013**, *132*, e1341–e1350. [CrossRef] [PubMed]
31. Millward, C.; Ferriter, M.; Calver, S.; Connell-Jones, G. Gluten- and casein-free diets for autistic spectrum disorder. *Cochrane Database Syst. Rev.* **2008**, *2*, CD003498. [CrossRef] [PubMed]
32. Bolte, E.R. Autism and Clostridium tetani. *Med. Hypotheses* **1998**, *51*, 133–144. [CrossRef]
33. Finegold, S.M.; Molitoris, D.; Song, Y.; Liu, C.; Vaisanen, M.-L.; Bolte, E.; McTeague, M.; Sandler, R.; Wexler, H.; Marlowe, E.M.; et al. Gastrointestinal Microflora Studies in Late-Onset Autism. *Clin. Infect. Dis.* **2002**, *35*, S6–S16. [CrossRef]
34. Pulikkan, J.; Mazumder, A.; Grace, T. Role of the Gut Microbiome in Autism Spectrum Disorders. In *Reviews on Biomarker Studies in Psychiatric and Neurodegenerative Disorders*; Guest, P.C., Ed.; Springer International Publishing: Cham, Switzerland, 2019; pp. 253–269, ISBN 978-3-030-05542-4.
35. Sharon, G.; Cruz, N.J.; Kang, D.-W.; Gandal, M.J.; Wang, B.; Kim, Y.-M.; Zink, E.M.; Casey, C.P.; Taylor, B.C.; Lane, C.J.; et al. Human Gut Microbiota from Autism Spectrum Disorder Promote Behavioral Symptoms in Mice. *Cell* **2019**, *177*, 1600–1618.e17. [CrossRef]
36. Strati, F.; Cavalieri, D.; Albanese, D.; De Felice, C.; Donati, C.; Hayek, J.; Jousson, O.; Leoncini, S.; Renzi, D.; Calabrò, A.; et al. New evidences on the altered gut microbiota in autism spectrum disorders. *Microbiome* **2017**, *5*, 24. [CrossRef] [PubMed]
37. Kang, D.-W.; Adams, J.B.; Gregory, A.C.; Borody, T.; Chittick, L.; Fasano, A.; Khoruts, A.; Geis, E.; Maldonado, J.; McDonough-Means, S.; et al. Microbiota Transfer Therapy alters gut ecosystem and improves gastrointestinal and autism symptoms: An open-label study. *Microbiome* **2017**, *5*, 10. [CrossRef]
38. Kang, D.-W.; Adams, J.B.; Coleman, D.M.; Pollard, E.L.; Maldonado, J.; McDonough-Means, S.; Caporaso, J.G.; Krajmalnik-Brown, R. Long-term benefit of Microbiota Transfer Therapy on autism symptoms and gut microbiota. *Sci. Rep.* **2019**, *9*, 5821. [CrossRef] [PubMed]
39. Masi, A.; DeMayo, M.M.; Glozier, N.; Guastella, A.J. An overview of autism spectrum disorder, heterogeneity and treatment options. *Neurosci. Bull.* **2017**, *33*, 183–193. [CrossRef]

40. de Theije, C.G.M.; Wu, J.; Koelink, P.J.; Korte-Bouws, G.A.H.; Borre, Y.; Kas, M.J.H.; da Silva, S.L.; Korte, S.M.; Olivier, B.; Garssen, J.; et al. Autistic-like behavioural and neurochemical changes in a mouse model of food allergy. *Behav. Brain Res.* **2014**, *261*, 265–274. [CrossRef] [PubMed]
41. de Theije, C.G.M.; van den Elsen, L.W.J.; Willemsen, L.E.M.; Milosevic, V.; Korte-Bouws, G.A.H.; da Silva, S.L.; Broersen, L.M.; Korte, S.M.; Olivier, B.; Garssen, J.; et al. Dietary long chain n-3 polyunsaturated fatty acids prevent impaired social behaviour and normalize brain dopamine levels in food allergic mice. *Neuropharmacology* **2015**, *90*, 15–22. [CrossRef]
42. Saunders, J.M.; Moreno, J.L.; Ibi, D.; Sikaroodi, M.; Kang, D.J.; Muñoz-Moreno, R.; Dalmet, S.S.; García-Sastre, A.; Gillevet, P.M.; Dozmorov, M.G.; et al. Gut microbiota manipulation during the prepubertal period shapes behavioral abnormalities in a mouse neurodevelopmental disorder model. *Sci. Rep.* **2020**, *10*, 4697. [CrossRef]
43. Wu, J.; de Theije, C.G.M.; da Silva, S.L.; Abbring, S.; van der Horst, H.; Broersen, L.M.; Willemsen, L.; Kas, M.; Garssen, J.; Kraneveld, A.D. Dietary interventions that reduce mTOR activity rescue autistic-like behavioral deficits in mice. *Brain Behav. Immun.* **2017**, *59*, 273–287. [CrossRef]
44. Le Roy, T.; Debédat, J.; Marquet, F.; Da-Cunha, C.; Ichou, F.; Guerre-Millo, M.; Kapel, N.; Aron-Wisnewsky, J.; Clément, K. Comparative Evaluation of Microbiota Engraftment Following Fecal Microbiota Transfer in Mice Models: Age, Kinetic and Microbial Status Matter. *Front. Microbiol.* **2019**, *9*, 3289. [CrossRef]
45. Stilling, R.M.; Moloney, G.M.; Ryan, F.J.; Hoban, A.E.; Bastiaanssen, T.F.; Shanahan, F.; Clarke, G.; Claesson, M.J.; Dinan, T.G.; Cryan, J.F. Social interaction-induced activation of RNA splicing in the amygdala of microbiome-deficient mice. *eLife* **2018**, *7*, e33070. [CrossRef]
46. Hoban, A.E.; Stilling, R.M.; Moloney, G.; Shanahan, F.; Dinan, T.G.; Clarke, G.; Cryan, J.F. The microbiome regulates amygdala-dependent fear recall. *Mol. Psychiatry* **2018**, *23*, 1134–1144. [CrossRef] [PubMed]
47. Luczynski, P.; Whelan, S.O.; O'Sullivan, C.; Clarke, G.; Shanahan, F.; Dinan, T.G.; Cryan, J.F. Adult microbiota-deficient mice have distinct dendritic morphological changes: Differential effects in the amygdala and hippocampus. *Eur. J. Neurosci.* **2016**, *44*, 2654–2666. [CrossRef]
48. Desbonnet, L.; Clarke, G.; Shanahan, F.; Dinan, T.G.; Cryan, J.F. Microbiota is essential for social development in the mouse. *Mol. Psychiatry* **2014**, *19*, 146–148. [CrossRef]
49. Buffington, S.A.; Di Prisco, G.V.; Auchtung, T.A.; Ajami, N.J.; Petrosino, J.F.; Costa-Mattioli, M. Microbial Reconstitution Reverses Maternal Diet-Induced Social and Synaptic Deficits in Offspring. *Cell* **2016**, *165*, 1762–1775. [CrossRef] [PubMed]
50. Neufeld, K.M.; Kang, N.; Bienenstock, J.; Foster, J.A. Reduced anxiety-like behavior and central neurochemical change in germ-free mice. *Neurogastroenterol. Motil.* **2011**, *23*, 255–264.e119. [CrossRef] [PubMed]
51. Arentsen, T.; Raith, H.; Qian, Y.; Forssberg, H.; Diaz Heijtz, R. Host microbiota modulates development of social preference in mice. *Microb. Ecol. Health Dis.* **2015**, *26*, 29719. [CrossRef]
52. Lionetti, E.; Castellaneta, S.; Francavilla, R.; Pulvirenti, A.; Tonutti, E.; Amarri, S.; Barbato, M.; Barbera, C.; Barera, G.; Bellantoni, A. Introduction of gluten, HLA status, and the risk of celiac disease in children. *N. Engl. J. Med.* **2014**, *371*, 1295–1303. [CrossRef]
53. Leonard, M.M.; Camhi, S.; Huedo-Medina, T.B.; Fasano, A. Celiac Disease Genomic, Environmental, Microbiome, and Metabolomic (CDGEMM) Study Design: Approach to the Future of Personalized Prevention of Celiac Disease. *Nutrients* **2015**, *7*, 9325–9336. [CrossRef]
54. Gotham, K.; Pickles, A.; Lord, C. Standardizing ADOS Scores for a Measure of Severity in Autism Spectrum Disorders. *J. Autism Dev. Disord.* **2009**, *39*, 693–705. [CrossRef]
55. Guthrie, W.; Swineford, L.B.; Nottke, C.; Wetherby, A.M. Early diagnosis of autism spectrum disorder: Stability and change in clinical diagnosis and symptom presentation. *J. Child. Psychol. Psychiatry* **2013**, *54*, 582–590. [CrossRef]
56. Wetherby, A.; Lord, C.; Woods, J.; Guthrie, W.; Pierce, K.; Shumway, S.; Thurm, A.; Ozonoff, S. The Early Screening for Autism and Communication Disorders (ESAC): Preliminary Field-Testing of An. Autism-Specific Screening Tool for Children 12 to 36 Months of Age. In Proceedings of the International Meeting for Autism Research, Chicago, IL, USA, 7–9 May 2009. Available online: https://www.researchgate.net/publication/268144139_The_Early_Screening_for_Autism_and_Communication_Disorders_ESAC_Preliminary_Field-Testing_of_An_Autism-Specific_Screening_Tool_for_Children_12_to_36_Months_of_Age (accessed on 15 October 2020).

57. Akshoomoff, N. Use of the Mullen Scales of Early Learning for the assessment of young children with Autism Spectrum Disorders. *Child. Neuropsychol.* **2006**, *12*, 269–277. [CrossRef] [PubMed]
58. Freeman, B.J.; Del'Homme, M.; Guthrie, D.; Zhang, F. Vineland Adaptive Behavior Scale Scores as a Function of Age and Initial IQ in 210 Autistic Children. *J. Autism Dev. Disord.* **1999**, *29*, 379–384. [CrossRef]
59. Harris, P.A.; Taylor, R.; Thielke, R.; Payne, J.; Gonzalez, N.; Conde, J.G. Research Electronic Data Capture (REDCap)-A metadata-driven methodology and workflow process for providing translational research informatics support. *J. Biomed. Inform.* **2009**, *42*, 377–381. [CrossRef] [PubMed]
60. Houser, B. Bio-Rad's Bio-Plex® suspension array system, xMAP technology overview. *Arch. Physiol. Biochem.* **2012**, *118*, 192–196. [CrossRef] [PubMed]
61. Wetie, A.G.N.; Wormwood, K.L.; Russell, S.; Ryan, J.P.; Darie, C.C.; Woods, A.G. A Pilot Proteomic Analysis of Salivary Biomarkers in Autism Spectrum Disorder. *Autism Res.* **2015**, *8*, 338–350. [CrossRef]
62. Curran, E.A.; Dalman, C.; Kearney, P.M.; Kenny, L.C.; Cryan, J.F.; Dinan, T.G.; Khashan, A.S. Association Between Obstetric Mode of Delivery and Autism Spectrum Disorder: A Population-Based Sibling Design Study. *JAMA Psychiatry* **2015**, *72*, 935–942. [CrossRef]
63. Tseng, P.-T.; Chen, Y.-W.; Stubbs, B.; Carvalho, A.F.; Whiteley, P.; Tang, C.-H.; Yang, W.-C.; Chen, T.-Y.; Li, D.-J.; Chu, C.-S.; et al. Maternal breastfeeding and autism spectrum disorder in children: A systematic review and meta-analysis. *Nutr. Neurosci.* **2019**, *22*, 354–362. [CrossRef]
64. Bailey, A.; Le Couteur, A.; Gottesman, I.; Bolton, P.; Simonoff, E.; Yuzda, E.; Rutter, M. Autism as a strongly genetic disorder: Evidence from a British twin study. *Psychol. Med.* **1995**, *25*, 63–77. [CrossRef]
65. Rosenberg, R.E.; Law, J.K.; Yenokyan, G.; McGready, J.; Kaufmann, W.E.; Law, P.A. Characteristics and concordance of autism spectrum disorders among 277 twin pairs. *Arch. Pediatrics Adolesc. Med.* **2009**, *163*, 907–914. [CrossRef]
66. Losh, M.; Adolphs, R.; Poe, M.D.; Couture, S.; Penn, D.; Baranek, G.T.; Piven, J. Neuropsychological profile of autism and the broad autism phenotype. *Arch. Gen. Psychiatry* **2009**, *66*, 518–526. [CrossRef]
67. Warren, Z.E.; Foss-Feig, J.H.; Malesa, E.E.; Lee, E.B.; Taylor, J.L.; Newsom, C.R.; Crittendon, J.; Stone, W.L. Neurocognitive and behavioral outcomes of younger siblings of children with autism spectrum disorder at age five. *J. Autism Dev. Disord.* **2012**, *42*, 409–418. [CrossRef]
68. Constantino, J.N. The quantitative nature of autistic social impairment. *Pediatric Res.* **2011**, *69*, 55R–62R. [CrossRef] [PubMed]
69. Gamliel, I.; Yirmiya, N.; Jaffe, D.H.; Manor, O.; Sigman, M. Developmental trajectories in siblings of children with autism: Cognition and language from 4 months to 7 years. *J. Autism Dev. Disord.* **2009**, *39*, 1131–1144. [CrossRef]
70. Pickles, A.; Starr, E.; Kazak, S.; Bolton, P.; Papanikolaou, K.; Bailey, A.; Goodman, R.; Rutter, M. Variable expression of the autism broader phenotype: Findings from extended pedigrees. *J. Child. Psychol. Psychiatry Allied Discip.* **2000**, *41*, 491–502. [CrossRef]
71. Constantino, J.N.; Todd, R.D. Intergenerational transmission of subthreshold autistic traits in the general population. *Biol. Psychiatry* **2005**, *57*, 655–660. [CrossRef]
72. Constantino, J.N.; Lajonchere, C.; Lutz, M.; Gray, T.; Abbacchi, A.; McKenna, K.; Singh, D.; Todd, R.D. Autistic social impairment in the siblings of children with pervasive developmental disorders. *Am. J. Psychiatry* **2006**, *163*, 294–296. [CrossRef] [PubMed]
73. Steer, C.D.; Golding, J.; Bolton, P.F. Traits contributing to the autistic spectrum. *PLoS ONE* **2010**, *5*, e12633. [CrossRef] [PubMed]
74. Ronald, A.; Happé, F.; Bolton, P.; Butcher, L.M.; Price, T.S.; Wheelwright, S.; Baron-Cohen, S.; Plomin, R. Genetic heterogeneity between the three components of the autism spectrum: A twin study. *J. Am. Acad. Child Adolesc. Psychiatry* **2006**, *45*, 691–699. [CrossRef] [PubMed]
75. Ronald, A.; Larsson, H.; Anckarsäter, H.; Lichtenstein, P. A twin study of autism symptoms in Sweden. *Mol. Psychiatry* **2011**, *16*, 1039. [CrossRef]
76. Geschwind, D.H. Autism: Many genes, common pathways? *Cell* **2008**, *135*, 391–395. [CrossRef]
77. Coleman, M.; Gillberg, C. *The Biology of the Autistic Syndromes*; Praeger: Westport, NY, USA, 1985; ISBN 0-275-91309-0.
78. Abrahams, B.S.; Geschwind, D.H. Advances in autism genetics: On the threshold of a new neurobiology. *Nat. Rev. Genet.* **2008**, *9*, 341. [CrossRef] [PubMed]

79. Hart, G.W.; Copeland, R.J. Glycomics hits the big time. *Cell* **2010**, *143*, 672–676. [CrossRef] [PubMed]
80. Wasilewska, J.; Klukowski, M. Gastrointestinal symptoms and autism spectrum disorder: Links and risks-a possible new overlap syndrome. *Pediatric Health Med. Ther.* **2015**, *6*, 153–166. [CrossRef] [PubMed]

Permissions

All chapters in this book were first published by MDPI; hereby published with permission under the Creative Commons Attribution License or equivalent. Every chapter published in this book has been scrutinized by our experts. Their significance has been extensively debated. The topics covered herein carry significant findings which will fuel the growth of the discipline. They may even be implemented as practical applications or may be referred to as a beginning point for another development.

The contributors of this book come from diverse backgrounds, making this book a truly international effort. This book will bring forth new frontiers with its revolutionizing research information and detailed analysis of the nascent developments around the world.

We would like to thank all the contributing authors for lending their expertise to make the book truly unique. They have played a crucial role in the development of this book. Without their invaluable contributions this book wouldn't have been possible. They have made vital efforts to compile up to date information on the varied aspects of this subject to make this book a valuable addition to the collection of many professionals and students.

This book was conceptualized with the vision of imparting up-to-date information and advanced data in this field. To ensure the same, a matchless editorial board was set up. Every individual on the board went through rigorous rounds of assessment to prove their worth. After which they invested a large part of their time researching and compiling the most relevant data for our readers.

The editorial board has been involved in producing this book since its inception. They have spent rigorous hours researching and exploring the diverse topics which have resulted in the successful publishing of this book. They have passed on their knowledge of decades through this book. To expedite this challenging task, the publisher supported the team at every step. A small team of assistant editors was also appointed to further simplify the editing procedure and attain best results for the readers.

Apart from the editorial board, the designing team has also invested a significant amount of their time in understanding the subject and creating the most relevant covers. They scrutinized every image to scout for the most suitable representation of the subject and create an appropriate cover for the book.

The publishing team has been an ardent support to the editorial, designing and production team. Their endless efforts to recruit the best for this project, has resulted in the accomplishment of this book. They are a veteran in the field of academics and their pool of knowledge is as vast as their experience in printing. Their expertise and guidance has proved useful at every step. Their uncompromising quality standards have made this book an exceptional effort. Their encouragement from time to time has been an inspiration for everyone.

The publisher and the editorial board hope that this book will prove to be a valuable piece of knowledge for researchers, students, practitioners and scholars across the globe.

List of Contributors

Karthikeyan Krishnamurthy, Michael K. Yeung and Yvonne M. Y. Han
Department of Rehabilitation Sciences, The Hong Kong Polytechnic University, Hong Kong, China

Agnes S. Chan
Department of Psychology, The Chinese University of Hong Kong, Hong Kong, China

Luca Pangrazzi, Luigi Balasco and Yuri Bozzi
Center for Mind/Brain Sciences (CIMeC), Neurodevelopmental Disorders Research Group, University of Trento, 38068 Rovereto, Italy

Gabriele Masi, Silvia Scullin, Antonio Narzisi, Pietro Muratori, Deborah Fabiani, Francesca Lenzi, Maria Mucci and Giulia D'Acunto
IRCCS Stella Maris, Scientific Institute of Child Neurology and Psychiatry, Calambrone, 56018 Pisa, Italy

Marinella Paciello
Faculty of Psychology, Università Telematica Internazionale Uninettuno, 00186 Rome, Italy

Ewa Pisula and Karolina Ziegart-Sadowska
Faculty of Psychology, University of Warsaw, Stawki 5/7, 00-183 Warsaw, Poland

G. Bradley Schaefer
University of Arkansas for Medical Sciences, Arkansas Children's Hospital, 1 Children's Way, Slot 512-22, Little Rock, AR 72202, USA

Sanae Tanaka
Division of Integrated Art and Sciences and Local Community Support, Research Center for Child Mental Development, Kanazawa University, Kanazawa 920-8640, Japan

Oko Arai and Aiko Komagome
The COI Site, Tokyo University of the Arts Tokyo 110-8714, Japan

Aya Iguchi-Sherry
Artlink Central, Scotland FK8 1EA, UK

Akiko Nagasaka
Department of Childhood Care and Education, Faculty of Social Work, Kinjo University, Hakusan 924-8511, Japan

Chiharu Tsuji, Teruko Yuhi and Haruhiro Higashida
Department of Basic Research on Social Recognition, Research Center for Child Mental Development, Kanazawa University, Kanazawa 920-8640, Japan

Kana Minami
Department of Basic Research on Social Recognition, Research Center for Child Mental Development, Kanazawa University, Kanazawa 920-8640, Japan
Department of Health Development Nursing, Institute of Medical, Pharmaceutical and Health Sciences, Kanazawa University, Kanazawa 920-0942, Japan

Maki Rooksby
Adverse Childhood Experiences (ACE) Lab, Institute of Health and Wellbeing, University of Glasgow, Glasgow G12 8RZ, UK
Social Brain in Action Lab, Institute of Neuroscience and Psychology, University of Glasgow, Glasgow G12 8QB, UK

Mitsuru Kikuchi
Department of Psychiatry and Neurobiology, Graduate School of Medical Science, Kanazawa University, Kanazawa 920-8640, Japan

Takahiro Tsuji
Department of Basic Research on Social Recognition, Research Center for Child Mental Development, Kanazawa University, Kanazawa 920-8640, Japan
Department of Ophthalmology, Faculty of Medical Sciences, University of Fukui, Fukui 910-1193, Japan

Annaëlle Charrier
Pôle Hospitalo-Universitaire de Psychiatrie de l'Enfant et de l'Adolescent (PHUPEA), Université de Rennes 1, Centre Hospitalier Guillaume-Régnier, 154 Rue de Châtillon, Rennes 35000, France

Bertrand Olliac
Pôle Universitaire de Psychiatrie de l'Enfant et de l'Adolescent, Centre Hospitalier Esquirol, Limoges 87025, France
INSERM, U1094, Tropical Neuroepidemiology, Limoges 87000, France

Pierre Roubertoux
Aix Marseille Université, INSERM, GMGF UMR_S 910, Marseille 13385, France

Sylvie Tordjman
Pôle Hospitalo-Universitaire de Psychiatrie de l'Enfant et de l'Adolescent (PHUPEA), Université de Rennes 1, Centre Hospitalier Guillaume-Régnier, 154 Rue de Châtillon, Rennes 35000, France
Laboratoire Psychologie de la Perception (LPP), Université Paris Descartes, CNRS UMR 8158, Paris 75270, France

Flavia Marino, Paola Chilà, Chiara Failla, Ilaria Crimi, Roberta Minutoli, Alfio Puglisi, Antonino Andrea Arnao, Gennaro Tartarisco, Liliana Ruta, David Vagni and Giovanni Pioggia
Institute for Biomedical Research and Innovation (IRIB), National Research Council of Italy (CNR), 98164 Messina, Italy

Jinhee Lee
Department of Psychiatry, Yonsei University Wonju College of Medicine, Wonju 26426, Korea

Min Ji Son and Jong Yeob Kim
Yonsei University College of Medicine, Seoul 03722, Korea

Chei Yun Son
Department of Psychological & Brain Sciences, Washington University in St. Louis, St. Louis, MO 63130, USA

Gwang Hun Jeong
College of Medicine, Gyeongsang National University, Jinju 52727, Korea

Keum Hwa Lee and Jae Il Shin
Department of Pediatrics, Yonsei University College of Medicine, Seoul 03722, Korea

Kwang Seob Lee
Severance Hospital, Yonsei University College of Medicine, Seoul 03722, Korea

Younhee Ko
Division of Biomedical Engineering, Hankuk University of Foreign Studies, Gyeonggi-do 17035, Korea

Jun Young Lee
Department of Nephrology, Yonsei University Wonju College of Medicine, Wonju 26426, Korea

Joaquim Radua
Early Psychosis: Interventions and Clinical-detection (EPIC) Lab, Department of Psychosis Studies, Institute of Psychiatry, Psychology & Neuroscience, King's College London, London SE5 8AB, UK
Mental Health Networking Biomedical Research Centre (CIBERSAM), 08036 Barcelona, Spain
Centre for Psychiatry Research, Department of Clinical Neuroscience, Karolinska Institute, 11330 Stockholm, Sweden
Institut d'Investigacions Biomèdiques August Pi i Sunyer (IDIBAPS), 08036 Barcelona, Spain

Michael Eisenhut
Department of Pediatrics, Luton & Dunstable University Hospital NHS Foundation Trust, Luton LU4ODZ, UK

Florence Gressier
CESP, Inserm UMR1178, Department of Psychiatry, Assistance Publique-Hôpitaux de Paris, Bicêtre University Hospital, 94275 Le Kremlin Bicêtre, France

Ai Koyanagi
Research and Development Unit, Parc Sanitari Sant Joan de Déu, Universitat de Barcelona, Fundació Sant Joan de Déu, CIBERSAM, 08830 Barcelona, Spain
ICREA, Pg. Lluis Companys 23, 08010 Barcelona, Spain
Instituto de Salud Carlos III, Centro de Investigación Biomédica en Red de Salud Mental, CIBERSAM, 28029 Madrid, Spain

Brendon Stubbs
Physiotherapy Department, South London and Maudsley NHS Foundation Trust, London SE5 8AZ, UK
Department of Psychological Medicine, Institute of Psychiatry, Psychology and Neuroscience, King's College London, London SE5 8AF, UK

Marco Solmi
Early Psychosis: Interventions and Clinical-detection (EPIC) Lab, Department of Psychosis Studies, Institute of Psychiatry, Psychology & Neuroscience, King's College London, London SE5 8AB, UK
Department of Neurosciences, University of Padua, 90133 Padua, Italy
Neurosciences Center, University of Padua, 90133 Padua, Italy

Theodor B. Rais
Department of Psychiatry, University of Toledo Medical Center, Toledo, OH 43614, USA

Andreas Kronbichler
Department of Internal Medicine IV, Medical University Innsbruck, Anichstraße 35, 6020 Innsbruck, Austria

Elena Dragioti
Pain and Rehabilitation Centre and Department of Health, Medicine and Caring Sciences, Linköping University, SE-581 85 Linköping, Sweden

Daniel Fernando Pereira Vasconcelos and Felipe Rodolfo Pereira da Silva
Laboratory of Histological Analysis and Preparation (LAPHIS), Federal University of the Parnaiba Delta, Parnaiba 64202-020, Brazil

Kalthoum Tizaoui
Department of Basic Sciences, Medicine Faculty of Tunis, Tunis El Manar University, 15 Rue Djebel Lakdar, Tunis 1007, Tunisia

André Russowsky Brunoni
University Hospital, University of São Paulo, São Paulo CEP 05508-000, Brazil
Service of Interdisciplinary Neuromodulation, Department and Institute of Psychiatry, University of São Paulo Medical School, São Paulo CEP 01246-903, Brazil
Laboratory of Neuroscience and National Institute of Biomarkers in Neuropsychiatry, Department and Institute of Psychiatry, University of São Paulo Medical School, São Paulo CEP 01246-903, Brazil
Department of Psychiatry and Psychotherapy, University Hospital, LMU Munich, 80336 Munich, Germany

Andre F. Carvalho
Centre for Addiction & Mental Health, Toronto, ON M6J 1H4, Canada
Department of Psychiatry, University of Toronto, Toronto, ON M5T 1R8, Canada

Sarah Cargnin and Salvatore Terrazzino
Department of Pharmaceutical Sciences and Interdepartmental Research Center of Pharmacogenetics and Pharmacogenomics (CRIFF), University of Piemonte Orientale, 28100 Novara, Italy

Andrew Stickley
The Stockholm Center for Health and Social Change (SCOHOST), Södertörn University, 141 89 Huddinge, Sweden
Department of Preventive Intervention for Psychiatric Disorders, National Institute of Mental Health, National Center of Neurology and Psychiatry, 4-1-1 Ogawahigashicho, Kodaira, Tokyo 187-8553, Japan

Lee Smith
The Cambridge Centre for Sport and Exercise Sciences, Anglia Ruskin University, Cambridge CB1 1PT, UK

Trevor Thompson
Department of Psychology, University of Greenwich, London SE10 9LS, UK

Paolo Fusar-Poli
Early Psychosis: Interventions and Clinical-detection (EPIC) Lab, Department of Psychosis Studies, Institute of Psychiatry, Psychology & Neuroscience, King's College London, London SE5 8AB, UK
OASIS Service, South London and Maudsley NHS Foundation Trust, London SE8 5HA, UK
Department of Brain and Behavioral Sciences, University of Pavia, 27100 Pavia, Italy

Laurent Pasquier, Léna Damaj, Sylvie Odent and Mélanie Fradin
Service de Génétique Clinique, Centre de Référence Maladies Rares Anomalies du Développement (Centre Labellisé pour les Anomalies du Développement de l'Ouest: CLAD Ouest), Hôpital Sud, Centre Hospitalier Universitaire de Rennes, 35200 Rennes, France

Cyrille Robert
Pôle Hospitalo-Universitaire de Psychiatrie de l'Enfant et de l'Adolescent (PHUPEA), University of Rennes 1 and Centre Hospitalier Guillaume Régnier, 35200 Rennes, France

David Cohen
Hospital-University Department of Child and Adolescent Psychiatry, Pitié-Salpétrière Hospital, Paris 6 University, 75013 Paris, France

Roberto Canitano
Division of Child and Adolescent Neuropsychiatry, University Hospital of Siena, 53100 Siena, Italy

Juliana Magdalon, Karina Griesi-Oliveira and Andréa L. Sertié
Hospital Israelita Albert Einstein, Centro de Pesquisa Experimental, São Paulo 05652-900, Brazil

Sandra M. Sánchez-Sánchez
Hospital Israelita Albert Einstein, Centro de Pesquisa Experimental, São Paulo 05652-900, Brazil
Departamento de Genética e Biologia Evolutiva, Instituto de Biociências, Universidade de São Paulo, São Paulo 05508-090, Brazil

Jacopo Troisi and Giovanni Scala
Theoreo srl spin off company of the University of Salerno, Via degli Ulivi, 3, 84090 Montecorvino Pugliano (SA), Italy

Reija Autio
Faculty of Social Sciences, Health Sciences Unit, Tampere University, Arvo Ylpön Katu 34, 33014 Tampere, Finland

Thanos Beopoulos, Manuel Gea and François Iris
Bio-Modeling System, 3, Rue De L'arrivee. 75015 Paris, France

Carmela Bravaccio
Department of Science Medicine Translationa University of Naples Federico II, Via Pansini 5, 80131 Naples, Italy

Federica Carraturo and Francesco Paolo Tuccinardi
Promete srl, Piazzale Tecchio 45, 80125 Napoli, Italy

Giulio Corrivetti
Azienda Sanitaria Locale (ASL) Salerno, Via Nizza, 146, 84125 Salerno (SA), Italy

Stephen Cunningham, Lokesh Joshi, Geraldine Leader and Arlene Mannion
National University of Ireland Galaway, University Road, Galaway, Ireland

Samantha Devane and Sarah Kadzielski
Massachusetts General Hospital, Fruit Street, 55, Boston, MA 02114, USA

Daniele Fallin and Christine Ladd-Acosta
John Hopkins School of Public Health and the Wendy Klag Center for Autism and Developmental Disabilities, 615 N. Wolfe St, Baltimore, MD 21205, USA

Serguei Fetissov
Laboratory of Neuronal and Neuroendocrine Differentiation and Communication, Inserm UMR 1239, Rouen University of Normandy, 25 rue Tesnière, 76130 Mont-Saint-Aignan, France

Antonio Giorgi
Medinok Spa, Via Palazziello, 80040 Volla (NA), Italy

Aletta Kraneveld, Lucia N. Peralta Marzal, Paula Perez Pardo and Naika Z. Prince
Division of Pharmacology, Utrecht Institute for Pharmaceutical Sciences, Faculty of Science, Utrecht University, Universiteitsweg 99, 3508 TB Utrecht, The Netherlands

Himanshu Kumar and Guus Roeselers
Danone Nutricia Research, Uppsalalaan, 12, 3584 CT Utrecht, The Netherlands

Elise Maximin, Laurent Naudon, Sylvie Rabot and Lea Roussin
Institut National de Recherche Pour L'agriculture, L'alimentation et L'environnement (INRAE), AgroParisTech, Micalis Institute, Université Paris-Saclay, 78350 Jouy-en-Josas, France

Alessandra Mezzelani and Luciano Milanesi
Consiglio Nazionale delle Ricerche (CNR), Piazzale Aldo Moro, 7, 00185 Roma, Italy

Christophe Roos
Euformatics, Tekniikantie, 02150 Espoo, Finland

Alessio Fasano
European Biomedical Research Institute of Salerno (EBRIS), Via S. de Renzi, 3, 84125 Salerno (SA), Italy

Index